Health Systems, Wealth and Societal Well-being

Assessing the case for investing in health systems

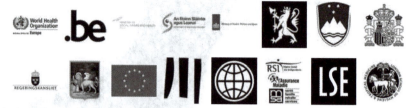

The European Observatory on Health Systems and Policies supports and promotes evidence-based health policy-making through comprehensive and rigorous analysis of health systems in Europe. It brings together a wide range of policy-makers, academics and practitioners to analyse trends in health reform, drawing on experience from across Europe to illuminate policy issues.

The European Observatory on Health Systems and Policies is a partnership between the World Health Organization Regional Office for Europe, the Governments of Belgium, Finland, Ireland, the Netherlands, Norway, Slovenia, Spain, Sweden and the Veneto Region of Italy, the European Commission, the European Investment Bank, the World Bank, UNCAM (French National Union of Health Insurance Funds), the London School of Economics and Political Science, and the London School of Hygiene & Tropical Medicine.

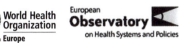

Health Systems, Health, Wealth and Societal Well-being

Assessing the case for investing in health systems

Edited by

Josep Figueras and Martin McKee

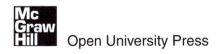

Open University Press

Open University Press
McGraw-Hill Education
McGraw-Hill House
Shoppenhangers Road
Maidenhead
Berkshire
England
SL6 2QL

email: enquiries@openup.co.uk
world wide web: www.openup.co.uk

and Two Penn Plaza, New York, NY 10121-2289, USA

First published 2012

A catalogue record of this book is available from the British Library

ISBN-13: 978-0-335-24430-0 (pb)
ISBN-10: 0-335-24430-0
eISBN: 978-0-335-24431-7

Library of Congress Cataloging-in-Publication Data
CIP data applied for

Typesetting and e-book compilations by
RefineCatch Limited, Bungay, Suffolk
Printed and bound in the UK by Bell & Bain Ltd, Glasgow

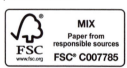

MIX
Paper from
responsible sources
FSC
www.fsc.org
FSC® C007785

The *McGraw·Hill* Companies

European Observatory on Health Systems and Policies Series

The European Observatory on Health Systems and Policies is a unique project that builds on the commitment of all its partners to improving health systems:

- World Health Organization Regional Office for Europe
- Government of Belgium
- Government of Finland
- Government of Ireland
- Government of the Netherlands
- Government of Norway
- Government of Slovenia
- Government of Spain
- Government of Sweden
- Veneto Region of Italy
- European Commission
- European Investment Bank
- World Bank
- UNCAM
- London School of Economics and Political Science
- London School of Hygiene & Tropical Medicine

The series

The volumes in this series focus on key issues for health policy-making in Europe. Each study explores the conceptual background, outcomes and lessons learned about the development of more equitable, more efficient and more effective health systems in Europe. With this focus, the series seeks to contribute to the evolution of a more evidence-based approach to policy formulation in the health sector.

These studies will be important to all those involved in formulating or evaluating national health policies and, in particular, will be of use to health policy-makers and advisers, who are under increasing pressure to rationalize the structure and funding of their health system. Academics and students in the field of health policy will also find this series valuable in seeking to understand better the complex choices that confront the health systems of Europe.

The Observatory supports and promotes evidence-based health policy-making through comprehensive and rigorous analysis of the dynamics of health care systems in Europe.

Series Editors

Josep Figueras is the Director of the European Observatory on Health Systems and Policies, and Head of the European Centre for Health Policy, World Health Organization Regional Office for Europe.

Martin McKee is Director of Research Policy and Head of the London Hub of the European Observatory on Health Systems and Policies. He is Professor of European Public Health at the London School of Hygiene & Tropical Medicine as well as a co-director of the School's European Centre on Health of Societies in Transition.

Elias Mossialos is the Co-director of the European Observatory on Health Systems and Policies. He is Brian Abel-Smith Professor in Health Policy, Department of Social Policy, London School of Economics and Political Science and Director of LSE Health.

Richard B. Saltman is Associate Head of Research Policy and Head of the Atlanta Hub of the European Observatory on Health Systems and Policies. He is Professor of Health Policy and Management at the Rollins School of Public Health, Emory University in Atlanta, Georgia.

Reinhard Busse is Associate Head of Research Policy and Head of the Berlin Hub of the European Observatory on Health Systems and Policies. He is Professor of Health Care Management at the Berlin University of Technology.

European Observatory on Health Systems and Policies Series

Series Editors: Josep Figueras, Martin McKee, Elias Mossialos, Richard B. Saltman and Reinhard Busse

Published titles

Regulating entrepreneurial behaviour in European health care systems
Richard B. Saltman, Reinhard Busse and Elias Mossialos (eds)

Hospitals in a changing Europe
Martin McKee and Judith Healy (eds)

Health care in central Asia
Martin McKee, Judith Healy and Jane Falkingham (eds)

Funding health care: options for Europe
Elias Mossialos, Anna Dixon, Josep Figueras and Joe Kutzin (eds)

Health policy and European Union enlargement
Martin McKee, Laura MacLehose and Ellen Nolte (eds)

Regulating pharmaceuticals in Europe: striving for efficiency, equity and quality
Elias Mossialos, Monique Mrazek and Tom Walley (eds)

Social health insurance systems in western Europe
Richard B. Saltman, Reinhard Busse and Josep Figueras (eds)

Purchasing to improve health systems performance
Josep Figueras, Ray Robinson and Elke Jakubowski (eds)

Human resources for health in Europe
Carl-Ardy Dubois, Martin McKee and Ellen Nolte (eds)

Primary care in the driver's seat
Richard B. Saltman, Ana Rico and Wienke Boerma (eds)

Mental health policy and practice across Europe: the future direction of mental health care
Martin Knapp, David McDaid, Elias Mossialos and Graham Thornicroft (eds)

Decentralization in health care
Richard B. Saltman, Vaida Bankauskaite and Karsten Vrangbæk (eds)

Health systems and the challenge of communicable diseases: experiences from Europe and Latin America
Richard Coker, Rifat Atun and Martin McKee (eds)

Caring for people with chronic conditions: a health system perspective
Ellen Nolte and Martin McKee (eds)

Nordic health care systems: recent reforms and current policy challenges
Jon Magnussen, Karsten Vrangbæk and Richard B. Saltman (eds)

Diagnosis-related groups in Europe: moving towards transparency, efficiency and quality in hospitals
Reinhard Busse, Alexander Geissler, Wilm Quentin and Miriam Wiley (eds)

Migration and health in the European Union
Bernd Rechel, Philipa Mladovsky, Walter Devillé, Barbara Rijks, Roumyana Petrova-Benedict and Martin McKee (eds)

Contents

Foreword

Member States in the WHO European Region are facing a formidable economic crisis that is also calling into question the sustainability of the European social welfare model as a whole and necessitating even greater cost–effectiveness of health systems. Policy-makers are being called on to account for each and every area of public expenditure and are expected to maximize value for money; indeed, the sizeable share of public money that is devoted to health and the ever-increasing cost pressures and demands to cut public expenditure put health systems at the heart of the policy debate. Consequently, the central message of this volume is very relevant, timely and welcome: health systems are not a drain on resources but an investment in health and wealth – that is, in the health of the population and in economic growth.

An earlier draft version of this volume served as background for the WHO European Ministerial Conference on Health Systems in Tallinn in 2008. It underpinned the deliberations of Member States as they elaborated the Tallinn Charter: Health Systems for Health and Wealth. The evidence contained in this volume illustrates how health constitutes a major component of societal well-being. It demonstrates that health has both a value in itself and a major impact on economic productivity and the economy as a whole. Moreover, it shows the contributions of health systems to health improvement, population health and equity: making a powerful case for investing in health systems.

These are not, however, arguments for a blank cheque. Investments in health system interventions need to be underpinned by evidence on performance, including impacts on overall population health gain and value for money. Importantly, they must also be set against investments in other sectors because a large share of the burden of disease is preventable through early interventions not only within but also outside the health system in sectors such as education, transport, housing or employment; all these areas influence the broader determinants of health. Investments in many of these public health interventions are best value in terms of both health gain and cost-effectiveness. Policy-makers should, therefore, be held accountable both for the operation of the health services and for the health leadership that they exercise across sectors to maximize the overall health of their populations.

The WHO Regional Office for Europe in this second decade of the new century is strengthening the work of the Tallinn Charter with its central message on the value of investing in health systems. This is being done by extending the fundamental principles of the Tallinn Charter to cover the strengthening and integration of public health within the health system and, where relevant, also in other sectors. Strengthening public health is also at the core of the new WHO European health policy, Health 2020, now under discussion in our Member States. The new policy argues for 'whole-of-government' and 'whole-of-society' approaches that will consolidate the ideals encompassed in health in all policies. This concept emphasizes the need to improve the integration of government activities with health and to reach out beyond government to engage patients and citizens, developing a responsive and inclusive approach to governance for health. The policy will be accompanied by a raft of evidence that underlines its rationale, most particularly around enabling implementation – a lynchpin for policy success. This includes a review of social determinants and the health divide in the European Region, pointing towards successful interventions, and studies on the economics of prevention and on effective tools to improve health governance. The current volume is, therefore, a welcome and timely addition to this arsenal.

Zsuzsanna Jakab
WHO Regional Director for Europe

Acknowledgements

This volume is part of a series of books by the European Observatory on Health Systems and Policies and was produced in close collaboration with the WHO Regional Office for Europe. An earlier draft of this volume was prepared for the WHO European Ministerial Conference on 'Health Systems, Health and Wealth' in 2008 in Tallinn, Estonia. Its constituent papers served to inform, and be informed by, conference presentations and discussions. In addition, the papers have been updated to reflect more recent debates on the subject as well as the comments and suggestions from external reviewers and the authors themselves who reviewed parts of the volume.

The editors are indebted to the chapter authors for their effort and enthusiasm, as well as their patience, as we went through a number of iterations of their papers, introducing our comments and those of external reviewers. We gratefully acknowledge the contribution of those who participated in a workshop held in Brussels to discuss directions and review contents of individual draft chapters of the volume. Those individuals involved were, in addition to the chapter authors, Claudia Bettina Maier, Willy Palm, Govin Permanand and Maria Cristina Profili. In addition we would like to acknowledge Nata Menabde, who was involved in editing the previous draft version of this volume, and Philip Berman, Richard Saltman, Antonio Durán and Claudia Bettina Maier who reviewed the whole volume. We are particularly indebted to Suszy Lessof who worked with us on the editing of the volume. We greatly benefited from her comments, suggestions and edits throughout the course of the work.

Finally, this book would not have appeared without the able and patient support of our head of publications, Jonathan North, and his collaborator Caroline White. Special thanks also go to the copy-editor , Jane Ward, and the production team at Open University Press.

About the authors

Sara Allin, Senior Researcher at the Canadian Institute for Health Information, with the Canadian Population Health Initiative, and an Assistant Professor at the School of Public Policy and Governance, at the University of Toronto, Canada.

Reinhard Busse, Associate Head of Research Policy and Head of the Berlin Hub of the European Observatory on Health Systems and Policies, and he is Professor of Health Care Management at the Berlin Technical University, Germany.

Antonio Durán, CEO at Técnicas de Salud, Sevilla, Spain, visiting Lecturer at the Andalusian School of Public Health, in Granada,Spain, visiting Lecturer at the Management Centre in Innsbruck, Austria, and Technical Adviser for the European Observatory on Health Systems and Policies, Brussels, Belgium.

David Evans, Department of Health Systems Financing at the World Health Organization, Geneva, Switzerland.

Dr Josep Figueras, Director, European Observatory on Health Systems and Policies, and Head, WHO European Centre for Health Policy, Brussels, Belgium.

Marina Karanikolos, Research Fellow at the European Observatory on Health Systems and Policies and the London School of Hygiene and Tropical Medicine, United Kingdom.

Anton E. Kunst, at the time of writing, was assistant professor at the Department of Public Health, Erasmus MC, the Netherlands. He now is an associate professor at the Department of Public Health, Academic Medical Center, Amsterdam, the Netherlands.

Joseph Kutzin, at the time of writing, was the Head of the Barcelona Office for Health Systems Strengthening, WHO Regional Office for Europe. He is now Coordinator, Health Financing Policy, World Health Organization Geneva, Switzerland.

Suszy Lessof, Director of Management at the European Observatory on Health Systems and Policies, Brussels, Belgium.

Johan P. Mackenbach, Professor and Chair, Department of Public Health, Erasmus MC, Rotterdam, the Netherlands.

José M. Martin-Moreno, Professor of Preventive Medicine and Public Health at the University of Valencia, Spain and Director of Programme Management at the WHO Regional Office for Europe, Copenhagen, Denmark.

David McDaid, Research Fellow in Health Policy and Health Economics at LSE Health and Social Care and the European Observatory on Health Systems and Policies at the London School of Economics and Political Science, London, United Kingdom.

Martin McKee, Professor of European Public Health at the London School of Hygiene & Tropical Medicine, United Kingdom, and Research Director at the European Observatory on Health Systems and Policies, London, United Kingdom.

Nata Menabde, WHO representative, India, Country Office of the World Health Organization, India.

Elias Mossialos, Professor of Health Policy at the London School of Economics and Political Science, Co-Director of the European Observatory on Health Systems and Policies and Director of LSE Health, and Minister of State, Greece.

Charles Normand, Edward Kennedy Professor of Health Policy & Management, University of Dublin Trinity College, Visiting Professor of Health Economics at the London School of Hygiene and Tropical Medicine, and Vice Chair of St James University Hospital Board in Dublin, Ireland.

Ellen Nolte, Director of the Health and Healthcare Policy Research Programme at RAND Europe, Cambridge, United Kingdom.

Irene Papanicolas, Lecturer in Health Economics at LSE Health, Department of Social Policy, the London School of Economics and Political Science, London, United Kingdom.

Amit Prasad, Technical Officer at the World Health Organization Kobe, Japan.

Lorenzo Rocco, Senior Lecturer of Economics at the University of Padova, Italy.

Richard B. Saltman, Associate Head of Research Policy at the European Observatory on Health Systems and Policies, and Professor of Health Policy and Management at the Rollins School of Public Health of Emory University in Atlanta, United States of America.

Regina Sauto Arce, Consultant at INFYDE (Información y Desarrollo, SL) in Bilbao, Spain.

Peter C. Smith, Professor of Health Policy at Imperial College Business School and the Centre for Health Policy, London, United Kingdom.

Marc Suhrcke, Professor in Public Health Economics at University of East Anglia, Norwich Medical School, United Kingdom.

Phyllida Travis, Health Systems Advisor at the World Health Organization, Geneva, Switzerland.

Nicole Valentine, Health Economist, Department of Ethics, Equity, Trade and Human Rights at the World Health Organization, Geneva, Switzerland.

Dr Ewout van Ginneken, Researcher, Berlin University of Technology, Berlin, Germany.

Mathias Wismar, Senior Health Policy Analyst, European Observatory on Health Systems and Policies, Brussels, Belgium.

List of tables, figures and boxes

Tables

Figures

Boxes

Abbreviations

These abbreviations are used throughout the book; others are defined by chapter

EU	European Union
EU15	EU Member States before May 2004
EU25	EU Member States after May 2004
EU27	EU Member States after January 2007
GDP	gross domestic product
HIV/AIDS	human immunodeficiency virus/acquired immunodeficiency syndrome
OECD	Organisation for Economic Co-operation and Development
R&D	research and development
WHO	World Health Organization

chapter one

Health systems, health, wealth and societal well-being: an introduction

Josep Figueras, Suszy Lessof,
Martin McKee, Antonio Durán
and Nata Menabde

Introduction

This book looks at health systems from a new perspective. It argues that they
are not, as is often believed, simply a drag on resources but rather are part
and parcel of improving health and achieving better economic growth. The
relationship between health systems, health and wealth is complex, but the
three are inextricably linked so that investing cost-effectively in health systems
can contribute to the ultimate goal of societal well-being (Figueras et al. 2009;
McKee et al. 2009).

The policy debate on health systems has been dominated in recent decades
by concerns about sustainability and the system's ability to fund itself in the
face of growing cost pressures. More recently, the economic crises that have
afflicted some countries have added to these concerns. Health expenditure in
many European countries has been growing at a faster rate than the economy,
accounting for an increasing percentage of gross domestic product (GDP) and
creating unease about the costs falling upon industry and thus its competitiveness in an increasingly globalized economy. Containing costs has, consequently, become a major priority for most health systems in the World Health
Organization (WHO) European Region and beyond. Typically, policy-makers
have sought to find a balanced combination of different strategies acting on
both the supply and demand sides of health services (Box 1.1).

There is, however, a new wave of thinking that seeks to re-examine the
long-standing focus on cost-containment. It draws on new understandings
of the interdependency between health and wealth, of the value attached to

Box 1.1 Cost-containment strategies

Policy-makers have, for years, sought to contain costs rather than invest in health systems. They have used a combination of strategies that act on the demand and the supply sides of health systems.

Demand-side strategies

Demand-side strategies have focused largely on shifting the cost of health care from statutory sources to health service users by increasing cost-sharing and/or by rationing access to publicly funded services. Consequently, in some countries, services (e.g. dentistry) have been taken out of the statutory benefits package or, more often, new, expensive types of care (e.g. anti-cancer drugs) have not been included but are payable 'out of pocket' or through voluntary health insurance. These measures are often highly regressive and tend to undermine social solidarity by decreasing access for those with the highest needs. However, policy-makers have often seen such measures as the only viable option in the face of ever-increasing upward pressure on public expenditure.

Supply-side strategies

Strategies acting on the supply side have tried to secure more or better value for money. They include the introduction of strategic purchasing, market mechanisms introducing competition between providers to improve efficiency, performance-related payments, health technology assessment, better integration between levels of care, and strengthening the role of primary care. These have commanded broad support among policy-makers and some have resulted in efficiency increases. However, they have not succeeded in containing overall costs.

health by citizens and societies, and of the role health systems play in improving health.

This re-examination of the contribution health makes and the value attached to it has been termed the 'health and wealth' debate (European Health Forum Gastein 2003; Council of Europe 2007; European Commission 2007). It has brought to the fore the interrelationships between health status, health systems and economic growth. Increasingly, better health is now hailed as a driver of economic growth. This is in no small part due to the seminal work of the Commission on Macroeconomics and Health (2001), which, while focusing on developing countries, did much to bring evidence of the impact of health on economic development to a global policy audience. Three more recent studies have further developed this approach, looking at the European Union (EU) Member States before May 2004 (EU15) (Suhrcke et al. 2005, the countries of central and eastern Europe and the former Soviet Union (Suhrcke et al. 2007), and the Russian Federation (Suhrcke, Rocco and McKee 2007). They have demonstrated its relevance to high- and middle-income countries, explored the pathways by which improved health leads to economic productivity in the European Region and illustrated the magnitude of its impact.

At the same time as the utilitarian 'case for health' has been strengthened, WHO Member States of the European Region have restated the fundamental value of health as a human right, most recently at a major ministerial conference held in Tallinn in 2008 (WHO Regional Office for Europe 2008). They have committed to the principles of universal access, equity and solidarity as core values of European societies in a number of pan-European policy initiatives (Council of Europe 1996; WHO Regional Office for Europe 2005; Council of the European Union 2006; European Commission 2007). Even in the midst of austerity programmes, most governments have sought to safeguard health spending as far as possible. Health is seen as a key indicator of social development and well-being, as well as a means to increasing social cohesion.

This shift in the debate, and with it our views on the value of health in our societies, has shed new light on the role of health systems and the challenges they give rise to. From this new perspective, health systems, to the extent that they produce health, can be seen to be a productive sector rather than a drain on our economies, which, in turn, forces a re-examination of concerns about financial sustainability (Thomson et al. 2009). Increased spending on effective health systems can be recast as a contribution to a bigger (and more productive) economy, as well as a way of achieving health improvement and higher levels of well-being, which themselves are desirable societal objectives. In the EU context, this has placed health systems firmly at the centre of measures to further the Lisbon Agenda and the subsequent EU 2020 Agenda, pursuing the twin goals of economic competitiveness and social cohesion (Council of the European Union 2000), and challenges the simplistic view that health expenditure is a threat to financial viability.

Some analysts have gone further in arguing that investing in appropriate health system interventions may result in reduced growth of health care expenditure in the future. The two Wanless Reports commissioned by the United Kingdom Treasury are a case in point. They examined the financial sustainability of health services in the United Kingdom and recommended further investment to strengthen the National Health Service (NHS) (Wanless 2002) and, in particular, its contribution to public health (Wanless 2004) as a means of achieving long-term sustainability. There is also considerable interest in ways that appropriately targeted interventions by health systems might mitigate the health (and expenditure) consequences of population ageing, when coupled with coordinated action on retirement age and pension policies. Effective investment can be instrumental in securing longer life expectancy and, crucially, longer lives in good health, by preventing and/or treating premature or avoidable morbidity. This has been termed 'compression of morbidity' (Fries 1980, 2003) and can already be observed in some European countries with well-developed health systems. This could create a virtuous health systems cycle by which healthier older people use fewer services, retire later and contribute to the economy for longer, drawing less from pension funds and generally reducing the potential challenge to sustainability (Rechel et al. 2009).

However, while these arguments create a strong case for maintaining investment in health systems, they are far from justifying additional funds. Especially at a time of economic recession, there are inevitable concerns about value for money and competing calls to use available funds to safeguard investment in other sectors, some of which may themselves contribute to health. Claims for health spending need to be seen in the context of substantial, and in many cases justified, concerns about the appropriateness of current health interventions and technical inefficiencies in many parts of Europe's health systems. In some countries, many treatments provided are not supported by evidence. At best they provide no benefit for the patient and at worst may do actual harm. Whichever is the case, such treatments waste scarce resources and have a substantial opportunity cost. There also needs to be consideration of the way in which priorities are set and resources allocated between alternative or competing interventions and programmes, so that the choice between expenditure on areas such as mental health, primary care, prevention, secondary care and so on is made on the basis of outcomes, with the goal of maximizing health gains. However, it is just as important to take into consideration the opportunity costs of investing in health services rather than acting on determinants of health through action in other sectors.

It is also important to recognize the growth in attention to the social determinants of health (Commission on Social Determinants of Health 2008) and the renewed emphasis on Health in All Policies (Ståhl et al. 2006; Health Ministerial Delegation of EU Member States 2007), which demonstrates that investment in the physical environment, education or transport systems may yield higher health returns than investment in health systems. By the same token, health policy-making must acknowledge that additional expenditure in other areas of government activity may result in higher societal well-being, which is, after all, the ultimate societal objective in most, if not all, countries of the European Region. Indeed, a recent analysis in European countries found that reductions in spending on social welfare had even greater effects, at least in the short term, than reductions in health care expenditure (Stuckler, Basu and McKee 2010). The case for health systems investment, therefore, needs to be supported by strong and transparent performance assessment, demonstrating cost-effectiveness as well as its strengths over other competing expenditure areas.

This book synthesizes the evidence linking health systems, health and wealth, undertaking a systematic exploration of the various issues involved and the interaction between them. Its main aim is to assist policy-makers as they assess the case for investing in health systems. An earlier version of this volume was prepared to support the proceedings of the WHO Conference on Health Systems, Health and Wealth (Tallinn, June 2008) which gave rise to the Tallinn Charter on 'Health Systems for Health and Wealth' (WHO 2009).

What is a health system?

Policy-makers who seek to lever investment for health or to assess the impact of investment in health systems over investment in other areas must be able to define and delineate what they mean by 'health system'. So, what is a health system? This question seems straightforward, yet there does not seem to be a simple answer. The definitions of health systems put forward by analysts and organizations vary enormously, especially in the way that health system boundaries are determined. At one end of the spectrum are narrow definitions that focus on medical care, with 'patients, clear exit and entry points and services regarding disease, disability and death'. At the other end are broad approaches that encompass all those determinants that contribute directly or indirectly to health. We need to find a balance between the narrowest definitions that cover curative services only and the all-embracing notion of a health system that includes everything which might improve well-being (not least housing, education and environment). This process of establishing a balance or 'manageable boundaries' is particularly important when it comes to making definitions operational, as well as for managing and overseeing health systems and their performance in practice.

Definitions and functions

The health system definition put forward by *The World Health Report 2000* (WHR2000) (World Health Organization 2000) forms (along with later work) the basis for our approach here. The WHR2000 defines a health system as 'all the activities whose primary purpose is to promote, restore or maintain health' (p. 5). This definition incorporates 'selected intersectoral actions in which the stewards of the health system take responsibility to advocate for improvements in areas outside their direct control, such as legislation to reduce fatalities from traffic accidents' (Murray and Evans 2003: 7).

This definition underpinned the Health Systems Assessment Framework (HSAF) (see Chapter 2), designed to enable review of the performance of health systems against three major societal goals (Box 1.2). Performance is then understood as the attainment of these goals relative to the resources invested in them, which, in turn, implies a fourth goal, namely efficiency or productivity. In order to achieve these goals, all health systems have to carry out four core functions, regardless of how they are organized or of the terminology they use (Box 1.2).

The HSAF, with its goals and functions, is presented in more detail in Chapter 2 and is used later in this book as the basis of discussion on health systems reforms and strategies (Chapter 9), and on measures to improve performance (Chapter 10).

This approach is taken further here. A health system includes, in practical terms, the following three items:

1. The delivery of (personal and population-based) health services, including primary and secondary prevention, treatment, care and rehabilitation
2. The activities to enable the delivery of health services, specifically the functions of finance, resource generation and stewardship
3. Stewardship activities aimed at influencing the health impact of 'relevant' interventions in other sectors, regardless of whether or not the primary purpose of those interventions is to improve health.

This approach relies on the understanding that the health system functions of financing, resource allocation and delivery relate directly to health services,

Box 1.2 Health system goals and functions

Goals

To improve:

- the health status of the population (both the average level of health and the distribution of health);
- the responsiveness to the nonmedical expectations of the population, including two sets of dimensions: respect for persons (patient dignity, confidentiality, autonomy and communication) and client orientation (prompt attention, basic amenities, social support and choice);
- fairness of financing (financial protection; i.e. avoidance of impoverishment as a consequence of health payments, along with equitable distribution of the burden of funding the system).

Functions

To achieve:

- financing (revenue collection, fund pooling and purchasing)
- resource generation (human resources, technologies and facilities)
- delivery of personal and population-based health services
- stewardship (health policy formulation, regulation and intelligence).

---

while the stewardship function (above all others) has an additional role in other sectors beyond health services, influencing the determinants of health.

Steering health systems: the role of government

The definition above asserts that the responsibility of those charged with oversight of health systems, typically ministries of health, extends beyond health care. It emphasizes the crucial message that they are accountable for exercising stewardship in other sectors to ensure that health objectives are considered in their policies – what has been termed Health in All Policies. The corollary is that it also acknowledges that the funding, provision and management of many health-relevant interventions are the responsibility of other sectors. The ministry of health, or equivalent has a stewardship function assessing performance across sectors and influencing the allocation of resources to maximize health gains and allocative efficiency. This means that ministries of health should be held accountable not only for health services but also for the stewardship they exercise over other sectors.

This approach, however, is more normative than descriptive. While it might be desirable that ministries exercise stewardship across sectors, in practice many share responsibility even for the formal health sector and have only limited authority beyond it. Furthermore, health ministries are often relatively weak, both technically and politically. Context is all important and the level of decentralization, models of finance or delivery, and the role of other actors, among other factors, all complicate the ministry's own role. Moreover, exercising influence across sectors is far from easy. It requires the ability to exert leverage, and there are not always the appropriate intersectoral tools, mechanisms or implementation capacity available. Nor is it easy to hold other ministries accountable for the health impact of their policies.

Nonetheless, despite the complexities of implementation and the normative nature of the assertion, a ministry of health must seek, in whatever way is appropriate in the context, to develop a central role in the governance of the health system and to influence health determinants in other sectors. This is not to say that that accountability for a population's health should fall solely on the ministry of health, rather, as noted, health governance is a whole government affair involving other ministries including the office of the prime minister who should ultimately be held accountable for the health of the population.

A conceptual framework

The case for health systems investment rests on the understanding that health systems are intricately linked to health and wealth. The relationships between them are complex and dynamic. This book, therefore, employs a conceptual framework that can guide policy-makers in articulating the links between issues, providing the backbone of this analysis (Figueras et al. 2009). The framework links health systems (as defined above) to health, wealth and societal well-being, with the causal, direct and indirect relationships between the key elements captured (at least in part) by the 'conceptual triangle' shown in Fig. 1.1.[1] It supports a systematic review of the issues and also, crucially, positions health system investment in a direct relationship with the ultimate goal of all social systems: societal well-being.

The notion of societal well-being requires some explanation. It is generally accepted that health, despite its importance to the public, is not viewed explicitly as the ultimate goal of organized societies. Rather, societies strive towards a

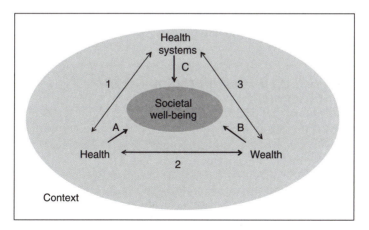

Figure 1.1 Health systems, health, wealth and societal well-being: a triangular relationship

positive and sustainable state of well-being. This is a multidimensional concept and a very difficult one to pin down, not least because so many disciplines and experts have used overlapping but slightly different language to explore it. For the present purposes, societal well-being stands for the total well-being of the entire society and touches on notions of happiness and quality of life. It can also be taken to reflect many other elements, such as quality of the environment, levels of crime, access to essential social services as well as the more religious or spiritual aspects of life. 'Societal well-being' has been chosen in preference to 'social welfare' to avoid any potential misunderstanding, as social welfare is also understood to be primarily about welfare services.

The understanding captured by the framework in Fig. 1.1 is that health systems contribute to societal well-being in three main ways. The relationships between health systems, health, wealth and societal well-being are indicated by 1–3 and A–C. First, and above all, health systems produce health (1), which is both a major and inherent component of well-being (A) and through its impact on wealth creation (2), an indirect (yet key) contributor to well-being (B). Second, although to a much lesser extent, health systems have a direct impact on wealth as a significant component of the economy (3), which again impacts on societal well-being (B). Third, health systems contribute directly to societal well-being because societies draw satisfaction from the existence of health services and the ability of people to access them, regardless of whether or not services are effective or indeed whether or not they are used (C). One final point must be raised here – that of context. Context refers to the country-specific social, economic, cultural and political environment in which the triangular relationship between health systems, health, wealth and societal well-being is embedded. Figure 1.1 seeks to reflect the importance of different contexts in determining the nature and the extent of the individual causal relationships shown.

There is a subset of relationships or 'lesser triangles' nested within the main triangle. These are not all of equal importance and not all are covered in equal detail here. Nonetheless, the most important are addressed in the subsections that follow, including health systems and their contribution to health and societal well-being; health's contribution to wealth and societal well-being; and health systems' impact on wealth.

Health systems: their contribution to health and societal well-being

In reality, this is the subset of relationships that is uppermost in the thinking of most health policy-makers. Most important of all is the impact that health systems have on health improvement (1 in Fig. 1.1). The impact of health systems on health includes all the goals and functions of the HSAF, outlined in Fig. 2.1 (p. 28), namely health (levels and equity), responsiveness and fairness of financing (financial protection and equity in the distribution of funding) that are not explicitly captured by the triangle. Later chapters look at the impact of health systems on some of these goals including health (Chapters 5 and 6), health inequalities (Chapter 7) and responsiveness (Chapter 8).

Others look at how health systems can be improved and efficiency maximized through strategies for reform (Chapter 9) and performance assessment (Chapter 10), recognizing not only that value for money is absolutely indispensable for sustained investment but also that there is a significant potential gap between the 'what health systems can do' of theoretical debate and the 'what they achieve', which policy-makers have to address when competing for resources.

It should also be noted that the relationship between health systems and health is bidirectional and that levels and patterns of ill health will feed back into the health system, shaping its priorities and the allocation of resources between interventions.

In addition to their impact on health, health systems make a direct contribution to societal well-being (C in Fig. 1.1) by virtue of the value that citizens attach to them as guarantors of health protection. The right to health protection is not to be understood as the right to be healthy. Most societies attach a distinct value simply to the fact that an organized health system exists and can be accessed – these are held to be truly important and are de facto a fundamental component of social cohesion and societal well-being (Council of Europe 1997; Council of the European Union 2006).

Health: its contribution to wealth and societal well-being

A second set of key relationships links health, wealth and well-being. These form the 'inner triangle' at the base of the main triangle in Fig. 1.1. They also encapsulate the argument at the heart of this book (see Chapter 4). The contribution of health to societal well-being can be characterized as taking two main forms. Health constitutes a major component of well-being in its own right (A in Fig. 1.1). Citizens draw satisfaction from living longer and healthier lives and value health regardless of whether or not they are economically productive. As already noted, health also plays an important role in increasing economic productivity and thus national income (2 in Fig. 1.1), which, in turn, makes a key contribution to the dimension of societal well-being (B). In addition, health has an impact on wealth (2 in Fig. 1.1) and may contribute to budgetary gains from savings on health expenditure. Any discussion that touches on wealth demands figures to be produced as evidence. Quantifying wealth and the value of health in economic terms is of course complex, not least because health is not a normal traded commodity. Some of the concerns surrounding the use of gross domestic product as a measure of wealth and societal well-being are outlined in Box 1.3. In that regard the 2009 report by 'The Commission on the Measurement of Economic Performance and Social Progress' (CMEPSP) established by Nicholas Sarkozy and chaired by Joseph Stiglitz shows the limits of GDP as an indicator of economic performance and social progress and suggests alternative and more relevant indicators and tools to measure social progress (Stiglitz et al. 2009).

While the focus of this analysis is on the impact of health on wealth, it should be noted that this relationship is also bidirectional. Wealth has a major effect on health in its own right, both collectively and individually. Its impacts are direct through the material conditions that improve biological survival and health, as well as indirect, through its effects on social participation and people's control

Box 1.3 Some concerns surrounding the use of gross domestic product per capita as a measure of wealth and well-being

There are at least three major sets of caveats relating to the use of GDP per capita both as a measure for wealth and as a proxy for societal well-being.

1. First, GDP per capita is no more than the sum of monetary transactions in the economy. It pays no attention to the use of resources and does not differentiate between expenditure that increases well-being, such as on many consumption goods, and that which diminishes it, such as the cost of clearing up pollution or responding to fear of crime. Yet the true purpose of economic activity is to maximize social welfare or societal well-being, not solely to produce goods.
2. It does not capture the important economic benefits from people who are not formally employed or paid but who provide significant support, for instance in terms of caring for older and younger people.
3. Finally, it pays no attention to those elements of the economy that are not linked to money, whether negative, such as pollution or fear of crime, or positive, such as happiness or, indeed, health itself. There are concerns about capturing the contribution of health to wealth too narrowly through foregone GDP income, which tends to privilege those in employment over the rest of the population. This can be partially addressed by translating the contribution of health to social welfare or societal well-being into economic terms and thus attributing a monetary value to health – and indeed, this is done routinely when individuals demand income premiums to undertake jobs associated with a risk of death. Following this approach, and in spite of the methodological challenges involved, a number of studies have calculated what is termed the value of statistical life through 'willingness to pay' (WTP) methodologies and developed 'full income' measures (Chapter 4).

over their life circumstances. It should be possible, then, to establish a virtuous cycle whereby better health improves economic performance and better economic performance improves health. This makes it all the more important that health systems exercise stewardship of relevant public health interventions and interventions in other sectors, as well as taking responsibility for seeking to address the socioeconomic determinants of health (Chapter 6).

Health systems: their contribution to wealth

The third relationship explored here, albeit far less significant, refers to the direct contribution of health systems to the economy (3 in Fig. 1.1), irrespective of their impact on health improvement. Health services are an important economic sector in many countries, often being the largest employer and playing a significant role as a driver of and consumer of technological innovation and research and development (R&D). A note of caution is needed at this point, as the sizeable impact of health systems on the economy does not alone create an automatic justification for investing in health systems, since investments in other sectors may yield better returns. Finally, as with the other relationships discussed, this 'third side of the triangle', linking health systems and wealth, is also bidirectional. There is a widely held view that health care spending increases inexorably with growth in national income but this is not supported by the available evidence (Parkin, McGuire and Yule 1987). The impact of economic growth on health care expenditure is, therefore, addressed in more detail in Chapter 3.

Finally, although we believe that it has valuable explanatory power, this conceptual framework must be treated with a degree of caution. There are certain issues to be considered that relate to its deceptively normative outlook, the strength of causality of its various relationships, the bidirectional nature of some of those relationships, the variation in meaning and terminology, the role of context and the values associated with societal well-being. These are outlined in Box 1.4.

This section has explored the complex interactions between the four components of a dynamic model (health systems, health, wealth and societal well-being). Clearly, this model cannot establish a set of quantitative functions or tools that will lead policy-makers automatically to the optimal investment decisions. Nor does it argue that increasing investment in health systems is automatically 'the right choice'. Rather, it constitutes a framework for policy-makers that will help them to balance the key elements in decision-making. While it acknowledges, on the one hand, the inexact nature and limitations of measurement, it also emphasizes, on the other hand, the need to measure, evaluate and assess performance in order to improve decision-making.

Objectives and structure

This book presents an analysis of the existing evidence on the impact of health systems on health, wealth and, ultimately, on societal well-being, with the overall aim of exploring the case for investing in health systems. This is developed by means of the following eight objectives.

1. To propose a conceptual framework to assess the relationship between health systems, health, wealth and well-being.
2. To propose a definition for health systems and a framework building on, and further developing, the WHO HSAF approach (Chapter 2).
3. To re-examine the impact of major cost pressures (Chapter 3).
4. To assess the contribution of health (level and distribution) on economic growth, health expenditure and societal well-being (Chapter 4).
5. To evaluate the impact of health systems on the goals of health, equity and responsiveness (Chapters 5–8).
6. To review the main health system reform strategies to improve performance (Chapter 9).
7. To outline the main approaches to measure performance (Chapter 10).
8. To draw policy lessons on making a case for investing in health systems (Chapter 11).

Box 1.4 Some concerns around the triangular relationship 'health systems, health, wealth and societal well-being'

The triangle shown in Fig. 1.1 is an effective graphical representation of the main relationships between health systems, health, wealth and societal well-being. However, as an image, it is almost deceptively simple and could be misleading. There are a number of caveats that need to be borne in mind.

1. While the model may come across as normative, it is positive/descriptive in its conception, describing a series of causal relationships but without any value judgement as to their relative importance or appropriateness. The only normative position refers to the achievement of societal well-being (the 'bubble' in the centre of the triangle) as the ultimate goal, a position that nonetheless commands widespread acceptance in most European societies.
2. Even when there is common ground about the importance of well-being, there are significant differences about what aspects are included (or indeed how to measure them), because this involves social preferences and underlying value judgements. What constitutes the maximization of welfare will, therefore, depend on the objectives and unstated ideals of a particular society.
3. The causal relationships between these components are not clear cut or linear, nor are they easily measurable. There needs to be a full discussion and proper exploration of the nuances, strength and nature of these links, as the triangle tends to imply that all the relationships have the same weight.
4. The context matters enormously – all the relationships in the triangle are context specific and depend on the particulars of, among other things, the understanding of societal well-being; the economic, social, cultural and political situation; and the model of health system organization in the given setting. It is therefore clear that the model will need to be applied with full consideration of how context will determine specific relationships, bearing in mind all that this implies for drawing conclusions and positing policy lessons that are relevant across countries.

The first of these objectives is the conceptual framework that constitutes the backbone of this book and which has already been explained. The remaining seven objectives are outlined in more detail in the following paragraphs.

Health systems framework

The second objective is to propose a health systems framework that builds on the WHO HSAF. This was introduced briefly above and is addressed in more detail in Chapter 2. An overview of the main health system definitions and typologies is followed by a detailed review of the definition, boundaries, functions and goals set out in WHR2000 on health systems performance (World Health Organization 2000). The chapter focuses particularly on the role of health systems in public health and intersectoral work and on the practical uses of the framework to facilitate improved performance. Chapter 2 concludes with a discussion of the implications of the framework for management, governance and accountability – for health ministries in particular.

Cost pressures

The third objective is to re-examine the actual impact of major external challenges on health systems, including the ageing of the population (the demographic transition), medical progress through new technologies, higher expectations, economic growth and higher relative prices for health care inputs. These are considered to push costs upwards and thus threaten financial sustainability. However, the effect of these challenges has not been well quantified nor have we fully understood the dynamics and the interplay between them. Chapter 3, therefore, re-examines and clarifies the role and impact of these drivers of health expenditure. Reviews of the role of each factor (ageing, new technologies, expectations, economic growth, price of inputs) are followed by the latest evidence on their combined impact on current and future (projected) health care expenditure. The chapter concludes with some policy lessons about how best to address those cost pressures.

Economic consequences of ill health

The book's fourth objective is to summarize the evidence on health's contribution to economic growth and thus societal well-being, which forms the basic tenet in the case for investing in health systems. Chapter 4 explores the evidence on the impact of health on wealth along three strands. The first examines health as a 'consumption good' – exploring (and quantifying in economic terms) the value that individuals and societies attribute to better health as a major component of societal well-being. The second takes a human capital approach – reviewing the impact of ill health on economic productivity and the economy as a whole. The third provides an examination of the economic consequences in terms of health care expenditure and social security benefits that stem from reduced morbidity and mortality.

Health systems impact

Fifth, and perhaps most significantly, Chapters 5–8 seek to reassess the evidence on the contributions of health systems to health improvement, population health, equity and responsiveness.

Chapter 5 provides an overall assessment of the role of health services in population health, first reviewing the current state of the art in methodologies for measuring their impact. These include the use of the inventory approach, amenable mortality and tracer condition indicators. The authors use some of these measures to quantify approximately the impact of health services in improving health status. In particular, they look at the contribution of amenable mortality to changing life expectancy and assess recent trends in a selection of European countries for which data exist. The authors also discuss how to identify the best buys (i.e. the most effective health service interventions available) bearing in mind the burden of disease in different parts of the European region, cost-effectiveness considerations and contextual differences in values and priorities.

Chapter 6 is a review of the evidence on the costs and effectiveness of a range of public health interventions within health and in other sectors – particularly as they act on the determinants of health. An overview of the economic argument for investment in public health and health-promoting interventions begins by briefly highlighting the nature of health problems in Europe. This illustrates that, at least in principle, a large share of the existing disease burden is preventable through early intervention. The authors highlight the case for the use of economic evaluation as a tool in the policy-making process. They also discuss the state of the cost-effectiveness evidence base, providing examples from different areas of public health and health promotion and focusing particularly on interventions delivered outside the health system.

This analysis supports the view that health systems impact on societal well-being by improving health and increasing equity and responsiveness. Chapter 7 assesses the extent to which health system interventions can address inequalities in health and thus promote equity. The authors aim to bring together the policy implications of the results of recent studies on health inequalities in European countries as well as those on the effectiveness of specific interventions and policies to tackle health inequalities. In particular, they look at interventions in three fields: (i) labour market and welfare policies, (ii) interventions and policies to improve health-related behaviours, and (iii) health service interventions and policies in both finance and delivery. This chapter also presents estimates of the economic implications of health inequalities in terms of overall economic performance, health care and social security expenditure and societal well-being. The impact on societal well-being includes direct damage to overall health as well as the value that societies attach to equity itself. This clearly highlights the dual roles of the health system as both a deliverer and a steward of health services and as a steward of health and equity in other relevant sectors.

Chapter 8 addresses the relationship between health services and responsiveness. The authors explore the basic concepts behind responsiveness and satisfaction and consider major methodological approaches and actors to measure them. They outline the results of various studies to compare the levels of satisfaction and responsiveness between different health systems and highlight the complexities when attempting to interpret them. This chapter concludes with a review of the impact of a range of health service strategies (such as increasing choice of provider or addressing waiting lists) aimed at improving responsiveness and a consideration of any trade-offs with efficiency and equity.

Health system reforms

Chapter 9 addresses the sixth objective in a review of the main reform strategies that have been adopted to improve health systems performance in countries of the European Region. This examination is grouped according to the four main functions of the health systems framework introduced previously: (i) delivery of health services (i.e. reforms that tackle appropriate and cost-effective delivery), (ii) resource generation (i.e. reforms that seek to ensure the right level and mix of inputs, particularly human resources, technology and capital), (iii) financing (i.e. reforms that focus on revenue collection and pooling, to improve sustainability and solidarity, and purchasing, with an emphasis on effective purchasing to improve allocative and technical efficiency), and (iv) stewardship and initiatives to strengthen governance, accountability and responsiveness.

Performance measurement

If reforms are to succeed and contribute to societal objectives, then policy-makers must be informed about their progress and effects. Performance measurement is central to the design, stewardship and implementation of reform strategies; therefore, the seventh objective is to outline the main approaches to measure health systems performance and link them with governance. Chapter 10 provides a synthesis of the main methodologies for assessing performance; it draws lessons for the implementation of performance measurement systems and puts forward policy recommendations to link measurement with governance mechanisms and the improvement of health systems.

Drawing the lessons

Chapter 11 provides some reflections on the implications of this study for policy-makers and for the case for investment in health systems. It draws a series of policy-relevant lessons from each one of the chapters of the study concluding that societies should invest in health systems as part of societal efforts to enhance health and wealth and achieve societal well-being, provided that they have the performance assessment systems in place to demonstrate the investments are cost effective.

Endnote

1 The conceptual triangle was developed in a seminar at the WHO Regional Office for Europe in Copenhagen in 2007, with the participation (in alphabetical order) of Rifat Atun, Antonio Durán, Josep Figueras, Joseph Kutzin, Nata Menabde and Elias Mossialos.

References

Commission on Macroeconomics and Health (2001) *Macroeconomics and Health: Investing in Health for Economic Development*. Geneva: World Health Organization, Commission on Macroeconomics and Health.

Commission on Social Determinants of Health (2008) *Closing the Gap in a Generation: Health Equity Through Action on the Social Determinants of Health: Final Report of the Commission on Social Determinants of Health*. Geneva: World Health Organization.

Council of Europe (1996) *European Social Charter (revised)*. [CETS No. 163, Art. 11.] Strasbourg: Council of Europe.

Council of Europe (1997) *Convention for the Protection of Human Rights and Dignity of the Human Being with regard to the Application of Biology and Medicine: Convention on Human Rights and Biomedicine*. [CETS No. 164, Art. 3.] Strasbourg: Council of Europe.

Council of Europe (2007) *Terms of Reference of the European Health Committee (CDSP)*. [Appendix 9 (Item 6.2b), Fact Sheet.] Strasbourg: Council of Europe (https://wcd.coe.int/ViewDoc.jsp?id=1119365&BackColorInternet=DBDCF2&BackColorIntranet=FDC864&BackColorLogged=FDC864, accessed May 2008).

Council of the European Union (2000) *The Lisbon European Council – An Agenda for Economic and Social Renewal for Europe: Contribution of the European Commission to the Special European Council in Lisbon, 23–24 March*. Brussels: Council of the European Union.

Council of the European Union (2006) *Council Conclusions on Common Values and Principles in European Union Health Systems*. [2006/C 146/01.] Brussels: Council of the European Union.

European Commission (2007) *White Paper. Together for health: A strategic approach for the EU 2008–2013*. [COM(2007)630 final.] Brussels: European Commission (http://ec.europa.eu/health/ph_overview/Documents/strategy_wp_en.pdf, accessed May 2008).

European Health Forum Gastein (2003) *Congress Report of the Sixth European Health Forum Gastein: Economic and Social Dimensions of Health*, Bad Gastein, 1–4 Oct.

Figueras, J., Lessof, S., McKee, M. et al. (2009) *Health Systems for Health, Wealth and Societal Well-being*. Copenhagen: WHO Regional Office for Europe on behalf of the European Observatory on Health Systems and Policies.

Fries, J.F. (1980) Ageing, natural death, and the compression of morbidity. *New England Journal of Medicine*, 303: 130–5.

Fries, J.F. (2003) Measuring and monitoring success in compressing morbidity. *Annals of Internal Medicine*, 139: 455–9.

Health Ministerial Delegation of EU Member States (2007) *Declaration on 'Health in All Policies': Health in All Policies: Achievements and Challenges*. [EU Ministerial Conference, Rome.] Brussels: European Commission and WHO Regional Office for Europe.

McKee, M., Suhrcke, M., Nolte, E. et al. (2009) Health systems, health, and wealth: a European perspective. *Lancet*, 373: 349–51.

Murray, C.J.L. and Evans, D.B. (2003) Health systems performance assessment: goals, framework and overview, in C.J.L. Murray and D.B. Evans (eds.) *Health Systems Performance Assessment. Debates, Methods and Empiricism*. Geneva: World Health Organization: 3–22.

Parkin, D., McGuire, A. and Yule, B. (1987) Aggregate health care expenditures and national income: is health care a luxury good? *Journal of Health Economics*, 6: 109–27.

Rechel, B., Doyle, Y., Grundy, E. and McKee, M. (2009) *How can health systems respond to population ageing?* Copenhagen: WHO Regional Office for Europe on behalf of the European Observatory on Health Systems and Policies (HEN-OBS Joint Policy Brief No. 10).

Ståhl, T., Wismar, M., Ollila, E., Lahtinen, E. and Leppo, K. (eds.) (2006) *Health in All Policies. Prospects and Potentials*. Helsinki: Ministry of Social Affairs and Health, under the auspices of the European Observatory on Health Systems and Policies.

Stiglitz, J., Sen, A. and Fitoussi, J. (2009) *Report by the Commission on the Measurement of Economic Performance and Social Progress*. http://www.stiglitz-sen-fitoussi.fr/en/index.htm (accessed 15 August 2011).

Stuckler, D., Basu, S. and McKee, M. (2010) Budget crises, health, and social welfare programmes. *British Medical Journal*, 341: 77–9.

Suhrcke, M., McKee, M., Sauto Arce, R., Tsolova, S. and Mortensen, J. (2005) *The Contribution of Health to the Economy in the European Union*. Brussels: European Commission.

Suhrcke, M., Rocco, L., McKee, M., Mazzuco, S., Urban, D. and Steinherr, A. (eds.) (2007a) *Economic Consequences of Non communicable Diseases and Injuries in the Russian Federation*. Copenhagen: WHO Regional Office for Europe on behalf of the European Observatory on Health Systems and Policies.

Suhrcke, M., Rocco, L. and McKee, M. (eds.) (2007b) *Health: A Vital Investment for Economic Development in Eastern Europe and Central Asia*. Copenhagen: WHO Regional Office for Europe on behalf of the European Observatory on Health Systems and Policies, http://www.euro.who.int/__data/assets/pdf_file/0003/74739/E90569.pdf (accessed 2 September 2010).

Thomson, S., Foubister, T., Figueras, J. et al. (2009) *Addressing Financial Sustainability in Health Systems*. Copenhagen: WHO Regional Office for Europe on behalf of the European Observatory on Health Systems and Policies (HEN-OBS Joint Policy Summary No. 1).

Wanless, D. (2002) *Securing Our Future Health: Taking a Long-term View: Final Report*. London: The Stationery Office.

Wanless, D. (2004) *Securing Good Health for the Whole Population: Final Report*. London: The Stationery Office.

WHO Regional Office for Europe (2005) *European Health for All Series*, No. 7: *The Health for All Policy Framework for the WHO European Region – 2005 Update*. Copenhagen: WHO Regional Office for Europe.

WHO Regional Office for Europe (2008) *The Tallinn Charter: Health Systems for Health and Wealth*. Copenhagen: WHO Regional Office for Europe, http://www.euro.who.int/document/E91438.pdf (accessed 2 September 2010).

World Health Organization (2000) *The World Health Report 2000. Health Systems: Improving Performance*. Geneva: World Health Organization. http://www.who.int/whr/2000/en/ (accessed 1 September 2010).

chapter two

Understanding health systems: scope, functions and objectives

Antonio Durán, Joseph Kutzin,
José M. Martin-Moreno and Phyllida Travis

Introduction

Recent years have seen a renewed interest in health systems, in all parts of the world. They are now recognized as playing a vital role in preventing disability and premature death. Yet there are also demands that they do so as efficiently as possible at a time when some countries are implementing deep cuts in public spending (WHO Regional Committee for Europe 2009).

Health systems pose many challenges to politicians. Advances in medical technology have raised expectations about what health systems can deliver, causing continuing upward pressure on costs. Ideas for reform hold out the promise of cost-containment but rarely manage to deliver. Outcomes achievable in theory are not always achieved in practice (Hsiao and Heller 2007).

Health ministers can be disadvantaged by the lack of clarity about the boundaries of the health system. Often clinicians by background, many ministers are frustrated by the apparent lack of mechanisms at their disposal to bring about change, while the political dimension of health policies (World Health Organization 2004) adds to the complexity (as they often assume responsibility for failure but may have little control over the actions necessary for success).

This chapter proposes a framework for understanding health systems and defining their objectives and functions. It offers a means to promote effective decision-making within countries but also facilitates comparisons that support learning from experiences elsewhere.

The starting-point, as discussed in Chapter 1, is *The World Health Report 2000* (WHR2000); (World Health Organization 2000). In order to operationalize it, we will now restate its main features; clarify areas of ambiguity, such as those related to boundaries; and expand upon it by filling in some of the spaces between broad goals and functions.

The structure of this chapter is as follows. The health system and its boundaries are defined initially, followed by an examination of the goals of the health system, differentiating broad goals and intermediate objectives and functions. This is followed by two sections looking at how to apply the framework to individual countries and how to incorporate essential public health functions into service delivery, resource generation, financing and stewardship. The next section explores outstanding issues (for ministries of health in particular) from the experience since the Report's publication. The concluding section reflects on the practical use of the health systems framework; it identifies some weaknesses that may need to be addressed but argues that, overall, it provides a strong basis to move forward.

Understanding and defining health systems

Main definitions

Terms such as health care system, health and health care services and health sector are used widely (Hogarth 1996; WHO Regional Office for Europe 1996; European Observatory on Health Systems and Policies 2000), but analysts and policy-makers define them in substantially different ways. In essence, the different names mainly reflect different understandings of the health system boundaries and, specifically what to include. They range from those that limit the terms to health care (doctors, nurses, hospitals, etc.) to an all-encompassing concept embracing any activity, resource and/or institution that results in health improvements. The treatment of a sick person is straightforward (health care) but the idea that health outcomes also depend on actions not directly focused on individuals who are already sick (thereby including the wider determinants of health) is more complex. In 1989, Duplessis et al. defined a health system as (italics added):

> . . . organizations providing health services (hospital, health care centers, professional officers, and public health services) and also other networks, sectors, institutions, ministries and organizations *which have a definite influence* on the ultimate objective of the system – health. Important in this respect are education, transportation, social services, housing, the food industry, etc.

We know that health is indeed the result of a number of factors, some of which are resistant to short-term measures (e.g. biology, climate), and others that are less so (e.g. personal behaviour, health care, food safety). If the definition of the health system is confined to health care alone, it will exclude interventions with great potential to improve health (such as policies in education, environmental protection and agriculture). However, the all-encompassing definition of Duplessis et al. (1989) is problematic (particularly from a policy or management perspective) because a social system (which includes health systems) is more usefully understood as 'an arrangement of parts and their interconnections that come together for a *purpose*' (von Bertalanffy 1968). If we consider that a system includes all factors that have an influence on a given outcome, then, on the one hand, there are no meaningful boundaries and no clarity on managerial roles or on responsibilities and accountability. On the other hand, the very narrow health care definition is unduly limiting, considering health promotion as outside the boundaries of the health system, for example, would generate unnecessary fragmentation and may even question the duty of doctors, nurses and health ministries to incorporate health promotion into their work.

The WHO definition

None of the definitions alluded to above is satisfactory. The WHR2000 definition, adopted here, sought to overcome such problems: 'a health system consists of all organizations, people and institutions producing actions whose primary intent is to promote, restore or maintain health'. This definition is now used by other organizations, such as the World Bank (2006) and the EU (European Commission 2007).

Traditionally, services have been defined by their place in the evolution of a disease (e.g. preventive, therapeutic, rehabilitative), by the technology involved (laboratory, radiological), by who delivers them (medical, nursing, surgical), or by the recipients of care (mother, child). The WHR2000 categorizes services in ways that are meant to be both generic (applicable across a wide variety of contexts) and managerially relevant. *Personal services* are those that are delivered to individuals on a one-to-one basis such as a surgical operation, a general practice consultation, individual counselling, immunizing a child or supporting a mother in feeding a child. *Population-based* services are those delivered to a group or an entire population; these include immunization campaigns, warning labels on cigarette packs and workplace health promotion.

As this categorization of services depends on the mode of delivery, it is driven by organizational and managerial concerns. Notably, personal services can include interventions that are not only curative but also preventive and promotional. These include interventions delivered to individual patients that also provide benefits to others (e.g. treatment of infectious disease). Population-based services are preventive and promotional but exclude individual treatment.

Health is influenced by the actions of sectors whose primary purpose is other than to produce health. Each day parliaments, private companies and individuals make decisions that affect health, for example on housing, labour or fiscal policies. These are not included in the definition of a health system but this should not prevent health authorities from seeking to influence them. In contrast, efforts to promote healthy public policies so as to influence health determinants that lie outside the health system are *health actions* whose *primary intent* is to promote, preserve or protect health. As such, they are part of the health system and health authorities should be held accountable for such actions. For example, interventions to promote a health-oriented trade policy fall inside the boundaries of the health system but the resulting trading activities do not. The same applies to efforts to promote measures that address the social and economic determinants of health (e.g. pensions, housing, agriculture, roads). This responsibility for influencing other sectors is one of the key dimensions of what is termed stewardship, within which the WHR2000 includes the 'incorporate[ion of] selected intersectoral actions in which the stewards of the health system take responsibility to advocate for improvements in areas outside their direct control, such as legislation to reduce fatalities from traffic accidents'.

The definition of a health system, therefore, includes:

- health services (personal and population based) and the activities to enable their delivery provided by finance, resource generation and stewardship functions;
- stewardship, which includes activities seeking to influence the positive health impact of other sectors – even though the primary purpose of those sectors is not to improve health.

The criterion of *primary intent* was employed in the WHR2000 for a specific reason: to create a definition that enabled comparison (and therefore ranking) of all the national health systems worldwide. Yet, when looking at the performance of an individual health system, this can create difficulties. For example, it is arguable whether the primary purpose of garbage collection, water sanitation or the construction of cycle paths is health related. For that reason, for the present purposes, we incorporate the additional pragmatic notion of *mandate*. This provides some flexibility to adapt the boundaries of the health system to national contexts. For example, water chlorination may be the responsibility of a district health team in one country and of other parts of local government in another. Pragmatically, the former would be viewed as being inside the health system but the latter would not. However, in both cases, health authorities have an interest in ensuring that such activities are performed correctly. As we will see below, this extension to the definition may create a problem of accounting (and in particular precludes the possibility of creating global health system rankings), but not of accountability.

Notably, not all factors that affect health (or even those that meet the primary intent criterion) are covered by the concept of *assigned responsibilities*, which considers which bodies are designated as 'in charge of health'. In many countries, the national health ministry does not even have direct responsibility for conventional health care services, which may be the responsibility of a range of non-state actors, such as health insurance funds and private providers, or may be devolved to regional tiers of government. Nevertheless, those services remain part of the health system for reasons of primary intent. The situation is further confused by the grouping of functions including health within governments. Thus, there are ministries of health and consumer affairs; ministries of health and social security; ministries of health, labour and social affairs; ministries of health, youth and sport, etc. The WHR2000 (p. 6) warned that the definition:

> . . . does not imply any particular degree of integration, nor that anyone is in overall charge of the activities that compose it. In this sense, every country has a health system however fragmented it may be among different organizations or however unsystematically it may seem to operate. Integration and oversight do not determine the system, but they may greatly influence how well it performs.

The authors of that definition had in mind something that could fit all countries, based only on functions and primary intent. As noted above, our decision to incorporate mandate is driven by the need to use this framework to support national decision-making rather than international comparisons. For this reason we distinguish (i) health services as the 'machinery' related to the delivery of personal and population-based interventions from (ii) other activities addressing the broad determinants of health, and (iii) health systems as defined above but incorporating some context-specific notion of mandate as well as primary intent.

Goals and functions of health systems

What should health systems try to achieve?

The normative dimension of the proposed framework concerns what health systems *should* try to achieve, in other words, their goals. The rationale of this book, on health systems, health, wealth and societal well-being derives from welfare economics and, more specifically, draws on a social welfare function in which health is an intrinsic component of welfare, most notably through the impact of good or bad health on incomes (see Chapter 4).

The WHR2000 used a similar approach, based on the notion of social systems and social goals (Murray and Frenk 2000). In this construction, health is one of several social systems (e.g. education, economic, political), each with a *defining goal* (i.e. the reason why the system exists). The defining goal of a health system is to improve health, although this may affect the defining goals of other systems (e.g. impacts on economic well-being; educational attainment). The health system also has other goals ('fairness in the financial contribution required to make the system work' and 'responsiveness of the system to the legitimate expectations of the population') contributing to social welfare. The WHR2000 considered both levels and distribution, setting the goals as:

- improving the health status of the population: the average level of health and equity in the distribution of health;
- improving both the average level and the distribution of system responsiveness when individuals come into contact with the health system: respect for persons (ensuring patient dignity, confidentiality and autonomy) and client (service-user) orientation (prompt attention, basic amenities and choice);
- improving fairness in financial contributions, incorporating both avoidance of impoverishment as a consequence of 'catastrophic' health payments and equitable distribution of the burden of funding the system.

A further important distinction was made between health system attainment and performance. Attainment refers to the level of progress towards each goal (or a weighted composite of all the goals). Performance refers to the level of attainment relative to what could be achieved given key contextual factors arising from outside the health system – the most obvious being a country's income level. For example, from this perspective, the fact that Norway attains better health status or greater fairness in financial protection than Tajikistan does not necessarily mean that Norway has a better-performing health system. Rather, the much higher income level in Norway suggests that it has far greater potential to attain better health or fairer financing. Performance, therefore, refers *to the gap between what is and what could be attained* and hence is a measure of overall health system efficiency (or the efficiency with which any particular goal is attained).

By means of slight modifications to enable a focus on individual systems (the WHR2000 approach was used initially to enable international comparisons of health system performance), the framework is used as the basis of a tool to improve health system performance. The need to create aggregate measures or composite indices is dispensed with since such measures do not readily inform decision-making at country level.

While maintaining the broad goals of WHR2000, relating to health and responsiveness (level and equity), 'fair financing' is disaggregated into the instrumental goals of improving financial protection and creating an equitable burden of funding the health system. The former, the extent to which people are protected from becoming economically impoverished as a consequence of their payments for health care, is central to the wider concept of health systems, health and wealth. This goal is probably the health systems most direct link to the wider anti-poverty agenda.

The fundamental goals need to be disaggregated in ways that can be used to analyse the performance of each national health system. Instrumental goals must be *generic* (i.e. sufficiently broad to be applicable to all countries) but specific, so that they can be operationalized by countries in their own specific circumstances: that is, generating objectives that are *actionable by policy*. Hence, an instrumental goal is one that is relevant to all countries and has a plausible link to one or more of the broad health system goals. Here, we define two such instrumental goals: (i) the elements of *effective coverage* and (ii) *technical efficiency*.

Effective coverage is defined as the probability that individuals will obtain a health care intervention if they need it and they will derive benefit from it (Shengelia et al. 2005). This concept incorporates objectives that are relevant to all systems, in particular: (i) narrowing the gap between an individual's need for a service and his/her awareness of that need (demand), (ii) narrowing the gap between an individual's need for a service and their use of that service (access), and (iii) maximizing health gain from the use of a service (quality).

It is not necessary to construct a composite measure of effective coverage to provide useful policy guidance; indeed, disaggregation into the component parts offers more relevant insights (see the example below) (Jakab, Lundeen and Akkazieva 2007). Hence, the instrumental goals of *improved health* and *equity in health* that can be derived from the concept of effective coverage are *utilization relative to the need for service* and *quality of care*. While the specific services needed to achieve these goals may vary across countries, the basic principles are relevant to all health systems.

Technical efficiency is distinct from the concept of overall health system efficiency (attainment of a mix of the goals relative to what could be attained). In simple terms, it means making the best use of available resources. This is instrumental in achieving all of the final goals in the sense that, by reducing waste, systems can attain better health, greater equity and better financial protection for a given total level of resources. As with effective coverage, the means of achieving technical efficiency are often specific to a country. In many countries of central and eastern Europe and the former Soviet Union, the quest for technical efficiency includes reducing the physical infrastructure. This reduces the share of total expenditures absorbed by fixed costs and enables a greater proportion of public spending to be used for consumable items such as drugs and medical supplies; in some cases, this can have beneficial effects on financial protection by reducing the need for patients to pay for these items out of their own pockets. In such contexts, therefore, we do not observe a trade-off between efficiency and equity; indeed, the consequences of inefficiencies appear to damage poor people more (Jakab 2007).

Health system functions

The framework described above goes beyond structural approaches to incorporate a *functional* perspective. By function, we mean a group of interdependent activities that every health system undertakes (in a positive, descriptive, non-normative sense) in order to achieve its goals. Four of these determine the way inputs are transformed into outputs and outcomes: (i) providing (personal and population) services, (ii) financing, (iii) generating resources, and (iv) providing stewardship of health services and related intersectoral actions. Each of these relate to a number of 'health system building blocks' such as human resources, technologies and information (World Health Organization 2007).

The first function used to pursue the goals of the health system is the production of health services. The *purposeful production of services* is at the core of all health systems. Services permeate the set of institutions, people and resources intended (mandated) to improve health; these include the doctor and nurse who treat a patient but also the trainer who provides health education and the producer of a television anti-tobacco campaign (Nolte and McKee 2004; see Chapter 5). Poor coordination between those involved leads to waste and inefficiency. The service production function encompasses decisions on what services should be produced, where such production should take place and how they should be managed. There is considerable evidence to guide countries to produce and manage health services that are accessible, affordable and acceptable.

The second health system function is financing: dealing with the sources, accumulation and allocation of funds used for the health system (revenue collection); pooling; and purchasing (the last is the allocation of resources from the pool to providers). By definition, all health systems fund personal care and public health measures that contribute to health improvements in individuals and populations. Countries employ a variety of arrangements that are part of the history of each health system; such arrangement modalities have been used to characterize models and types of health system (e.g. Bismarck, Semashko and Beveridge) but they are not intrinsically important to the achievement of health system goals. Moreover, many countries are combining funding sources, pooling arrangements and the basis for entitlement in new ways, illustrating that while the labels attached to these models may retain some political value, they add little conceptually to the understanding and analysis of health financing arrangements that is needed for effective policy-making.

The third vital health system function relates to the identification, creation and development of the resources required to produce health services and to build a health system: knowledge, staff, facilities and technology. Given the labour-intensive nature of health services, human resources are the most important input to any health system; appropriate mechanisms for training, deployment and retention are essential to avoid inadequate skill mix and brain drain. Effective services demand modern equipment and technologies for both personal (pharmaceuticals and consumable medical goods) and population-based services (communication/information and organization of health technologies). Also, now that medical technologies are challenging the historical foundations of hospital care and moving towards 'boundary-less hospitals' (Braithwaite et al. 1995), countries need to rethink the ways in which they invest in capital (Rechel et al. 2009).

Finally, the *stewardship* function is the ensemble of activities aimed at ensuring that health actions (including intersectoral measures) have a clear direction and are carried out in ways that maximize the likelihood of achieving the systems goals. The WHO2000 defined stewardship (p. 136) as 'the careful and responsible management of the well-being of the population': protecting the public interest with regard to health issues. For conceptual (and hence operational) clarity, it is useful to disaggregate stewardship into three specific dimensions: (i) formulating and coordinating health policy, (ii) exerting influence, and (iii) collecting and using intelligence to assure quality.

While the goals of the health system are normative and value-driven (i.e. what health systems *should* try to achieve), the functions are positive (i.e. a value-free descriptive tool); every health system performs the functions described above, whether or not they are recognized or explicit. However, this does not mean that it is not possible to attempt a more normative approach by describing the ideal; for example, good health financing responds to the health priorities of a country while providing the right incentives to improve the performance of health professionals. Good purchasing, in particular, should link resource allocation to information on providers' performance and/or the health needs of the population being served. Similar reasoning could be applied to the characteristics of the other functions (good resource generation, good service production, etc.).

Because of its overriding importance to the performance of the system, we note some elements of good health stewardship. They apply to all interventions with a significant impact on health, regardless of their primary purpose. These elements are *steering* (leading and providing vision, rather than managing all operations), *governing* (ensuring clear rules and good use of resources) and ensuring *accountability* (for both performance outcomes and fair/reasonable processes). A good steward is guided by goals, values and evidence to encourage structural microsystems (primary health care centres, hospitals, etc.) to respond to individual and societal needs with appropriate personal and population services while modulating the relationships between stakeholders (e.g. the health insurance market). In a context of transparency and accountability, the steward should also provide leadership and priorities to sectors beyond the health system in order to enhance their health impact. The steward should be able to target *action*, based on intelligence that seeks to understand (i) all the factors that influence health (i.e. the determinants), (ii) which factors emanating from outside the system are amenable to change, and (iii) who holds the mandate for relevant activities.

Such distinctions between positive and normative analysis of functions are essential at country level: the 'goodness' characteristics help to assess how well a particular system is performing each function. However, these can only be justified by plausible links to the system goals (the purchasing and stewardship examples above are based on the assumption that good purchasing and proper regulation lead to better access, improved coverage and quality of care, which, in turn, lead to better health).

Each individual health system function is important, as is their interconnectedness – how the parts of the health system fit together. Each function is linked with all the others. For example, as noted above, some health promotion services are personal (e.g. administering vaccine to an infant) and some are population based (implementing a radio campaign). Both require specific resources and funds in order for these to become health interventions delivered to individuals or the community. Decisions on which services to produce, in what numbers and under which regulatory conditions, are influenced by the priorities of the health system concerned. An understanding of the wider interconnectedness between health and other sectors is essential to enable health system stewards to lead multisectoral health-promoting actions.

Applying the framework to individual countries

The fundamental and instrumental goals and functions described above are generic in the sense that they apply to all health systems. Figure 2.1 provides a simplified illustration of these. Such a broad portrayal is merely the starting-point for systematic reforms of a health system in any particular country. The framework becomes operational when the goals and objectives are translated into the national context and then strategies are developed to (re-)organize the functions to achieve these objectives.

This framework can be used to support national decision-making in two related ways: (i) in development of a coherent, goal-oriented health reform strategy, and (ii) for performance assessment and monitoring. Both involve working backwards from the broad goals to identify country-specific objectives that are measurable and *actionable* by policy.

This is illustrated by a recent analysis of measures to reduce the toll of ill health resulting from hypertension in Kyrgyzstan (Jakab, Lundeen and Akkazieva 2007). The analysis began by applying the elements of effective coverage to diagnose the nature of the problem within the country. This informed the definition of an overall objective: to identify the percentage of people with hypertension whose blood pressure is being controlled. In turn, this led to the definition of three more specific objectives: (i) improving people's awareness of their hypertension status (measured as the percentage of the adult population with hypertension who are aware of their status), (ii) ensuring that those diagnosed with hypertension are prescribed appropriate medications (percentage of those with hypertension taking treatment for their condition), and (iii) ensuring that

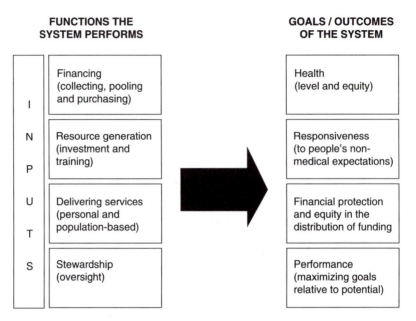

Figure 2.1   Health Systems Assessment Framework: functions and goals

Source: Courtesy of Phyllida Travis.

treatment is effective (that people's hypertension is controlled: percentage of those who took medication during the past 24 hours whose blood pressure is under control). Each of these was measured in a household survey.

The next step in applying the framework is to work forwards from the functions in order to identify a range of possible policy interventions (i.e. reforms) that might contribute to these objectives. The functional framework helps to ensure a comprehensive approach. Continuing with the example of the Kyrgyzstan hypertension study, this analysis led to a series of policy recommendations based on the following functions:

Population-based service interventions: to improve population awareness and knowledge; to provide the population with understandable and valid information about the importance of regular hypertension measurement, in an attempt to increase the number who are aware of their condition; to provide information on hypertension and its consequences; to promote medication adherence; and to improve understanding of the benefits of using generic drugs.

Personal health care service interventions: to improve physician adherence to guidelines (particularly to reduce the number of patients who take medication intermittently because doctors advise that it is taken only at times of crisis); and to implement continuous education programmes, guidelines and quality improvement processes.

Financing interventions: to improve access and financial protection; extend population coverage of the existing outpatient drug benefit scheme; and attempt to increase the use of generic medicines.

Resource generation interventions: to improve quality on a sustainable basis and to emphasize appropriate and inappropriate medication practices in medical training.

Stewardship: to ensure overall coherence, sufficient resources and priority for addressing hypertension; develop a renewed cardiovascular diseases strategy; and use existing analyses to attract donor funds, currently heavily weighted towards communicable diseases. Also, to undertake further analysis (generating intelligence) of the demand for generic drugs compared with proprietary hypertension medication; on the impact of medication choice on the continuity of treatment; and to improve understanding of prescribing, dispensing and consumption patterns.

This example illustrates how the framework can support a systematic approach to understanding poor health system performance and in designing a comprehensive policy response.

The framework may also be used to support analysis of a single health system function. This involves defining intermediate objectives associated with a particular function by considering the goals that it is likely to influence as well as the means or *pathways* by which this can occur. For the health financing function (Kutzin 2008), for example, the final goals are the same as those for the entire health system. For financial protection and equity in finance, the health financing subsystem has a direct impact on the goal (Fig. 2.2). Financing is hypothesized to affect other health system goals through

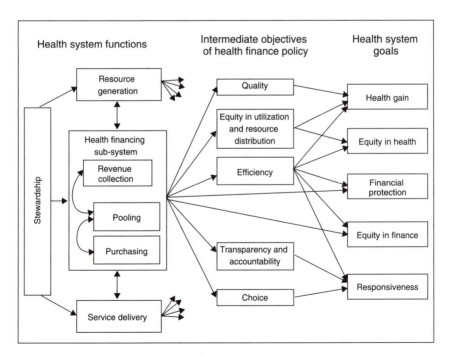

Figure 2.2   Intermediate objectives and goals for the health finance function

Source: Adapted from Kutzin 2008.

intermediate objectives with a plausible link to both the function and the goals. This helps to define specific intermediate objectives for this function (middle column), while noting (at the far left) that the financing subsystem does not operate in isolation.

The process of translating the generic framework to a specific country context requires considerable time and effort but is not conceptually complex. Indeed, it can be a relatively simple, linear process of moving from global goals to concrete, measurable objectives. As this translation process continues, it provides a mechanism for stakeholder engagement as well as movement towards objectives amenable to policy action (e.g. reducing infant mortality per se does not lend itself directly to a discrete number of strategies, but increasing immunization coverage does). This is the real purpose of this (or any) framework – to provide a means to organize thinking in a comprehensive, coherent manner that provides a basis for action.

The health systems framework and public health

As with 'health system', the term 'public health' has had a number of conflicting or differing definitions. A decade ago the problem was well summarized by Julio Frenk (1999) as follows.

> Historically, the term public health has been used with multiple and often equivocal meanings. I have been able to identify at least five major connotations that have been used at various times. The first equates the adjective 'public' to governmental action, that is, the public sector. The second is somewhat broader, since it includes not only government programmes but also the participation of the organized community, that is to say, 'the public'. The third identifies public health with 'non-personal health services' – that is, services that cannot be appropriated by a specific individual, since they are targeted at the environment (e.g. sanitation) or the community (e.g. mass health education). The next is slightly broader, since it adds a series of personal preventive services for vulnerable groups (for example, maternal and child care programmes). Finally, the expression 'public health problem' is often used, particularly in non-technical language, to refer to diseases that are particularly frequent or dangerous . . . As a field of action through professional practice, the modern conception of public health comprises the systematic efforts being made to identify health needs and to organize comprehensive services with a well-defined population base. It thus encompasses the information required for characterizing the conditions of the population and the mobilization of resources necessary for responding to such conditions through the health system.

Winslow's original definition of public health in 1920 was slightly rephrased by WHO's European Office in order to incorporate explicitly the health protection dimension of public health (including occupational health and food safety). Public health is thus defined as 'The science and art of protecting health, preventing disease, and promoting health (with the goal of prolonging and improving life) through the organized efforts and informed choices of society, public and private organizations, communities and individuals' (Adshead et al. 2008).

In 1998, the Pan American Health Organization, the US Centers for Disease Control and Prevention and the Latin American Center for Health Systems Research formulated the Essential Public Health Functions (EPHF) (Pan American Health Organization/World Health Organization 1998). These are understood to be the core areas of public health for which governments are ultimately responsible (ministries of health do not necessarily have to implement and finance them directly, rather they are achieved through other government agencies, community and nongovernmental organizations or the private sector, among others.) The EPHF comprises a checklist of 11 operations that attempt to capture the role of national health authorities in public health and for which standards should be established.

Strictly speaking, the EPHF is not an alternative framework of analysis. Rather it is a mission statement or a checklist of operations that good health systems should perform. These EPHFs can be incorporated in the health systems framework as normative aspects of *goodness* (things that should be done) within specific health system functions. In particular, the 11 EPHFs can be categorized as follows.

1. *Monitoring, evaluation and analysis of health status:* this belongs to the intelligence dimension of stewardship.
2. *Surveillance, research and control of risks and threats to public health:* these are population-based services.
3. *Health promotion:* this is part of service delivery, within both personal and population services.
4. *Social participation in health:* this can be seen as an intermediate objective, a means to an end (policy approach) or even a reflection of underlying values.
5. *Development of policies and institutional capacity for public health planning and management:* this is part of the health policy formulation and coordination dimension of stewardship, and possibly of the human resources for health dimension of resource generation.
6. *Strengthening public health regulation and enforcement capacity:* this is another element of the stewardship function (exerting influence).
7. *Evaluation and promotion of equitable access to necessary health services:* this is a managerial component of both the stewardship (intelligence) and the service production functions.
8. *Human resource development and training in public health:* this is a key aspect of the resource generation function.
9. *Quality assurance in personal and population-based health services:* this is part of the service delivery function.
10. *Research in public health:* this is part of the intelligence dimension of stewardship.
11. *Reduction of the impact of emergencies and disasters on health:* this is an objective linked to the functions of stewardship and service delivery.

Implementing the framework

Policy and managerial issues

The proposed health systems definition and framework provides a set of boundaries, functions and goals that should facilitate policy and managerial action, performance measurement and accountability. In practice, however, a number of implementation challenges remain.

It is very difficult to assess the performance of a system when its main goal (health) is influenced strongly by external factors and activities with impacts that are difficult to disentangle from that of the health system. Other chapters in this book and the recent European Observatory volume on performance measurement further illustrate the complexities in accounting for such external factors (Smith et al. 2009).

It can also be difficult to operationalize the health system goals in practice. For example, while what constitutes good stewardship is understood in general terms, to determine the precise and measurable characteristics of good stewardship in a particular country and assess its contribution to health system goals is far more challenging.

Accounting for 'all health system activities, organizations and institutions whose primary intent/mandate is to improve health' under each of the functions poses another major technical challenge. With the financing function, for instance, total health system expenditure should be calculated by adding together health service expenditure with expenditure from activities (in other sectors) whose primary intent is to improve health, such as enforcing seat-belt legislation, road safety or water quality control. Moreover one should also include other *health actions* such as the costs incurred by citizens and service users at individual or small group levels in improving or preserving health. This includes self-care and personal health education or the costs of informal care within families. In practice, however, figures for health system expenditure include little more than public (and to varying degrees, private) expenses incurred by personal and population-based interventions provided through the formal health system.

A further issue is that of accountability (Brinkerhoff 2004). The formal responsibilities of health ministries vary enormously. The concept of stewardship implies that the health ministry is at the helm – accountable for the operation and impact of health services, for advocating healthy public policy and for exercising stewardship in other sectors to ensure that health implications are considered in all public policies. This envisages that the health ministry should be held accountable for influencing primary intent actions in other sectors. Clearly, this is not the reality in most countries. Even responsibility for the formal health care sector is often distributed among different tiers of government with different ministries and agencies, such as insurance funds, professional bodies and provider associations. Many health ministries have a low status in the political hierarchy. In some countries where health financing is based on insurance, health ministries have barely developed the capacity to exercise more than the most basic influence on health care. There are many examples where intersectoral action to promote health has originated in other ministries, such as those of finance, education or transport, with the health ministry following later or, worse, declining to cooperate in initiatives it views as properly belonging to it. Hence, it is inappropriate to argue that health ministries could or should take responsibility for implementing *all* activities included under the health system definition, as their ability to do so, or to exercise leadership to get things done, depends on a number of other factors.

One final major challenge in implementing the framework is the quality of available data needed to assess performance and inform decision-making. Few countries have sufficiently reliable, population-based data to operationalize and measure the many variables included in this framework. For example, health service utilization data are surprisingly scarce and often incomplete in many countries, and, of course, there are few data on the impact of intersectoral actions.

All things considered, however, the advantages of adopting the health systems framework outnumber the problems. What is important, when applying it, is to consider the *specific political and institutional contexts with a clear understanding of the differences between political and managerial responsibilities.*

Implications for research

There is a need for more experience in the implementation of the framework in different countries. In particular, there is a need for better understanding of the impact of the political context within which health systems operate. A World Bank strategy paper (World Bank 2006) rightly warned against presenting health outcomes as the mere product of a set of physical inputs, human resources, organizational structures and managerial processes – hence seeing health system reforms as mere mechanistic adaptations. Instead, health systems should be seen as complex *adaptive* (Plsek, Wilson and Greenhalgh 2001) (rather than mechanical) systems. This would focus efforts on working with political actors and other stakeholders towards achieving specific objectives rather than on producing an overdetailed set of managerial arrangements and incentives. There is a large arsenal of research on organizational architecture and change management, originated mostly in the commercial sector, that can usefully be applied and adapted to the public sector (Roberts 2004; Roberts et al. 2004; Shortell and Kaluzny 2006).

There is also a need for more research on mapping institutional accountability. This would include, for instance, a review of the responsibilities and accountabilities of ministries of health, examining their particular roles, functions and organizational structures.

The same applies to the need to map political values (as well as their inherent trade-offs), which are often used in debates to justify policy instruments (McKee 2008). For example, the EU Member States committed to a set of common values and principles (Council of the European Union 2006). The health systems framework analysed here is rooted in a series of values translated into a series of goals and objectives, as is the Tallinn Charter with its values of equity, solidarity and participation (WHO Regional Office for Europe 2008). There is a need to make these values explicit in any analysis and ascertain whether they are reflected in the objectives of the health system.

Conclusions

This chapter has defined a health system as the ensemble of organizations, institutions and resources that are mandated (within the political and institutional map of a country) to produce actions whose primary intent is to improve, maintain or restore health. While recognizing that the national diversity of approaches to health system organization reflects cultural, historical, economic and policy influences, it has taken the normative position that all health systems should pursue some combination of goals and objectives, as follows.

Health systems should reduce the burden of illness, impairment and disabilities among a population in an equitable way and through processes that are deemed to be responsive to individual preferences. In combination with other public policies, they should offer social protection against catastrophically costly illness and promote economic growth by enhancing human capital and, thereby, labour force participation and productivity, as a means to economic development.

All health systems perform a set of core functions, namely the provision of personal and population services, financing, resource generation and stewardship. The analysis of health determinants is a fundamental part of the stewardship function that extends beyond describing and decrying those determinants such as poverty to analysing whether these causes are amenable to change, identifying who can bring about such change and trying to influence them.

The concept of the health system framework offers a useful policy perspective. Using the fight against tobacco as an example, in addition to diagnosing and treating diseases that result from smoking, health workers should also provide anti-tobacco advice during consultations (personal services), supported by population services such as public education campaigns. Recent experience in many countries has shown that such measures are not enough to fight the scourge of tobacco, and action at many other levels is needed, including (for example) epidemiological research to provide the evidence to convince smokers to quit, warning labels on cigarette packs, advertising bans, taxation of cigarettes, trading standards enforcement, thwarting attempts by the tobacco industry to circumvent marketing restrictions, and bans on smoking in public places. Some of these actions would be taken by health authorities (ministries, regional and local health bodies, etc.) but others by a wide range of ministries, agencies and institutions.

As ultimate stewards of population health, governments (usually through their health ministries) should decide where their limited resources will have the most impact. Such decisions will be influenced by national politics and will have to balance often competing agendas. The long-term impact of tobacco control is often not as attractive as the short-term, politically appealing impact of a new cancer treatment centre. A strong public health focus is important.

This chapter has shown that the health systems framework offers a generic tool that can be adapted to support decision-making and analysis. The proposed framework brings together in a coherent way the positive (*what is* – the functions that all health systems perform) and normative (*what should be* – the goals that all health systems should strive to achieve given the constraints of available resources) aspects. Overall, the health systems framework offers a solid conceptual basis to understand health systems. The challenge is to generate further experience of using it in different settings.

References

Adshead, F., et al. (2008) *Strengthening Public Health Capacity and Services of the Health Systems in Europe: Focusing on the essential dimensions of Public Health.* Internal draft document elaborated by a Working Group sponsored by the WHO Regional Office for Europe, 2008.

Braithwaite, J., Lazarus, L., Vining, R.F. and Soar, J. (1995) Hospitals: to the next millennium. *International Journal of Health Planning and Management,* 10: 87–98.

Brinkerhoff, D.W. (2004) Accountability and health systems: toward conceptual clarity and policy relevance. *Health Policy and Planning,* 19(6): 371–9.

Council of the European Union (2006) *Council Conclusions on Common Values and Principles in European Union Health Systems* (2006/C 146/01). Brussels: Council of the European Union.

Duplessis, P., Dab, W., McCarthy, M. and Portella, E. (eds.) (1989) *Public Health and Industrialized Countries.* Quebec: Les Publications du Quebec.

European Commission (2007) *Health Systems Impact Assessment Tool.* Brussels: European Commission.   http://ec.europa.eu/health/ph_overview/co_operation/high_level/health_systems_en.htm (accessed 1 September 2010).

European Observatory on Health Systems and Policies (2000) *The Observatory's Health Systems Glossary.* Copenhagen: WHO Regional Office for Europe. http://www.euro.who.int/observatory/glossary/toppage (accessed May 2008; being updated, September 2010).

Frenk, J. (1999) What's in a name? *Bulletin of the World Health Organization,* 77(2): 101, http://www.who.int/bulletin/archives/77(2)101.pdf (accessed 2 September 2010).

Hogarth, J. (1996) *Glossary of Health Care Terminology.* Copenhagen: WHO Regional Office for Europe.

Hsiao, W. and Heller, P.S. (2007) *What Should Macroeconomists Know about Health Care Policy?* working paper 07/13. Washington, DC: International Monetary Fund.

Jakab, M. (2007) An empirical evaluation of the Kyrgyz health reform: does it work for the poor? PhD Thesis, University of Harvard.

Jakab, M., Lundeen, E. and Akkazieva, B. (2007) *Health System Effectiveness in Hypertension Control in Kyrgyzstan,* Bishkek: Health Policy Analysis Unit, Center for Health System Development http://www.hpac.kg/images/pdf/PRP44.E.pdf (accessed 15 September 2010).

Kutzin, J. (2008) *Health Financing Policy: A Guide For Decision-makers.* (Policy Research Paper No. 44) Copenhagen: WHO Regional Office for Europe (Health Financing Policy Paper 2008/1).

McKee, M. (2008) Solidarity in a unified Europe, *European Journal of Public Health,* 18(1): 2–4.

Murray, C.J.L. and Frenk, J. (2000) A framework for assessing the performance of health systems. *Bulletin of the World Health Organization,* 78(6): 717–31.

Murray, C.L.M. and Evans, D.B. (eds.) (2003) *Health Systems Performance Assessment; Debates, Methods and Empiricism.* Geneva: World Health Organization.

Nolte, E. and McKee, M. (2004) *Does Health Care Save Lives? Avoidable Mortality Revisited.* London: Nuffield Trust.

Pan American Health Organization/World Health Organization (1998) *Essential Public Health Functions (EPHF)*. World Health Statistics Quarterly, 51(1): 44–54, http://www.paho.org/English/DPM/SHD/HP/EPHF.htm (accessed 2 September 2010).
Plsek, P., Wilson, E. and Greenhalgh, T. (2001) Complexity science, the challenge of complexity in health care: *British Medical Journal,* 323: 625–8.
Rechel, B., Wright, S., Edwards, N., Dowdeswell, N.and McKee, M. (eds.) (2009) *Investing in Hospitals of the Future.* Copenhagen: WHO Regional Office for Europe on behalf of the European Observatory on Health Systems and Policies.
Roberts, J. (2004) *The Modern Firm.* New York: Oxford University Press.
Roberts, M., Hsiao, W., Berman, P. and Reich, M. (2004) *Getting Health Reform Right,* Oxford: Oxford University Press: 60–7.
Shengelia, B., Tandon, A., Adams, O.B. and Murray, C.L.M. (2005) Access, utilization, quality and effective coverage: an integrated conceptual framework and measurement strategy. *Social Science and Medicine,* 61: 97–109.
Shortell, S.M. and Kaluzny, A.D. (2006) *Health Care Management; Organisation Design and Behaviour.* Clifton Park, NY: Thomson Delmar Learning.
Smith, P.C., Mossialos, E., Papanicolas, I. and Leatherman, S. (eds.) (2009) *Performance Measurement for Health System Improvement: Experiences, Challenges and Prospects.* Cambridge: Cambridge University Press.
von Bertalanffy, L. (1968) *General System Theory: Foundations, Development, Applications.* New York: George Braziller.
WHO Regional Committee for Europe (2009) *Fifty-ninth Session of the Regional Committee for Europe: Health in Times of Global Economic Crisis – Implications for the WHO European Region,* Copenhagen, 14–17 September. Copenhagen: WHO Regional Office for Europe. http://www.euro.who.int/__data/assets/pdf_file/0006/66957/RC59_edoc07.pdf (accessed 1 September 2010).
WHO Regional Office for Europe (1996) *WHO Conference on Europe Health Care Reforms: Proceedings of the conference,* Ljubljana, Slovenia, 17–20 June. Copenhagen: WHO Regional Office for European, http:wholibdoc.who.int/euro/1994-97/EUR_ICP_CARE_01_02_01.pdf (accessed 29 September 2011).
WHO Regional Office for Europe (2008) *The Tallinn Charter: Health Systems for Health and Wealth.* Copenhagen: WHO Regional Office for Europe, http://www.euro.who.int/document/E91438.pdf (accessed 2 September 2010).
Winslow, C.E.A. (1920) The untilled fields of public health. *Science,* 51: 23–33.
World Bank (2006) *What is a Health System? Briefing to CODE,* strategy note annex F. Washington, DC: World Bank.
World Health Organization (2000) *The World Health Report. 2000, Health Systems: Improving Performance.* Geneva: World Health Organization: 1–44, http://www.who.int/whr/2000/en/ (accessed 1 September 2010).
World Health Organization (2004) *Poverty Reduction Strategy Papers: Their Significance for Health: Second Synthesis Report,* WHO/HDP/PRSP/O4.1. Geneva: World Health Organization: 15–17.
World Health Organization (2007) *Everybody's Business: Strengthening Health Systems to Improve Health Outcomes – WHO's Framework for Action.* Geneva: World Health Organization.

chapter three

Re-examining the cost pressures on health systems

Reinhard Busse, Ewout van Ginneken and Charles Normand

Introduction

Policy-makers and lay-people alike realize that health care costs have risen considerably and are under continuing upward pressure. However, myths and misunderstandings often shape any debate as the underlying factors, their effects and interactions may not be well understood. Ageing, or (more broadly) the demographic transition, is the most often cited driver, although higher expenditure can also be driven by economic growth and resulting higher incomes, medical progress through innovation and new technologies, health care organization and financing, higher relative prices for health care inputs and the increasing expectations of citizens. This chapter reviews recent research and evidence in order to provide an assessment of the present and potential future impacts of these drivers on health expenditure.

Before a more detailed examination of the evidence from studies on the different drivers, it is useful to clarify the different (but closely related) concepts of health care costs, expenditure and public or quasi-public spending. Higher expenditure may result from higher unit costs for the existing volume of services or from increases or changes in patterns of service use. Public or quasi-public funding agencies (including social health insurance funds) typically focus more on their own expenditure and may be less concerned about costs to patients and their families. Macroeconomic policy-makers may be concerned about the extent to which health spending (by anyone) may crowd out spending on other investments contributing to increased economic growth. The policy debate is not always clear about what are the main concerns.

The first, and largest, section of this chapter examines the role of the main drivers of health expenditure outlined above. It also includes data on the relative impact of the various drivers (see particularly Table 3.1). The latest evidence on current projections regarding future health care expenditures is presented and assessed in the second section. The chapter concludes with a summary of our findings and their policy implications.

Drivers of health expenditure growth

When examining the determinants of health expenditure, international literature groups itself roughly around the following 'culprits':

- ageing and demographic change
- economic growth and higher income
- new technologies and medical progress
- organization and financing of health care systems
- higher relative prices for health care inputs
- increasing expectations of populations.

These determinants are addressed below in light of recent evidence. This chapter focuses primarily on external cost pressures, and so the organization and financing of the system are not discussed here.

Ageing and demographic change

There is a widespread belief that health care costs rise steeply with age. Services for elderly people absorb between 35% and 50% of total health expenditure (Jacobzone 2003). This concern is heightened because European populations are likely to change dramatically in the next decades, as shown in various projections undertaken by the EU (Economic Policy Committee of the European Commission 2006, 2009), Organisation for Economic Co-operation and Development (OECD) (2006) and the World Bank (Chawla, Betcherman and Banerji 2007).

In their 2009 projection for the period 2008–2060, the Economic Policy Committee of the European Commission highlighted three major demographic trends in the 27 Member States in 2007 (EU27):

Fertility rates. These are projected to remain well below the natural replacement rate (growing only moderately from 1.52 births per woman in 2008 to 1.64 by 2060).

Life expectancy at birth. This is projected to rise by 8.5 years for men (from 76 to 84.5 years) and by 6.9 years for women (from 82.1 to 89) over the next five decades.

Inward migration. Between 2008 and 2060, this will add 59 million people, contributing to a still growing population (by around 5% from 495 million in 2008 to 520 million in 2060 – with the gain concentrating in most EU15 countries, while Germany, Greece and the new Member States would lose inhabitants), differentiating the 2009 projection from its 2006 predecessor (Economic Policy Committee of the European Commission 2006), which had predicted a fall by almost 1% in the EU25 until 2050.

These trends will result in dramatic changes in the age structure of the population. The working age population (15–64 years) is projected to fall by 15% between 2010 and 2060. In contrast, the population aged 65+ will rise sharply until 2060 (by 76 million or 78%). More significantly, the numbers in the very old age groups (above 80 years) will rise even more rapidly (from 22 million in 2008 to 61 million in 2060). The old-age dependency ratio (the number of people aged ≥65 relative to those aged 15–64) is projected to more than double, reaching 53.5% in 2060. Assuming no change in the current age of retirement, EU countries will thus move from the current situation of four people of working age for every elderly citizen to a ratio of two to one by 2050 (Economic Policy Committee of the European Commission 2009).

In the same way, a World Bank study (Chawla, Betcherman and Banerji 2007) contains very striking projections for the countries of central and eastern Europe and the Commonwealth of Independent States. By 2025, the median age will rise by 10 years in about half of these countries and the population will shrink in 18 of the 28 countries in this region. The population of the Russian Federation fell from 149 to 143 million between 1990 and 2005 and is projected to fall even further – to 111 million by 2050. The share of the population and the absolute number of people over the age of 65 will continue to rise, reaching one person in every five in most of the region's countries by 2025. The combination of rapidly ageing and relatively poor populations is unique to these countries.

Both ageing per se and new treatment options will have a significant impact on the health needs of the population and related patterns of disease. These needs are likely to increase and are certain to change, requiring changes to the organization and structure of health systems. For example, as higher numbers of people live to over 80 and 90 years, more people will need long-term health care services and specialized social services.

Ageing and health care financing

Ageing poses two (potential) sets of pressures for financing of the health care system: (i) decreasing income, and (ii) increasing utilization and health service expenditure. The former is a particular concern since the total dependency ratio will rise (i.e. fewer persons will bear the lion's share of funding the system). In other words, intergenerational transfers from the younger to the older genera-tions (which generally contribute less) will continue to increase. Although an increase in retirement age may ease funding problems, it is unlikely that this will completely address the problem of high intergenerational transfers, which some authors consider to be a form of inequity (Breyer and von Schulenburg 1987).

Health care utilization and costs are even more difficult to project than future dependency ratios. Current per capita expenditure on health care increases with age: that is, a larger proportion of older people will substantially increase health care costs if this relationship remains unchanged. The current relationship between age and health care expenditure is shown in Fig. 3.1.

Conversely, older people are now healthier than ever and will most likely be even healthier in the future (see discussion on longevity hypotheses below). At any given age, being healthier than the previous generation may well result in fewer health care needs and reduce utilization, or (at least) postpone it,

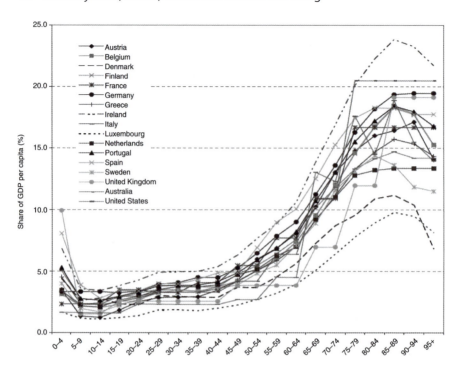

Figure 3.1 Public spending on health in each age group, share of gross domestic product (GDP) per capita

Source: Organisation for Economic Co-operation and Development 2006.

in so doing shifting the cost-by-age curve to the right. Therefore, the simple belief that an ageing population is automatically leading to increased health expenditure is being questioned by a growing body of evidence that suggests a more complicated picture. Increased age may be a useful indicator of the health status of a particular population but it is not the cause. A number of interrelated issues need to be considered as possible explanatory factors. The most relevant of these are (i) the relationship between increasing life expectancy, morbidity and health care expenditure; and (ii) the cost of dying or, rather, proximity to death (rather than age).

Compression of morbidity versus expansion of morbidity

The main question is whether increased and increasing life expectancy (rather than high age) will increase or decrease morbidity and thus health expenditure. Three theories have emerged over the last 30 years.

Compression of morbidity hypothesizes that morbidity and disability will gradually be compressed at very old age and the years spent with disability and disease will decrease (Fries 1980, 1983, 1989, 1993). Furthermore, humankind is approaching its genetically determined lifespan limit although life expectancy still grows. This second part of the hypothesis is contentious and has been rejected by several authors (Doblhammer and Kytir 2001; Oeppen and Vaupel 2002; Robine, Jagger and van Oyen 2005). Some recent approximately linear patterns of increasing life expectancy in developed countries suggest that we remain some way from any genetically determined limit to survival (White 2002).

Expansion of morbidity (Gruenberg 1977; Verbrugge 1984; Olshansky et al. 1991) is a much bleaker hypothesis. In line with popularly held belief, this argues that as life expectancy increases, older people become more vulnerable to chronic diseases. This results in more time spent in ill health, based on the following assumptions: (i) medical interventions prolong the survival of people with chronic illness but do not improve their health state; (ii) increased survival means that a larger part of the population is elderly and more vulnerable to chronic disease; and (iii) chronic disease can act as a risk factor for other illnesses.

Dynamic equilibrium can be seen as a compromise between the expansion and compression scenarios. Proposed by Manton and colleagues (Manton 1982; Manton, Stallard and Corder 1995), it suggests that healthy life expectancy grows at the same rate as total life expectancy (*healthy ageing*) and the number of years spent in ill health remains constant. However, it is important to note that as the years in ill health remain constant, the time spent in ill health decreases as a share of total life expectancy.

Although there is no critical body of evidence for any of these three hypotheses, a certain picture emerges. Studies that measured morbidity in terms of self-reported health or health-related quality of life, for example in Austria (Doblhammer and Kytir 2001), Denmark (Bronnum-Hansen 2005) or Germany (Dinkel 1998), tend to confirm the compression of morbidity hypothesis. However, this does not necessarily translate into lower health care expenditure in each age group as other factors (such as increased medical possibilities to treat healthier older persons; increased expectations of older persons) may outweigh potential savings.

Given the methodological complexities (such as measuring changes in morbidity, technological possibilities, expectations and differences in health systems), studies in this area are likely to remain difficult. Most studies that project future health care spending, such as those by the Economic Policy Committee of the European Commission (2006, 2009), the OECD (Organisation for Economic Co-operation and Development 2006) or the World Bank (Chawla, Betcherman and Banerji 2007) (see discussion below), encompass multiple scenarios that incorporate these hypotheses.

Proximity to death, not age per se

Fuchs (1984) was the first to point out that the relationship between age and health care utilization (or costs) is biased by the fact that the percentage of people in their last year of life increases rapidly with age, and that this is a period when people use more services. He hypothesized that if mortality in all age groups above 65 were constant, health care costs with age would also be constant. If this is true, then the attention of policy-makers and scientists is being diverted from more significant causes of health expenditure growth.

This view was first supported by Medicare data for citizens aged 65+ in the United States, which also demonstrated two additional complicating factors. First, health care costs for persons in their last year of life reach a maximum at about the age of 70 (later shown to be even lower in other countries) after which it falls with increasing age. Second, health care costs for the group of survivors rise until the age of about 85 and then fall with increasing age (Lubitz and Riley 1993). The marginal increase in lifetime costs associated with an additional year of life decreases as the age at death rises (Lubitz, Beebe and Baker 1995). However, these studies left a number of questions unanswered on the generalizability of these findings given the particular characteristics and incentives in the American health system.

Nevertheless, studies from other countries such as Canada (Roos, Montgomery and Roos 1987; McGrail et al. 2000), the Netherlands (van Vliet and Lamers 1998), Switzerland (Zweifel, Felder and Meiers 1999; Zweifel, Felder and Werblow 2004), Germany for statutory health insurance (Busse, Krauth and Schwartz 2002) and for private health insurance (Niehaus 2006) and France (Dormont, Grignon and Huber 2006) have generally confirmed the findings from the United States and have extended this knowledge to younger age groups. Using Italian data, Aprile (2004) confirmed that the costs of death tend to decline steadily after young and prime ages. More recently, Niehaus (2006) analysed German private health insurance data for deceased persons over a 10-year period prior to death. These were highest for persons dying between 50 and 60 years of age. Evidence from all available sources thus suggests that the costs of dying decline with older age, as older people tend to be treated less intensively as they near death (Raitano 2006).

On the basis of the Medicare data, Stearns and Norton (2004) concluded that 'time to death' should be included as an explanatory variable in individual health care expenditure. This was underscored by a study carried out by Zweifel, Felder and Werblow (2004) based on Swiss data, which covered a broad age range (from 30 years onwards) as well as a range of components of health care expenditure. Using the same Swiss data set, Werblow, Felder and Zweifel (2007) also concluded that most components of health care expenditure are driven not by age but by 'closeness to death'.

More recently, attention has turned to individual components of health care expenditure, such as ambulatory care, hospital care, drugs and, perhaps most importantly, long-term care. Spillman and Lubitz (2000) found a continuing shift from acute to long-term care late in life in Medicare data from the United States. They concluded that ageing is the main driver of the demand for long-term care, leaving the acute sector unaffected. This is supported by the finding that nursing-care costs in the last year of life rise with age, and this rise almost offsets falling hospital-care costs (Scitovsky 1994; McGrail et al. 2000).

Seshamani and Gray (2004a,b) found that proximity to death is strongly associated with hospital costs for as long as 15 years before death, with age playing a much smaller role. Furthermore, younger decedents do not only incur higher costs shortly before death, but the peaks in hospital days for persons in their last year of life are shifting to younger age groups (Liao et al. 2000; McGrail et al. 2000).

A recent study from Denmark showed a clear rise in the costs of drugs prescribed in primary care as people approach the end of life (Kildemoes et al. 2006). However, age, per se, had no effect on the cost of general practitioners when controlling for time to death (O'Neill et al. 2000). Dormont, Grignon and Huber (2006) studied the age effect on health care expenditure, controlling for health status, in a French data set. They found that pure age effects vanish with ambulatory care and pharmaceutical and hospital expenditures and concluded that changes in clinical practice are more important drivers, most of which can be ascribed to technological innovation.

All these theories related to the cost of death imply that longevity gains will lead to more years in good health (i.e. healthy ageing and rightward shifts to the cost curve for survivors), progressively postponing the age-related increase in expenditures (Organisation for Economic Co-operation and Development 2006). However, Gerdtham (1993), using Swedish data, pointed out that health care expenditure per capita had risen much faster in older than in younger age groups. This is supported by data from other countries, in seeming contradiction to the last-year-of-life effect and requires further explanation.

Taken together this evidence seems to underline Fuchs' hypothesis on the cost of dying. This is well illustrated in Fig. 3.2, which shows that the effect of dying accounts for an ever-increasing share of average costs by age: around one-third of lifetime costs for persons aged 95+ are attributable to events related to death. This high percentage is primarily a consequence of the large proportion of people in this age group who are dying, and not because of the higher costs of dying incurred by each deceased person. If this is deducted (i.e. by calculating only the costs of survivors) the increase by age is more moderate and shows a more pronounced peak.

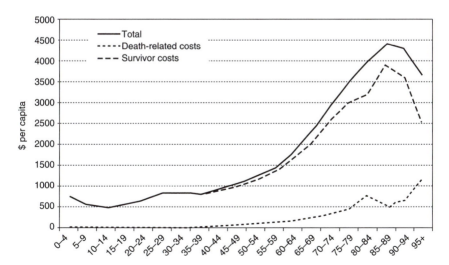

Figure 3.2   Expenditure per capita in each age group, separating the costs of dying from overall health care costs

Source: Organisation for Economic Co-operation and Development 2006.

The Survey of Health, Ageing and Retirement in Europe (SHARE) (Santos-Eggimann, Junod and Cornaz 2005) included 20,000 continental Europeans older than 50 years. Research using these data confirmed what was seen with Medicare data in the United States: higher utilization among older people (for ambulatory medical consultations, medication, hospital admissions and surgery) peaked at around 80–85 years before falling again.

However, even increasing life expectancy will only postpone death. The key question is whether the lower costs of dying at older age will offset the additional costs incurred during the longer period in good health, when some care is likely to be needed. There are few data regarding this issue. A calculation using German data showed that the number of days spent in hospital over the whole lifespan are directly proportional to the number of years lived, as the higher numbers of hospital days for (surviving) older people are compensated by lower numbers of hospital days in the last years of life (compared with younger decedents) (Busse, Krauth and Schwartz 2002). If these findings can be generalized to other countries and health care sectors, ageing would not increase health care costs – an average person who lived for 88 years rather than 80 would simply incur 10% higher lifelong costs. The costs per year of life would remain constant.

The role of ageing in health care expenditure

These findings are underlined by the OECD analysis of past trends in health expenditure, which reveals that ageing explains only a very small part (one tenth on average) of the total increase in health expenditure over the period 1970–2002 (Table 3.1). In European countries it ranges from virtually zero in Luxembourg to an average of 0.7% per year in Italy. In OECD countries, the age effect averages around 0.4%, significantly less than both the income (2.5% average annual growth) and the residual effect (1.5% average annual growth). These calculations confirm Gerdtham's (1993) earlier data from Sweden, which showed that changes in population ageing accounted for only 13% of the total increase in health care expenditure during the period 1970–1985.

The results from the studies cited above are supported by a cross-country perspective that takes account of the percentage of the population aged over 65 and the health expenditure as a percentage of GDP. As shown in Fig. 3.3, the percentage of older people in a country correlated only very weakly with the percentage of GDP spent on health in 1980. By 2004, the link had vanished. That this analysis no longer shows any effect may also reflect the relative unimportance of 65 years as an age cut-off point. In other words, given the discussion above on the compression of morbidity, the cut-off point should probably have been moved upwards reflecting higher life expectancy and better health.

Four main preliminary conclusions can be drawn from this review of the evidence:

- time of death is a more important explanation of health care expenditures than age
- cost of dying declines with age and is higher for those who die prematurely

Table 3.1 Decomposing growth in public health spending[a]: average expenditure growth rates per year 1971–2002[b]

Country	Age effect	Income effect[c]	Residual (i.e. other factors)	Total spending
Australia (to 2001 only)	0.5	1.7	1.7 (1.4)[d]	4.0 (3.6)[d]
Austria	0.2	2.5	1.5 (0.0)[d]	4.2 (2.2)[d]
Belgium (from 1995 only)	0.4	2.2	0.6	2.9
Canada	0.6	2.1	0.4 (0.6)[d]	3.1 (2.6)[d]
Czech Republic (from 1993 only)	0.4	2.8	−0.4	2.7
Denmark	0.2	1.6	0.1 (−0.5)[d]	1.9 (1.3)[d]
Finland	0.6	2.4	0.5 (0.2)[d]	3.4 (2.6)[d]
France	0.3	1.9	1.6 (1.0)[d]	3.9 (2.8)[d]
Germany	0.3	1.6	1.9 (1.0)[d]	3.7 (2.2)[d]
Greece (from 1987 only)	0.4	2.1	0.8	3.4
Hungary (from 1991 only)	0.3	2.8	−1.5	1.5
Iceland	0.1	2.7	3.2 (1.9)[d]	6.1 (3.5)[d]
Ireland	0.0	4.4	0.9 (−1.0)[d]	5.3 (3.9)[d]
Italy (from 1988 only)	0.7	2.2	−0.1	2.1
Japan (to 2001 only)	0.6	2.6	1.8 (1.1)[d]	4.9 (3.8)[d]
Republic of Korea (from 1982 only)	1.4	6.0	2.4	10.1
Luxembourg (from 1975 only)	0.0	3.3	0.7 (−0.1)[d]	4.2 (3.8)[d]
Mexico (from 1990 only)	0.7	1.7	2.4	4.5
Netherlands (from 1972 only)	0.4	2.0	0.9 (0.3)[d]	3.3 (2.6)[d]
New Zealand	0.2	1.2	1.4 (1.0)[d]	2.9 (2.7)[d]
Norway	0.1	3.0	2.2 (1.5)[d]	5.4 (4.0)[d]
Poland (from 1990 only)	0.5	3.2	0.6	3.1
Portugal	0.5	2.9	4.4 (2.8)[d]	8.0 (5.9)[d]
Slovakia (from 1997 only)	0.5	4.2	−1.5	2.1
Spain	0.4	2.4	2.5 (0.8)[d]	5.4 (3.4)[d]
Sweden	0.3	1.6	0.7 (−0.4)[d]	2.5 (1.5)[d]
Switzerland (from 1985 only)	0.2	0.9	2.9	3.8
Turkey (from 1984 only)	0.3	2.1	8.3	11.6
United Kingdom	0.1	2.1	1.5 (1.0)[d]	3.8 (3.4)[d]
United States	0.3	2.1	2.7 (2.6)[d]	5.1 (4.7)[d]
Average	*0.4 (0.3)[d]*	*2.5 (2.3)[d]*	*1.5 (1.0)[d]*	*4.3 (3.6)[d]*

Source: Organisation for Economic Co-operation and Development 2006.
Notes: [a]Total public health spending per capita; [b]Longest overlapping period available given (see years behind country name) if 1971–2002 is not available; [c]Assuming an income elasticity of health expenditure equal to one; [d]Average annual growth rate for the period 1981–2002 only; data for age and income effect not shown for individual countries as they are in line with 1971–2002 figures.

- when people live longer, this implies that the average costs of dying will decline
- utilization rates (and, therefore, acute health care expenditures) do not increase continuously with age; rather they peak at around 80–85 years and then start to fall.

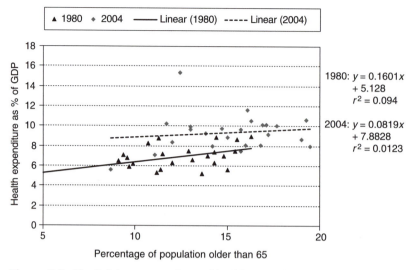

Figure 3.3   The link between ageing and health expenditure

Source: Authors' own calculations based on Organisation for Economic Co-operation and Development (various years).

Although the evidence is not yet sufficient to accept conclusively any of the longevity theories, the case in support of the dynamic equilibrium theory is most persuasive: a constant time spent in ill health or, in other words, a declining percentage of the average lifespan spent in ill health. However, survey data also provide some support for the compression of morbidity scenario: shorter periods in ill health as life expectancy increases. However, this does not necessarily translate into lower expenditure, as other factors (such as medical progress or increased expectations) may lead to higher utilization rates for healthier persons.

Economic growth and higher income

It seems logical that health care costs increase in line with a country's economic growth (or rather, its GDP). With an increasing GDP, health care personnel are better paid, health care facilities have more sophisticated medical technologies available and the population is likely to have higher expectations. Income or economic growth is, therefore, widely regarded to be the main non-demographic driver (Barros 1998; Docteur and Oxley 2003; Organisation for Economic Co-operation and Development 2006).

While health care expenditures seem substantial, it should be remembered that increasing expenditures in line with income (or GDP) growth alone would keep health expenditure as a percentage of GDP constant; that is, only the other factors produce an increase above GDP growth and, therefore, a higher share of it.

Consequently, it is interesting to know whether increasing income/GDP acts as a cost driver beyond the additional resources produced: whether the growth in health care expenditure is in line with the growth in GDP or whether this expenditure may even increase less steeply than the GDP.

Many studies since the 1960s have examined this relationship between GDP and health care expenditure (income elasticity) by trying to establish whether demand for health care, and thus expenditure, increases *more than proportionally* as income rises. In economic terms, this would imply that health care is a luxury good. Alternatively, health care may be a necessity good if demand increases *less than proportionally* as income rises. Most studies have used inadequate cross-sectional designs; others used pooled data (i.e. from several countries and several points in time), and a few used proper longitudinal designs (Murillo, Piatecki and Saez 1993; Kanavos and Yfantopoulos 1999). It has not been settled whether health care is a luxury (elasticity greater than one) or a necessity (elasticity between zero and one) (Organisation for Economic Co-operation and Development 2006). However, the studies suggest that there may be a correlation between the level of analysis and the measured income elasticity. Generally speaking, the higher the level of aggregation (e.g. national versus individual, macro versus micro) the higher the estimated income elasticity of health care spending. Getzen (2000) argued that, as the income elasticity varies with the level of analysis, health care is both a necessity and a luxury. With insurance, individual income elasticities are typically near zero, while national health expenditure elasticities are commonly greater than one. Furthermore, the high income elasticities found in macro-level studies may result from the failure to control true price effects (Organisation for Economic Co-operation and Development 2006), particularly in cross-sectional designs.

Studies with designs that were more methodologically sound produced more mixed results. They suggest that growth in GDP is closely related to health expenditure growth but may not be the determining factor and cannot explain the variations. The increased implementation of cost-containment policies could explain the apparent decrease in estimated elasticity since the beginning of the 1980s (Herwarts and Theilen 2003; Economic Policy Committee of the European Commission 2009). More recent studies using pooled time-series cross-section data and a wider range of explanatory variables suggest elasticities around or below one (Gerdtham and Löthgren 2002; Freeman 2003).

The OECD calculations (Table 3.1) are, therefore, based on the assumption that income growth leads to an equivalent growth in health care expenditure. According to these calculations, public health expenditures in OECD countries in the period 1971–2002 (1981–2002) grew by 4.3% (3.6%) per year. Almost two-thirds of this – 2.5% (2.3%) – was accounted for by income effects (assuming income elasticity equal to one) and 0.4% (0.3%) by demographics (Table 3.1).

The remaining (residual) health care expenditure growth is often ascribed to technology and medical progress and increases in the relative prices of health care goods. The residual growth is higher for the extended period 1971–2002 (1.5% annually) than for 1981–2002 (1%). This reflects the implementation of cost-containment policies in the 1980s and 1990s that sought to curb the strong residual growth (Organisation for Economic Co-operation and Development 2006). Data in Table 3.1 show that this cost-containment effect may be attributed mainly to European countries where the residual increase since 1981 is visibly smaller (e.g. Germany, Portugal, Spain), no longer existing

(Austria) or even negative (e.g. Denmark, Ireland, Sweden). No effect can be observed in countries such as Australia, New Zealand or the United States. The European countries were pursuing austerity measures agreed in the Maastricht Treaty in preparation for the single currency at this time.

In conclusion, it should be taken for granted that health care expenditure grows in line with economic growth; that is, policy-makers should not expect that health care costs will rise less than their GDP. Where this has happened in the decade from the mid 1990s (e.g. in Hungary, Slovakia (Table 3.1) or Estonia), they should critically examine whether underinvestment in health care has led to lower population health (than otherwise achievable) and, therefore, less economic growth.

Changes in technologies and medical progress

It is often asserted that new technologies and medical progress (such as new drugs and medical devices; organizational innovations) drive up the costs of health services. Conventional economic thinking suggests that advances in technology in themselves should reduce the costs of any given package of care (in the same way that advances in computing technology have lowered the costs of computing) (Normand 1998). However, this overlooks the fact that the relationship between progress and costs is more complicated because the 'product' is also changing through advances in technology (i.e. computers are much more powerful now).

The relationship between changes in medical technologies and health care expenditure is even more complicated as medical progress can have multiple effects. To disentangle them, it is crucial to distinguish (i) between effects on the provision of a particular service to an individual patient and effects on overall costs, and (ii) between costs (or rather health care expenditure) and value for money (or cost-effectiveness).

New technologies such as drugs can be expensive but may have the potential to reduce the need for hospital admission (e.g. the use of preventive medication in asthma management) or allow safe earlier discharge (e.g. as a result of modern antibiotics). Minimally invasive surgery may take longer than conventional surgery, but with the right preparation and support the patient recovers more quickly and spends less time in hospital. Some medical advances reduce the unit costs of providing particular treatments and may also reduce the need for continuing the treatment altogether. For example, the discovery that acid-related ulcers may be healed by eliminating a gastric bacterium has reduced the need for long-term drug therapy for peptic ulcers.

In other instances, new technologies (e.g. in diagnostic imaging) are additions and their costs must be added to those of the existing technology. Other technical and medical progress may (and often does) provide opportunities for new effective interventions and thus may raise total costs. In the same way, the availability of more effective (and potentially lower cost) treatments may create or increase demand and thus total costs. In some other instances, technological progress could lower the demand for future health care if early or less-invasive treatments improve health status and reduce future health care needs that may have higher linked costs. Conversely, it can increase future health needs by increasing the survival probabilities of people with chronic or multiple health conditions.

In general, medical innovations in the last decades have improved effectiveness and (frequently) lowered unit costs but often have not reduced overall costs at aggregate level. There are a number of reasons for this. On a positive note, medical innovations have extended the scope and range of treatments available, addressed previously unmet health needs and extended the quality and length of life. Less appropriately, some treatment has been extended to a wider set of indications even when this does not add to the overall health gain of society. This is the case when new technologies offer only marginal improvements over previous therapies and when medical progress is applied inappropriately, for example to patients or conditions where there is no extra marginal effect or real cost benefit (Weisbrod 1991). This is typically associated with perverse supply-side economic incentives such as skewed payment systems that create supplier-induced demand. In addition, this technology-push effect is encouraged by the propensity to pay for those innovations among governments and sickness funds.

The increasing tendency for funding agencies to apply economic criteria as a hurdle for new technologies suggests that there will be increasing reluctance to support innovations that bring limited advantage (Cohen, Stolk and Niezen 2007). However, it is currently beyond the scope of most health care systems to control indications for the use of new treatments. Even if technologies are assessed in medical trials, their subsequent use often includes other patient groups (Jacobzone 2003). Policy-makers are, therefore, advised to examine whether this approach should be extended beyond a yes/no decision. The use of (new) technologies could be steered by tying reimbursement to certain patients or defined by a particular indication, level of severity or similar. This will require smart use of documentation and information systems in order to avoid lengthy and resource-intensive control mechanisms.

Demand-side factors (i.e. treatable morbidity and/or patient expectations) also affect the extent to which new technologies are adopted into routine practice and may even spur research and innovation (Feldstein 1977; Goddeeris 1984; Pauly 1986). Thus, in some instances higher costs cause technical progress rather than vice versa.

How important is this factor in explaining expenditure increases? Clearly, it is hard to untangle the interplay between these mechanisms and determine their net effect on costs. This is illustrated by the fact that many studies use a residual approach, estimating more easily identifiable factors (e.g. demographics, income, growth in GDP) and then ascribe residual growth to technology. In addition, study results also depend on the scope and design of the research and whether total health care expenditures or components of health care spending (ambulatory care, hospital care, household spending, etc.) are included. Consequently, results vary significantly and must be treated cautiously.

Newhouse (1992) presented a health expenditure growth analysis for the United States (1950–1989). He concluded that about 50% of the increase in costs could not be explained by traditional factors and was attributable to progress. The estimation by Barros (1998) was 30%. A study by Shactman et al. (2003) attributed 43% of growth to new technologies in American hospitals; Hay (2003) found a 19% growth in inpatient expenditures at state level in the United States to be a result of hospital technology; Goethgebeur et al. (2003) estimated a 22% contribution to growth in overall health care spending between 2001 and 2002.

Although the evidence on the impact of adopting technical and medical developments is not clear cut, it suggests that increased utilization has outweighed unit cost savings (Economic Policy Committee of the European Commission 2006) and is, therefore, a significant but controllable driver on the rise of health care costs and expenditures. This is further supported by various literature reviews (Chernew et al. 1998; Docteur and Oxley 2003; Goetghebeur et al. 2003; Pammolli et al. 2005; Organisation for Economic Co-operation and Development 2006). However, the aforementioned decrease in the residual over time in many (particularly European) countries indicates that medical progress does not necessarily lead to higher health care expenditure.

This suggests that the policy focus should shift from the cost of technological developments per se towards ensuring that new technologies are appropriate and cost-effective. Health systems need to become more effective in managing the continuing challenge presented by the introduction of new technologies – identifying and adopting those that offer real benefits while discouraging the less cost-effective. Health technology assessment programmes aim to ensure that significant new medical advances are assessed properly before widespread uptake and that specialist advice is available to help clinicians to make best use of them (Velasco Garrido et al. 2008). It is important to note that the primary objective of health technology assessment is to improve the effectiveness and cost-effectiveness of health systems, even if costs increase (at least in the short-term) when new and effective technologies are added to the benefit basket.

Relative prices/costs

The relative prices of key components of health care expenditures (e.g. wages, capital investments and drug prices) are a frequently cited but not well-quantified influence on expenditure growth. There are good reasons to expect wages in health care to rise more rapidly than productivity, since a considerable part of the services provided has the characteristics of a handicraft industry (Baumol 1995). Labour productivity growth is generally slower than for other industries, as relatively little health care provision lends itself to labour-saving technical developments. Workers in industries with high productivity growth enjoy higher rewards, and increases in wages are needed to retain good workers in the health sector (Baumol 1995). In addition, the high income elasticities found in macro-studies may result from the failure to control true price effects (Organisation for Economic Co-operation and Development 2006). Baumol's model of unbalanced growth (Baumol 1967, 1993) identified nominal wage growth in excess of productivity growth as the main determinant of the rise in health care expenditure. This is supported by the 2008 study of Hartwig, which found empirical evidence in 19 OECD countries that health care expenditure is indeed driven by wage increases that exceed the productivity growth in the general economy.

Policy-makers should carefully examine whether productivity growth within health care can be brought in line with general economic growth. Medical technology that can contribute to such a development should be adopted in order to avoid the effect of an above-average growth of labour costs. In some areas (particularly long-term care, mental health and palliative care), this will not be possible in the foreseeable future and relatively increasing labour costs will drive up health care expenditure in these sectors. If inputs other than labour (e.g. drug prices) increase more rapidly than GDP, policy-makers should critically evaluate whether such increases are justified. The growing role of economic evaluation of (new) drugs testifies that countries have taken up this challenge.

Increased expectations

The need for health services to respond increasingly to people's expectations and concerns is frequently cited as a factor in increasing health care costs. The importance of a responsive health system is undisputed and supported by empirical evidence (see Chapter 8 on responsiveness). For example, in a survey of patients from 10 EU Member States by the International Alliance of Patients' Organizations, respondents rated timely access to the best treatment and information, the right to participate in decisions at the individual patient level, and patient involvement in policy-making among their top priorities (International Alliance of Patients' Organization 2006). However, it is much less clear whether people's expectations are increasing measurably or whether such an increase in expectations leads to higher health care costs. Several arguments suggest that this is (and will be) an increasingly important factor.

As countries and their citizens become richer, they develop higher expectations of the range of treatments and the quality of services available. Richer countries can afford to offer more and newer technologies and provide more opportunities for their delivery. Manufacturers of drugs and medical devices may push for such a development by means of lobbying and support from patients' groups (see below).

Health policy-makers in many, if not most, countries have ensured sufficient responsiveness in health care systems through greater choice of both primary care and hospital providers and of purchasers in some countries. This may have contributed to the significance of this pressure on growth, particularly if increased choice is introduced at the cost of less gatekeeping: that is, if citizens can act directly on their higher expectations by visiting specialists and demanding particular (new) technologies.

To our knowledge, no robust quantitative studies have assessed the impact of expectations. This may be because of the methodological problems of the overlap with other factors such as increased incomes, technical developments and the organization of the system (e.g. gatekeeping versus free access to specialists). Arguably, the observed higher expenditures in countries using a social health insurance system (rather than a tax-funded system) are the result of systems that are more responsive to people's expectations (Chapter 8). However, health care expenditure growth rates in countries with social health insurance have been smaller (Table 3.1), possibly reflecting some catching-up in tax-funded systems.

There are few data on the exact degree to which expectations impact on health care costs. Nevertheless, it is clear that they pressurize health care professionals and decision-makers to adopt the latest available medical innovations and a broader range of services and to implement more choice. Patients have become more involved in the choice of treatment and can now access an almost limitless amount of medical information through the Internet. Patients in some countries (e.g. the Netherlands) are empowered by an emphasis on consumer choice and have patient organizations that find ways to exert influence in the decision-making process. A newer development in Europe (but well known in the United States) is patient groups funded by pharmaceutical and medical technology companies. Although this might seem a strange alliance, it is a logical partnership between two actors with a shared interest – access to the newest treatments (which benefits patients) for which positive reimbursement decisions (which benefit the pharmaceutical industry) are prerequisite. However, this relationship often has an information asymmetry, which the industry could use to distort the reimbursement debate. Policy-makers are, therefore, well advised to inform citizens and engage them in the policy-making progress, for example by inviting them to participate and by providing funding for patients' organizations. This will enable a common understanding to be reached and will encourage realistic expectations of the cost-effectiveness of treatments and the sustainability of health systems.

Forecasting future health care expenditure

Since the mid 1980s, several cross-country studies have sought to forecast future expenditures on health care. In Europe, most were carried out by national governments, the OECD, the European Commission and the World Bank. With methodological progress, these projections have become more sophisticated and increasingly cover demographic as well as non-demographic factors. The aim of this section is to briefly outline some of the results and particularly to discuss some of the methodological complexities.

The OECD projections for the period 2005–2050 include separate examinations of long-term care and health care (Organisation for Economic Co-operation and Development 2006). The drivers for health care encompass demographic factors and non-demographic factors. The exercise does not seek to disentangle the non-demographic factors but adopts two scenarios: (i) cost-pressure (expenditure growth 1% per year faster than income) and (ii) cost-containment (expenditure growth eliminated by the end of 2050). This approach is similar to the various scenarios in the Wanless Reports (2002, 2004) in the United Kingdom.

Demographic factors are also included in the prediction for long-term care. This is likely to rise as the proportion of older people increases but will be mitigated to a certain extent by 'healthy ageing'. Non-demographic factors assume that expenditures are likely pushed up by relative prices of long-term care. This increases in line with average productivity growth in the economy because the scope for productivity gains is more limited.

These projections result in a cost-pressure scenario in which the average health care and long-term care spending across OECD countries is projected to almost double from close to 7% of GDP to 13% by 2050. The cost-containment scenario estimates growth to increase from 7% to 10% by 2050 (Table 3.2). Non-demographic factors (including technology and relative prices) exert

Table 3.2 Projections by the OECD for public spending on health and long-term care 2005–2050 – cost pressure and cost-containment scenarios

	Health care			Long-term care			Total		
	2005	2050		2005	2050		2005	2050	
		CP	CC		CP	CC		CP	CC
Australia	5.6	9.7	7.9	0.9	2.9	2.0	6.5	12.6	9.9
Austria	3.8	7.6	5.7	1.3	3.3	2.5	5.1	10.9	8.2
Belgium	5.7	9.0	7.2	1.5	3.4	2.6	7.2	12.4	9.8
Canada	6.2	10.2	8.4	1.2	3.2	2.4	7.3	13.5	10.8
Czech Republic	7.0	11.2	9.4	0.4	2.0	1.3	7.4	13.2	10.7
Denmark	5.3	8.8	7.0	2.6	4.1	3.3	7.9	12.9	10.3
Finland	3.4	7.0	5.2	2.9	5.2	4.2	6.2	12.2	9.3
France	7.0	10.6	8.7	1.1	2.8	2.0	8.1	13.4	10.8
Germany	7.8	11.4	9.6	1.0	2.9	2.2	8.8	14.3	11.8
Greece	4.9	8.7	6.9	0.2	2.8	2.0	5.0	11.6	8.9
Hungary	6.7	10.3	8.5	0.3	2.4	1.0	7.0	12.6	9.5
Iceland	6.8	10.7	8.9	2.9	4.4	3.4	9.6	15.2	12.3
Ireland	5.9	10	8.2	0.7	4.6	3.2	6.7	14.5	11.3
Italy	6.0	9.7	7.9	0.6	3.5	2.8	6.6	13.2	10.7
Japan	6.0	10.3	8.5	0.9	3.1	2.4	6.9	13.4	10.9
Republic of Korea	3.0	7.8	6.0	0.3	4.1	3.1	3.3	11.9	9.1
Luxembourg	6.1	9.9	8.0	0.7	3.8	2.6	6.8	13.7	10.6
Mexico	3.0	7.5	5.7	0.1	4.2	3.0	3.1	11.7	8.7
Netherlands	5.1	8.9	7.0	1.7	3.7	2.9	6.8	12.5	9.9
New Zealand	6.0	10.1	8.3	0.5	2.4	1.7	6.4	12.6	10.0
Norway	7.3	10.7	8.9	2.6	4.3	3.5	9.9	15.0	12.4
Poland	4.4	8.5	6.7	0.5	3.7	1.8	4.9	12.2	8.5
Portugal	6.7	10.9	9.1	0.2	2.2	1.3	6.9	13.1	10.4
Slovakia	5.1	9.7	7.9	0.3	2.6	1.5	5.4	12.3	9.4
Spain	5.5	9.6	7.8	0.2	2.6	1.9	5.6	12.1	9.6
Sweden	5.3	8.5	6.7	3.3	4.3	3.4	8.6	12.9	10.1
Switzerland	6.2	9.6	7.8	1.2	2.6	1.9	7.4	12.3	9.7
Turkey	5.9	9.9	8.1	0.1	1.8	0.8	6.0	11.7	8.9
United Kingdom	6.1	9.7	7.9	1.1	3.0	2.1	7.2	12.7	10.0
United States	6.3	9.7	7.9	0.9	2.7	1.8	7.2	12.4	9.7
Average	*5.7*	*9.6*	*7.7*	*1.1*	*3.3*	*2.4*	*6.7*	*12.8*	*10.1*

Source: Organisation for Economic Co-operation and Development (2006).
Notes: CP: Cost pressure; CC: Cost containment.

significant upward pressure on long-term care expenditures and form the most important driver.

The results in Table 3.2 show significant variation among European countries. In the cost-containment scenario, countries expected to experience increases in health expenditure of more than 4% include countries that are ageing rapidly (Italy, Spain), those expected to see dramatic changes in their population structure (Slovakia) and those with currently low labour participation that are likely to face substantial increases in the demand for formal long-term care (Italy, Ireland, Spain). Sweden is in an advanced phase of its ageing process and already spends a relatively high share of its GDP on health. Therefore, Sweden only shows an increase of 1.5% to reach 10.1% in 2050 (i.e. the OECD average for 2050).

In its 2009 impact of ageing projection exercise for the EU27 2008–2060, the European Commission looked at the effects on pensions, health care, long-term care, education and unemployment transfers (Economic Policy Committee of the European Commission 2009). Multiple scenarios capturing all demographic and non-demographic factors were developed, distinguishing between health and long-term care. The working group on ageing populations scenario takes account of the effects of ageing, the health care status of elderly citizens and the income elasticity of demand. Under this 'reference' scenario (i.e. that to be considered most likely), the EU Member States will expect an average increase of public expenditures on health care of 1.5% of GDP. For most, the figure will be between 1% and 2% (with a few outliers: Bulgaria, Cyprus and Sweden <1%; the Czech Republic, Malta and Slovakia <2%). The average figure is 1.1% for long-term care, with wider variation between countries, ranging from almost 0% to 4.7%. The combined effects of health care and long-term care range from 1.3% to 5.8% of GDP until 2060. The projections show that non-demographic factors are relevant drivers of spending.

The World Bank study *From Red to Gray* (Chawla, Betcherman and Banerji 2007) used the same approach as the European Commission study (Economic Policy Committee of the European Commission 2009) and sought to shed some light on future spending in the countries of central and eastern Europe (which includes some EU Member States) and the newly independent states of the European part of the former Soviet Union. The study contains four health-expenditure scenarios (pure ageing, constant morbidity, compressed morbidity, and pure ageing adjusted for death-related costs) and two long-term care scenarios (pure ageing and constant disability), all based on different basic assumptions related to the longevity scenarios.

All these studies should be interpreted with caution. All the projections are based on various assumptions regarding utilization levels (usually assumed to be constant but may change when new technologies become available or the benefit package is broadened or narrowed), age-related public expenditures on health- and death-related costs (which may not be available, particularly in non-EU Member States), and GDP growth rates. The last is an important determinant but is very hard to forecast, as explained above, particularly in transition countries. This can be illustrated by the projections for the new EU Member States included in both the European Commission (Economic Policy Committee of the European Commission 2006) and the World Bank (Chawla,

Betcherman and Banerji 2007) studies. Although both organizations used the same approach, the World Bank used different data sources and made different assumptions (e.g. regarding future population and health spending). This produced widely diverging results: in its version of the pure-ageing scenario for EU Member States, the World Bank projected lower changes in health expenditure as a percentage of GDP between 2010 and 2050, for example Lithuania (−0.30% versus +0.6%) and the Czech Republic (+0.18% versus +1.5%), than did the European Commission. The main cause of these huge variations lies in the widely different projections of GDP growth rates (i.e. level, fluctuating or constant) in the two studies (Chawla, Betcherman and Banerji 2007). As the experience of the 2008 recession has shown, this is an area of intrinsic uncertainty.

Pragmatic policy-making should simply assume that health care expenditure growth is at least in line with GDP growth. There is also a modest additional effect from demography (as shown above, less than 0.5% annually in the past) and other effects (medical progress, relative prices, increased expectations) that are all more amenable to policy-makers' actions. If the latter can be managed successfully (e.g. by achieving efficiency gains wherever possible, such as in diagnostic imaging or by replacing inpatient treatment with ambulatory procedures), and allowing for any necessary increase in labour costs (e.g. in long-term care), then the combined effect of these factors does not need to be larger than zero. Taken together, these results show that countries should expect growth in health care expenditure to be somewhere between the two OECD projections.

Conclusions: policy implications

The review in this chapter enables some conclusions and policy lessons to be drawn.

Ageing explains only a small part of increasing health care expenditures. Income growth as well as new technologies/medical progress, relative costs and other difficult-to-quantify determinants have made a larger contribution to increases in health care expenditures over the past few decades.

The observed stagnating, and in some cases falling, level in utilization rates at older ages (after around 80 years of age) shows that policy-makers may have to refocus their attention. There is an increasing number of much older people (80+ years) but this may not have as many financial implications for health care as has often been suggested, unlike long-term care where the relationship with age is much clearer. Instead, policy-makers should be aware that increased numbers of people aged 65–79 years will require greater resources than they may have anticipated (while long-term care costs for them will decrease). This also challenges the belief that longer life expectancy automatically results in higher total lifetime expenditures. Longer life expectancy decreases death-related costs, which, in turn, offsets the added health costs incurred as a result of the gains in life expectancy. Policy-makers should, therefore, focus on establishing an effective health system with active policies to facilitate healthy ageing, enabling older people to remain economically active (Doyle et al. 2009).

Evidence suggests that proximity to death is a more important predictor for increasing health care expenditures than ageing. Time to death should, therefore, be included in ageing studies that aim to project future health care costs (as in the projections reviewed here). However, good data on spending in each age group are prerequisites for achieving a meaningful analysis and projection. Countries should ensure the collection of such data as they are not always available in Europe (particularly in some central and eastern European and former Soviet countries).

The policy focus should be on adopting cost-effective technology and ensuring appropriate use (i.e. technology is given only to those with the 'right', positively evaluated, indication) rather than absolute costs of technological innovations. Policy action should, therefore, encourage and incorporate the use of health technology assessment programmes in its reimbursement systems and aim to develop innovative policies that control the indications and appropriate use of these new treatments.

Policy-makers should strive to engage citizens and patient groups in an independent debate on evidence and to enable their participation in the decision-making process. Also, the provision of funding would enable better organized patient groups, which could then contribute effectively to the policy debate (rather than a fragmented landscape or patient groups funded by industry). The aim of this debate should be to reach a common understanding and ensure realistic expectations of the cost-effectiveness of treatments and the sustainability of health systems.

References

Aprile, R. (2004) *How to Take Account of Death-Related Costs in Projecting Health Care Expenditure – Updated Version*. Rome: Ragioneria Generale Dello Stato.

Barros, P.P. (1998) The black box of health care expenditure growth determinants. *Health Economics*, 7: 533–44.

Baumol, W.J. (1967) Macroeconomics of unbalanced growth: the anatomy of urban crisis. *American Economic Review*, 57(3): 415–26.

Baumol, W.J. (1993) Health care, education and the cost disease: a looming crisis for public choice. *Public Choice*, 77(1): 17–28.

Baumol, W.J. (1995) *Health care as a handicraft industry*. London: Office of Health Economics.

Breyer, F. and von Schulenburg, M. (1987) Voting on social security: the family as decision-making unit. *Kyklos*, 40(4): 529–47.

Bronnum-Hansen, H. (2005) Health expectancy in Denmark, 1987–2000. *European Journal of Public Health*, 15(1): 20–5.

Busse, R., Krauth, C. and Schwartz, F.W. (2002) Use of acute hospital beds does not increase as the population ages: results from a 7-year cohort study in Germany. *Journal of Epidemiology and Community Health*, 56(4): 289–93.

Chawla, M., Betcherman, G. and Banerji, A. (2007) *From Red to Gray: The Third Transition of Aging Populations in Eastern Europe and the Former Soviet Union*. Washington, DC: World Bank.

Chernew, M.E., Hirth, R.A., Sonnad, S.S., Ermann, R. and Fendrick, A.M. (1998) Managed care, medical technology, and health care cost growth: a review of the evidence. *Medical Care Research Review*, 55(3): 259–88; discussion 289–97.

Cohen, J., Stolk, E. and Niezen, M. (2007) The increasingly complex fourth hurdle for pharmaceuticals. *PharmacoEconomics*, 25(9): 727–34.

Dinkel, R.H. (1998) Demographische Entwicklung und Gesundheitszustand. Eine empirische Kalkulation der Healthy Life Expectancy für die Bundesrepublik auf Basis von Kohortendaten, in H. Häfner (ed.) *Gesundheit – unser höchstes Gut?* Berlin: Springer: 61–83.

Doblhammer, G. and Kytir, J. (2001) Compression or expansion of morbidity? Trends in healthy-life expectancy the elderly Austrian population between 1978 and 1998. *Social Science and Medicine*, 52: 385–91.

Docteur, E. and Oxley, H. (2003) *Health-Care Systems: Lessons from the Reform Experience*, working paper no. 9. Paris: Organisation for Economic Co-operation and Development.

Dormont, B., Grignon, M. and Huber, H. (2006) Health expenditure growth: reassessing the threat of ageing. *Health Economics*, 15: 947–63.

Doyle, Y., McKee, M., Rechel, B. and Grundy, E. (2009). Meeting the challenge of population ageing. *British Medical Journal*, 339: 892–4.

Economic Policy Committee of the European Commission (2006) *The Impact of Ageing on Public Expenditure: Projections for the EU-25 Member States on Pensions, Healthcare, Long-Term Care, Education, and Unemployment Transfers (2004–50)*. Brussels: Directorate-General for Economic and Financial Affairs of the European Commission.

Economic Policy Committee of the European Commission (2009) *The 2009 Ageing Report: Economic and Budgetary Projections for the EU-27 Member States (2008–2060)*. Brussels: Directorate-General for Economic and Financial Affairs of the European Commission.

Feldstein, M. (1977) Quality change and the demand for hospital care. *Econometrica* 45: 1681–1702.

Freeman, D.G. (2003) Is health care a necessity or a luxury? Pooled estimates of income elasticity from US state-level data. *Applied Economics*, 35(5): 495–502.

Fries, J.F. (1980) Ageing, natural death, and the compression of morbidity. *New England Journal of Medicine*, 303: 130–5.

Fries, J.F. (1983) The compression of morbidity. *Milbank Quarterly*, 61: 397–419.

Fries, J.F. (1989) The compression of morbidity: near or far? *Milbank Quarterly*, 67: 208–32.

Fries, J.F. (1993) Compression of morbidity: life span, disability, and health care costs. *Facts and Research in Gerontology*, 7: 183–90.

Fuchs, V.R. (1984) Though much is taken: reflections on ageing, health, and medical care. *Milbank Quarterly*, 62: 143–66.

Gerdtham, U.G. (1993) The impact of ageing on health care expenditure in Sweden. *Health Policy*, 24: 1–8.

Gerdtham, U.-G. and Löthgren, M. (2002) New panel results on cointegration of international health expenditure and GDP. *Applied Economics*, 34: 1679–86.

Getzen, T.E. (2000) Health care is an individual necessity and a national luxury: applying multilevel decision models to the analysis of health care expenditures. *Journal of Health Economics*, 19(2): 259–70.

Goddeeris, J.H. (1984) Insurance and incentives for innovation in medical care. *Southern Economic Journal*, 51: 530–9.

Goetghebeur, M.M., Forrest, S. and Hay, J.W. (2003) Understanding the underlying drivers of inpatient cost growth: a literature review. *American Journal of Managed Care*, 9: 3–12.

Gruenberg, E.M. (1977) The failure of success. *Milbank Quarterly*, 55: 3–24.

Hartwig, J. (2008) What drives health care expenditure? Baumol's model of 'unbalanced growth' revisited. *Journal of Health Economics*, 27(3): 603–23.

Hay, J.W. (2003) Hospital cost drivers: an evaluation of 1998–2001 state-level data. *American Journal of Managed Care*, 9: SP13–SP24.

Herwarts, H. and Theilen, B. (2003) The determinants of health-care expenditure: testing pooling restrictions in small samples. *Health Economics*, 12(2): 113–24.

International Alliance of Patients' Organization (2006) *A Survey of Patient Organizations' Concerns. Perceptions of Healthcare.* New York: Consensus Research Group for the International Alliance of Patients' Organization, http://www.patientsorganizations.org/attach.pl/751/343/Patient%20Survey%20Report.pdf (accessed 7 September 2010).

Jacobzone, S. (2003) Ageing and the challenges of new technologies: can OECD social and healthcare systems provide for the future? *Geneva Papers on Risk and Insurance*, 28(2): 254–74.

Kanavos, P. and Yfantopoulos, J. (1999) Cost containment and health expenditure in the EU: a macroeconomic perspective, in E. Mossialos and J. Le Grand (eds.) *Health Care Cost Containment in the European Union.* Aldershot: Ashgate: 155–98.

Kildemoes, H., Christiansen, T., Gyrd-Hansen, D., Kristiansen, I. and Andersen, M. (2006) The impact of population ageing on future Danish drug expenditure. *Health Policy*, 75(3): 298–311.

Liao, Y., McGee, D.L., Cao, G. and Cooper, R.S. (2000) Quality of the last year of life of older adults: 1986 vs 1993. *Journal of the American Medical Association*, 283: 512–18.

Lubitz, J.D. and Riley, G.F. (1993) Trends in Medicare payments in the last year of life. *New England Journal of Medicine*, 328: 1092–6.

Lubitz, J.D., Beebe, J. and Baker, C. (1995) Longevity and Medicare expenditures. *New England Journal of Medicine*, 332: 999–1003.

Manton, K.G. (1982) Changing concepts of morbidity and mortality in the elderly population. *Milbank Quarterly*, 60: 183–244.

Manton, K.G., Stallard, E. and Corder, L. (1995) Changes in morbidity and chronic disability in the US elderly population: evidence from the 1982, 1984 and 1989 National Long Term Care Surveys. *Journal of Gerontology: Social Sciences*, 50(4): S194–S204.

McGrail, K., Green, B., Barer, M.L., Evans, R.G., Hertzman, C. and Normand, C. (2000) Age, costs of acute and long term care and proximity to death: evidence for 1987/88 and 1994/95 in British Columbia. *Age and Ageing*, 29: 249–53.

Murillo, C., Piatecki, C. and Saez, M. (1993) Health care expenditure and income in Europe. *Health Economics*, 3: 127–38.

Newhouse, J. (1992) Medical care costs: how much welfare loss? *Journal of Economic Perspectives*, 6: 3–21.

Niehaus, F. (2006) *Alter und steigende Lebenserwartung – Eine Analyse der Auswirkungen auf die Gesundheitsausgaben.* Köln: Wissenschaftliches Institut der PKV.

Normand, C. (1998) Ten popular health economic fallacies. *Journal of Public Health Medicine*, 20(2): 129–32.

Oeppen, J. and Vaupel, J.W. (2002) Broken limits to life expectancy. *Science*, 296: 1029–31.

Olshansky, S.J., Rudberg, M.A., Carnes, B.A., Cassel, C.K. and Brody, J.A. (1991) Trading off longer life for worsening health. *Journal of Aging and Health*, 3: 194–216.

O'Neill, C., Groom, L., Avery, A., Boot, D. and Thornhill, K. (2000) Age and proximity to death as predictors of GP care costs: results from a study of nursing home patients. *Health Economics*, 9: 733–8.

Organisation for Economic Co-operation and Development (2006) *Projecting OECD Health and Long-term Care Expenditures: What are the Main Drivers?* Working paper no. 477. Paris: Organisation for Economic Co-operation and Development.

Organisation for Economic Co-operation and Development (various years) *OECD Health Data.* Paris: Organisation for Economic Co-operation and Development.

Pammolli, F., Riccaboni, M., Oglialoro, C., Magazzini, L., Baio, G. and Salerno, N. (2005) *Medical Devices, Competitiveness and Impact on Public Health Expenditure: Study Prepared for the Directorate Enterprise of the European Commission*. Florence: University of Florence, http://www.cermlab.it/_documents/MD_Report.pdf (accessed 7 September 2010).

Pauly, M.V. (1986) Taxation, health insurance, and market failure in the medical economy. *Journal of Economic Literature*, 24: 629–75.

Raitano, M. (2006) *The Impact of Death-related Costs on Health-Care Expenditure: A Survey*, research report no. 17. Brussels: European Network of Economic Policy Research Institutes, http://www.enepri.org/files/Publications/RR17.pdf (accessed 7 September 2010).

Robine, J.M., Jagger, C. and van Oyen, H. (2005) Interpreting national evidence on the evolution of morbidity and disability prevalence over time and perspectives for extended healthy life expectancy, in *Proceedings of the Joint EU–OECD Workshop*, 21–22 February 2005.

Roos, N.P., Montgomery, P. and Roos, L.L. (1987) Health care utilization in the years prior to death. *Milbank Quarterly*, 65: 231–54.

Santos-Eggimann, B., Junod, B. and Cornaz, S. (2005) Health services utilisation in older Europeans, in A. Börsch-Supan, A. Brugiavini, H. Jürges, J.P. Mackenbach, J. Siegrist and G. Weber (eds.) *Health, Ageing and Retirement in Europe: First Results from SHARE*. Mannheim: Mannheim Research Institute for the Economics of Aging: 141–9.

Scitovsky, A.A. (1994) The high cost of dying revisited. *Milbank Quarterly*, 72(4): 561–91.

Seshamani, M. and Gray, A.M. (2004a) Ageing and health care expenditure: the red herring argument revisited. *Health Economics,* 13: 303–14.

Seshamani, M. and Gray, A.M. (2004b) A longitudinal study of the effects of age and time to death on hospital costs. *Journal of Health Economics*, 23(2): 217–35.

Shactman, D., Altman, S.H., Eilat, E., Thorpe, K.E. and Doonan, M. (2003) The outlook for hospital spending: rapid growth is likely to persist. *Health Affairs*, 22(6): 12–26.

Spillman, B. and Lubitz, J. (2000) The effect of longevity on spending for acute and longterm care. *New England Journal of Medicine*, 342: 1409–15.

Stearns, S.C. and Norton, E.C. (2004) Time to include time to death? The future of health care expenditure predictions. *Health Economics*, 13: 315–27.

van Vliet, R.C. and Lamers, L.M. (1998) The high costs of death: should health plans get higher payments when members die? *Medical Care*, 36: 1451–60.

Velasco Garrido, M., Børlum Kristensen, F., Palmhøj Nielsen, C. and Busse, R. (eds.) (2008) *Health Technology Assessment and Health Policy-making in Europe: Current Status, Challenges and Potential*. Copenhagen: WHO Regional Office for Europe on behalf of the European Observatory on Health Systems and Policies.

Verbrugge, L.M. (1984) Longer life but worsening health? Trends in health and mortality of middle-aged and older persons. *Milbank Quarterly*, 62: 475–519.

Wanless, D. (2002) *Securing Our Future Health: Taking a Long-term View: Final Report*. London: The Stationery Office.

Wanless, D. (2004) *Securing Good Health for the Whole Population: Final Report*. London: The Stationery Office.

Weisbrod, B. (1991) The health care quadrilemma: an essay on technological change, insurance, quality of care and cost containment. *Journal of Economic Literature*, 29: 523–52.

Werblow, A., Felder, S. and Zweifel, P. (2007) Population ageing and health care expenditure: a school of 'red herrings'? *Health Economics*, 16(10): 1109–26.

White, K.M. (2002) Longevity advances in high-income countries, 1955–96. *Population and Development Review*, 28(1): 59–76.

Zweifel, P., Felder, S. and Meiers, M. (1999) Ageing of population and health care expenditure: a red herring? *Health Economics,* 8: 485–96.

Zweifel, P., Felder, S. and Werblow, A. (2004) Population ageing and health care expenditure: new evidence on the red herring. *Geneva Papers on Risk and Insurance: Issues and Practice,* 29(4): 653–67.

chapter four

Economic costs of ill health in the European Region

Marc Suhrcke, Regina Sauto Arce,
Martin McKee and Lorenzo Rocco

Introduction

All else being equal, greater wealth makes it easier to live a healthy life, both at the individual and the population level. Greater personal wealth allows us to choose healthy diets, live in healthy places, take exercise and access effective health care when needed. Is the opposite also true? Does better health lead to greater wealth, either for an individual or a society? The WHO Commission on Macroeconomics and Health (2001) addressed this question several years ago. Noting that politicians have long pursued economic growth by investing in physical infrastructure – such as roads, railways and, more recently, telecommunications – and in human resources, through education, the Commission presented the case for making similar investments in health. However, it said little of Europe. The Commission focused instead on the urgent public health crises facing sub-Saharan Africa, a region ravaged by cycles of disease and poverty. That focus was entirely justified as an initial attempt to understand the relationships between health and the economy, but left unanswered how this issue plays out in the WHO European Region. This chapter reviews some of the research that addresses this unanswered question.

Since the Commission published its report, a significant amount of work addressing the question has been undertaken in the European Region.[1] In response, public discourse on the economic consequences/costs of ill health (or the economic benefits of good health) has been handicapped by considerable confusion about what people mean by the term. This chapter seeks to address three different economic cost concepts, noting that without an a priori definition of the cost concept at issue, no meaningful debate can ensue. Figure 4.1 introduces the overall concept of these costs and suggests the outline for the chapter.

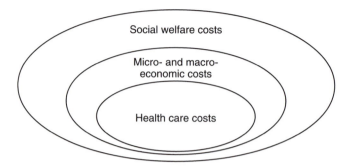

Figure 4.1 Three concepts of economic costs

The chapter comprises three main sections followed by some concluding remarks. The first discusses research findings concerning the broadest or most relevant concept: social welfare costs. From a welfare economic perspective, there is no doubt about what the true cost concept is: the value individuals attribute to better health. However, since health lacks the explicit market price that characterizes standard goods and services, extra effort is required to elicit the value people attribute to health. This is neither straightforward nor easy and may seem controversial, but the concept is widely accepted among economists.

The second section looks at a narrower but more widely used concept of economic costs as two categories: the micro- and macroeconomic costs of ill health. A number of questions arise: taking the micro perspective, 'Does illness reduce the likelihood that a person will be in work?', and at the macro level, 'Do improvements in a country's health promote its economic growth?' On balance, there is a greater consensus on the evidence and importance of microeconomic costs than macroeconomic ones.

Narrowing the focus even more, the third section looks at how ill health affects spending on health care. Policy-makers have long sought to know whether investing in health now will reduce health care expenditure in the future. For instance, a highly controversial (and heavily criticized) report commissioned by a tobacco company suggested that smoking benefited the public finance balance in the Czech Republic because the behaviour killed people off before they became old, unproductive and costly through extended illness (Arthur D. Little International 2000). By contrast, the claim that better health, primarily achieved by more prevention, would help to reduce future health expenditures is not infrequently put forward in political debates around health care reform (Leonhardt 2007). The truth lies somewhere between the extremes, and a number of partly countervailing factors determine the net effect.

It is beyond the scope of the discussion here to examine the costs and benefits of specific interventions to improve health. Instead, the focus will be on different measures of the costs of ill health (or, conversely, the benefits of good health). The important policy implications number at least three. First, the estimates of the costs of ill health can be thought of as the upper limit of the economic benefits that interventions could generate. Second, by showing how ill health can reduce social welfare, slow the economies of both individuals and entire countries and (possibly) exert upward pressure on health expenditures, it may be possible to capture the attention of policy-makers outside the health system. Third, while better health often produces tangible micro- and macroeconomic benefits and may reduce future costs of health care, these are very small compared with the full economic benefit of improved health, which is the monetary value people attribute to better health. Policy-makers should, therefore, be encouraged to factor welfare costs into their economic evaluations of health improvements. Failure to do so risks understating the true economic benefits derived from health interventions.

A broad perspective: social welfare costs

Conventional measures of the economic progress of nations have important limitations. The most common measure, GDP per capita, is the sum of monetary transactions in an economy. It excludes those elements that do not have a market price, such as environmental or health benefits (the health care inputs included in the measurement of GDP represent only a small share of the true value of health). Yet the true purpose of economic activity is to maximize social welfare, and the production of market goods and services is a mere means to that end as well as an (imperfect) proxy for social welfare. The concept of social welfare captures the utility people derive from being alive and healthy. The challenge then becomes that of quantifying social welfare gains attributable to health in monetary terms so that they become comparable to GDP measures, a challenge accepted by key international economic organizations such as the International Monetary Fund (Haacker 2004) and the World Bank (Laxminarayan et al. 2007).

While not captured in GDP, health is highly valued. When asked hypothetically what they would be willing to pay for better health, people propose large amounts, so they do have some idea of its value. Yet, while high, its value is not infinite, since people do not give up everything in exchange for better health. (This refers to situations where people face marginal trade-offs between health and other goods, not the far less representative situation where people face immediate death, which would probably yield a willingness to pay whatever one has.)

Much of the reservation about putting a monetary value on life and health stems from a misunderstanding of what such a value actually means. In fact, economists cannot – and do not seek to – place a monetary value on any identified person's life. Instead, they are valuing comparatively small changes in the risk of mortality, a very different matter. Although less elegant, it would be more appropriate to say 'the value of small mortality risk reductions' than 'the value of life'. While normally no one would trade his or her life or health for money, most people weigh safety against cost in choosing safety equipment or against time when crossing a busy street. Those contemplating a dangerous job, such as mining, will demand a wage premium in return for accepting greater risk. People demonstrably act as if life were not priceless and, in making these choices, are implicitly putting a price on (attributing a value to) changes in the risk of mortality.

One way to make the value attributed to health more explicit is by measuring the extent to which one is willing to trade health for those things that have a price. So-called willingness-to-pay (WTP) methods do precisely that, by analysing either how people act or how they answer certain questions. In 'revealed-preference studies', economists infer WTP from the premiums people implicitly demand for accepting more hazardous jobs or from the sums they pay for safety-enhancing products, such as seat-belts and smoke detectors. Knowing these premiums and the risks associated with them makes it possible to calculate the 'value of a statistical life', which can then be used to place a value on changes in the risk of mortality.

Clearly, the task of determining empirically a price for small changes in mortality risk is challenging, if not heroic (and far more can be said both in favour and against the approach than there is space for here). Nevertheless, many studies have now done so (Viscusi and Aldy 2003), inferring WTP for those small changes in mortality risk in labour markets or purchases of safety equipment. Others use an approach termed 'contingent valuation methodology', where survey respondents are asked how much they would pay to reduce their risk by a certain amount.

While WTP approaches have been refined and improved recently, considerable variation remains in the estimates obtained and there is considerable uncertainty (expressed as wide confidence intervals) around any mean estimate. Caution is appropriate when using these estimates (and in using adequate sensitivity analysis), but this is no reason to abandon the quest for more accurate measurement of this very meaningful concept. It is reasonable to believe that further improvements in both methodologies and data sources will narrow the degree of uncertainty around the estimates.

These approaches were first developed when Usher (1973) introduced the value of mortality reductions into national income accounting. He used the concept of 'full income' to capture the sum of the value of growth in GDP and the value of years of life expectancy gained. The initial study applied this concept to six political entities (Canada, Chile, France, Japan, Sri Lanka and Taiwan) and covered the middle decades of the twentieth century. In the higher-income states, about 30% of the growth in full income was attributable to declines in mortality. More recently, studying the United States, Nordhaus (2003) found that the economic value of increases in longevity in the last century roughly equalled the growth measured in non-health goods and services. Cutler and Richardson (1997), Miller (2000), Costa and Kahn (2003), Viscusi and Aldy (2003) and Crafts (2005) have produced similar results.

For our studies on Europe, we adopted the same general approach as used in this work to estimate the monetary worth of increases in life expectancy between 1970 and 2003 in selected European countries.[2] Conceptually, one can then measure the monetary value of health gains by the amount of money people would require to forego these gains. In other words, what income would someone living with a 2003 income and life expectancy require to be willing to live with the life expectancy that prevailed in 1970? The additional income he or she would require is a measure of the monetary value of the additional life-years gained between the two years.

Based on previously developed models (Becker, Philipson and Soares 2005; Soares 2007) and adopting the same fairly standard assumptions and parameters from those models, utility functions can be specified for two hypothetical individuals born in 1970 and 2003. These models incorporate, among other factors, life expectancy and GDP per capita in the corresponding years. The calculations generating the value of the additional life-years are very detailed and so are not reported here.[3] The difference in lifetime values, and thus the required compensation, is in column 6 of Table 4.1. This value can then be divided by the extra years of life expectancy over the period (column 7) to yield an annual figure, and it can then be expressed in relation to 2003 GDP per capita in order to reveal its size (column 8). These percentages vary between 29% and 38% of GDP per capita and illustrate the substantial value attributed to health gains in Europe, a value far exceeding each country's national health expenditures.

Table 4.2 presents the results of the same calculations for several of the countries in central and eastern Europe (CCEE) and the Commonwealth of Independent States (CIS) for a much shorter period, 1990–2003. Data for both life expectancy and real GDP have only been available for an appreciable number of countries since 1990. As some countries experienced a decrease in life expectancy between 1990 and 2003, they are associated with negative amounts for the monetary value of health gains, which represent a welfare loss.

Clearly, this exercise is a somewhat simplified calculation of the welfare gains from longer life, and it ignores the additional welfare gains from reduced or postponed morbidity that would accompany the reduction in mortality. Ideally,

Table 4.1 Monetary value of life-expectancy gains in selected European countries, 1970–2003

Country (1)[a]	Life expectancy at birth (years)		Real GDP per capita (PPP$)		Monetary value		
	1970 (2)	2003 (3)	1970 (4)	2003 (5)	Life-expectancy gains (PPP$) (6)	Gains per life year gained (PPP$) (7)	(7) as % of 2003 GDP per capita (8)
Austria	70.02	78.93	3,020	30,094	87,986	9,875	33
Finland	70.40	78.72	2,897	27,619	74,037	8,899	32
France	72.93	79.44	3,659	27,677	54,741	8,409	30
Greece	73.82	78.93	1,613	19,954	29,085	5,692	29
Ireland	70.75	78.28	1,934	37,738	95,450	12,676	34
Netherlands	73.71	78.80	3,542	29,371	45,426	8,925	30
Norway	74.17	79.71	3,015	37,670	64,398	11,624	31
Spain	72.88	79.78	2,313	22,391	45,312	6,567	29
Sweden	74.83	80.37	4,019	26,750	42,705	7,708	29
Switzerland	73.24	80.81	5,222	30,552	69,794	9,220	30
Turkey	54.15	68.70	927	6,772	37,796	2,598	38
United Kingdom	71.95	78.45	3,189	27,147	55,106	8,478	31

Source: WHO Regional Office for Europe (2007) for life expectancy and real GDP per capita.
Notes: [a]Countries were chosen on the basis of data availability for both life expectancy and real GDP in 1970 and 2003; PPP$: Purchasing power parity in US$.

Table 4.2 Monetary value of life-expectancy gains in selected countries of central and eastern Europe and the Commonwealth of Independent States, 1990–2003

Country (1)[a]	Life expectancy at birth (years)		Real GDP per capita (PPP$)		Monetary value		
	1990 (2)	2003 (3)	1990 (4)	2003 (5)	Life-expectancy gains (PPP$) (6)	Gains (loss) per life year gained (lost) (PPP$) (7)	(7) as % of 2003 GDP per capita (8)
Albania	72.61	75.77	3,000	4,584	3,157	999	22
Armenia	72.08	73.08	4,741	3,671	777	777	21
Azerbaijan	71.35	71.93	3,529	3,617	454	783	22
Belarus	71.25	68.53	5,727	6,052	−4,329	1,592[b]	26[b]
Bulgaria	71.48	72.39	4,700	7,731	1,873	2,059	27
Czech Republic	71.53	75.4	11,531	16,357	18,978	4,904	30
Estonia	69.94	71.78	6,438	13,539	7,741	4,207	31
Georgia	72.97	72.00	4,572	2,588	−466	480[b]	19[b]
Kazakhstan	68.81	65.89	4,716	6,671	−5,658	1,938[b]	29[b]
Kyrgyzstan	68.82	67.91	3,520	1,751	−279	306[b]	17[b]
Latvia	69.54	70.95	6,457	10,270	4,331	3,072	30
Lithuania	71.55	72.24	4,913	11,702	2,353	3,410	29
Republic of Moldova	68.64	68.07	3,896	1,510	−139	243[b]	16[b]
Poland	71.01	74.74	4,900	11,379	12,088	3,241	28
Romania	69.79	71.32	2,800	7,277	3,053	1,996	27
Russian Federation	69.28	64.94	7,968	9,230	−12,559	2,894[b]	31[b]
Tajikistan	70.03	72.78	2,558	1,106	363	132	12
Ukraine	70.54	67.83	5,433	5,491	−3,894	1,437[b]	26[b]
Uzbekistan	69.71	70.36	3,115	1,744	189	290	17

Source: WHO Regional Office for Europe (2007) for life expectancy and real GDP per capita.
Notes: [a]Countries were chosen on the basis of data availability for both life expectancy and real GDP in 1970 and 2003; [b]Loss of welfare; PPP$: Purchasing power parity in US$.

the findings would be based on direct estimates derived from European WTP studies, rather than from data calibrated for a model; however, this is not yet possible because of the scarcity of country-specific data. That said, the actual figures are unlikely to deviate much from the results suggested above, so if only a fraction of these life expectancy gains results from health interventions, the 'true' social productivity of spending on health (via the health system and other sectors that affect health) may have been many times greater than that of other forms of investment.

A more limited perspective: micro- and macroeconomic costs

This section examines two more-tangible but less-holistic types of economic consequences, which differ from each other in perspective: those that affect individual and household economies (microeconomic consequences) and those that affect national economies (macroeconomic consequences).[4] The former are important for individuals, most of whom may be unaware of the extent to which avoidable ill health affects different dimensions of their economic well-being. The latter hold promise for policy-makers, and particularly those outside the health sector, particularly in finance ministries. Understanding macroeconomic consequences and their causes may encourage policy-makers to consider investment in health as one way (of several) to achieve their economic objectives.

Before discussing the findings of research on these types of consequences and how they are examined through research, a simple framework is presented that shows how, in principle, health might affect economic outcomes. This can be expressed as an aggregate production:

$$Y = A \times F(KhL)$$

where Y is output or GDP, A is 'total factor productivity' (TFP), F is a production function of K, physical capital, L, labour, and h, the quality of labour or human capital. Growth in TFP, also called the Solow residual, represents output growth not accounted for by the growth in the other relevant inputs (here labour and physical capital). The TFP is a measure of how efficiently all inputs combined are used in a production process. Technology, monetary shocks and the political system all affect TFP.

Put simply, GDP grows only with increases in the level of TFP (A), in the aggregate level of physical capital (K) and/or the quality or quantity of labour (hL). Hence, if health is to affect economic output, it has to affect one or more of these factors. In principle, this could happen through three pathways: productivity, labour supply or education.

Healthier individuals could reasonably be expected to achieve greater *labour productivity*: to produce more output per hour worked. On the one hand, their productivity could be increased by their enhanced physical and mental activity. On the other, more physically and mentally active individuals could make better and more efficient use of technology, machinery and equipment (Currie and Madrian 1999). Labour productivity is typically measured by wages and/or earnings (the terms wages and earnings are used interchangeably here, although strictly speaking there is a difference: the wage rate is the price of one unit of labour, for instance an hour, while earnings comprise an individual's entire income from labour over a period of time, often a year). However, wages or earnings may also differ between individuals with different health conditions as a result of discrimination, entirely unrelated to reasons of productivity.

Somewhat counter-intuitively, economic theory predicts an ambiguous impact of health on *labour supply*. The ambiguity results from two effects, which may offset each other. On the one hand, if poor health reduces wages through lower productivity, workers might compensate for the lower economic return on their time by taking more leisure (substitution effect): they derive more value from leisure than income. On the other hand, falling wages over their lifetimes could push individuals to work more hours or years (income effect). Which effect becomes more important in a given set of circumstances thereby becomes an empirical question (Currie and Madrian 1999).

Human capital theory suggests that people with more and better education will be more productive (and obtain higher earnings). If children attain higher educational status, lose less time from school and are less likely to drop out because of better health, then improved health in youth would increase future productivity. Moreover, as improved health leads to longer life, healthier individuals will have more incentive to invest in their education and training, as they will be able to harvest the associated benefits for a longer period (Strauss and Thomas 1998).

Returning to the production function, health can (in principle) also have a direct effect on TFP. The aggregate productivity of an economy depends, among other things, on the business and research activities that citizens undertake. Evidence suggests that ill health can negatively affect these decisions (McCain and Mustard 1999), although more empirical work is needed. It has also been suggested that significant benefits from investment in health-related R&D can spill over to the larger economy (Box 4.1).

Box 4.1 Health-related research and development and its contribution to the broader economy

The health sector creates intensive demands for R&D: in 2003, 19.5% of domestic R&D expenditure by government and higher education sectors in the EU 25 countries (Member States from 1 May 2004) was in medical sciences (Eurostat 2008). This rate was exceeded only by natural sciences (34%) and engineering and technology (23%). Economists widely agree that investment in R&D contributes to economic growth (via its impact on total factor productivity).

Looking at R&D in general, research has documented spillovers of R&D expenditure beyond the firm, industry or country where the R&D took place (Griliches 1992; Nadiri 1993). Spillover refers to 'the impact of the discovered ideas or compounds on the productivity of the research endeavours of others' (Griliches 1992). Many developed countries have an explicit policy goal of increasing R&D expenditures. In fact, the EU's revised Lisbon Agenda had the goal of spending 3% of GDP on R&D by 2010. By analogy, it could be argued that R&D in the health sector could spill over to other productive sectors in an economy, contributing to its wider productivity. If true, this spillover advantage from health-related R&D could benefit an economy even if it failed to improve health.

Evidence from other sectors suggests that such a possibility seems highly plausible. To date, however, evidence is scant that health-related R&D has economy-wide benefits in Europe or globally. One exception is a study of the United States, which estimated that just 10 biomedical discoveries derived from publicly sponsored health research, and adopted by industry for purposes other than health services, generated an additional US$ 92 billion (€57 billion) annually (Silverstein, Garrison and Heinig 1995). Another study indicated that the considerable applications of biotechnology in non-health sectors (e.g. developments in plant genetics and food production, using bacteria to clean up oil spills, and organic compounds with novel industrial applications) may also reflect the economy-wide impact of health-related R&D (Pardes et al. 1999). Nevertheless, more research examining the extent to which health-related R&D benefits productivity at large, in particular in Europe, is clearly needed.

At an individual or population level, health may affect not just income but also how it is used, whether for consumption, savings or investment. Healthier individuals can reasonably expect to live longer and to have a longer time horizon. Their propensity to save for the future may be higher than that of individuals in poor health. A healthy workforce can also increase the incentive for business investment. High health care costs can also drive a household to sell productive assets, thereby exposing it to a greater poverty risk. In sum, a population experiencing a rapid increase in life expectancy may be expected – other things being equal – to save and invest more. This should also contribute to the likelihood of investing in physical capital (Bloom, Canning and Graham 2003).

Microeconomic costs

Here the microeconomic impact of health on the labour market is examined as a potential determinant of earnings and of various indicators of labour supply. The labour market is unarguably a key determinant of economic performance at micro- and macro-levels. Lower labour productivity and labour supply are recognized as among the prime reasons why Europe's economy lags behind that of the United States. The analysis here focuses on the labour market because this is where most empirical findings have been accumulated, partly because of the nature of existing data sets. However, this focus should not be seen as devaluing other microeconomic channels. A brief discussion of health's impact on education and savings has been published elsewhere (Suhrcke et al. 2005).

Over recent years, evidence on the labour market consequences of health has grown significantly, albeit from a low base. Most of this new research focuses on individual countries, although the European Community Household Panel (ECHP) and the more recent Survey on Health, Ageing and Retirement in Europe (SHARE) enable important new cross-country analyses in Europe. Microeconomic findings from research are increasingly also available for the eastern European countries (Suhrcke, Rocco and McKee 2007; Mete 2008). Research into the labour market consequences of health falls into two categories: one examining the impact of health indicators (e.g. chronic illness) and the other examining the impact of risk factors (e.g. smoking). The former is the main focus here (but see Box 4.3 below). Most, but not all, studies confirm theoretical prediction that ill health will lower earnings. While definitional and methodological differences among studies lead to quite different estimates of the size of the impact, it is possible to gain some idea of its magnitude.

Box 4.2   Methodological challenges in assessing the causal impact of health on the labour market and attempted solutions

At least three methodological challenges complicate measurement of the extent to which health affects income.

1. It is plausible that the relationship between health and employment or earnings acts in both directions: health may affect employment and employment may affect health. Such bidirectional causality creates problems for the most common econometric technique for this assessment, OLS estimation.
2. Health measurement is subject to systematic bias, particularly when self-assessed.
3. Available data sets may exclude crucial variables (e.g. individual preferences on time and risk), either because they were not investigated or are unobservable.

The studies reviewed here have generally tried to address one or more of these challenges.

Most work in this area uses cross-sectional data and employs various forms of instrumental variable techniques. These techniques require finding valid instruments that are uncorrelated with the error term and predict well the endogenous variables for each equation. Some studies use panel data, allowing the application of, for example, different versions of fixed and random effects models. Others use OLS estimation, defending this by assuming (or testing – to some extent – for) the exogeneity of the health measure (Jones 2007).

More studies have examined the effect of health on labour supply, particularly among older workers, presumably because it is easier to measure employment than earnings in household surveys. (A few look at earnings and supply simultaneously.) This type of research must overcome some methodological challenges (Box 4.2).

Health as a determinant of earnings

True labour productivity is relatively easy to measure in economies where the output derives from manual work, such as agriculture and mining. While more difficult to measure in economies where the output derives from non-manual work, in a competitive market the wage rate should equal marginal productivity, so that rate is typically used as a proxy for productivity. Based on the New Keynesian theory of downward-rigid or 'sticky' wages, the wage rate can correctly be used as a proxy for productivity only above a minimum level. Below that level, wages are unrelated to actual productivity (Mankiw, Gregory and Weil 1992).

To the best of our knowledge, the only study that has examined the impact of ill health on earnings using a European multicountry survey is Gambin's discussion paper in 2005, although her primary interest was in the potential differential impact of health on wages by gender. Using the eight waves of the ECHP covering 1994–2001 for 14 European countries, she found somewhat mixed results: overall, relationships were identified significant more often for men than for women. For both sexes, she obtained the most significant coefficients through pooled ordinary least squares (OLS) estimation rather than through random effects or fixed effects estimation. This suggests that the associations she observed may not reflect the impact of health on wages but rather the reverse.

Other single-country studies, often using national surveys that were part of the ECHP, find more robust impacts of health on earnings/wages. For instance, one study examined how self-assessed general and psychological health affected hourly wages – differently for males and females – by using longitudinal data from six waves of the British Household Panel Survey (Contoyannis and Rice 2001). The results suggest that poorer 'psychological health' (a variable the authors defined) led to a decrease in hourly wages for males, while excellent self-assessed health increased hourly wage for females.[5]

Jäckle (2007) used the German Socioeconomic Panel covering 1995–2005 to estimate men's and women's reduced-form wage equations, augmented by a variable measuring health satisfaction. He found that good health raised wages: a 10% increase in health satisfaction enhanced women's (hourly) wages by approximately 0.14–0.47% and men's by about 0.09–0.88%.[6]

Lechner and Vazquez-Alvarez (2004) used data from the same survey and for the years 1984–2001. Applying a matching model, they compared groups of people who were disabled with those without disability; both groups were the same in respect of other variables. They found that non-disabled people earn as much as DM 6200 (€3100) more annually than those with one definition of disability and as much as DM 10,700 (€5350) more than those with more severe disability. This statistically significant difference represents earnings gaps of approximately 16% and 20%, respectively. Measured as per capita disposable household income, the difference is less but still significant, with at most a gap of DM 2500 (€1250).

Turning to eastern Europe, we have analysed the potential impact of health on wages in the Russian Federation (Suhrcke, Rocco and McKee 2007). We used both cross-sectional analyses of successive waves of the Russian Federation Longitudinal Monitoring Survey (RLMS) and the much larger, but one-off, National Survey of Household Welfare and Program Participation (NOBUS). Both an instrumental variable estimate and longitudinal analyses were applied, taking advantage of the panel dimension of the RLMS.

In the RLMS analysis, individual self-reported health status and the reported number of workdays missed through illness were used as a proxy for health. In both, medically diagnosed diseases were used as instrument for self-reported health indicators. Good health (compared with less than good health) was found to increase the wage rate by 22% for women and 18% for men. Similarly, a workday missed through illness reduced the wage rate by 3.7% for men and by 5.5% for women.[7]

Self-reported health status was used as a proxy for health for the NOBUS data,[8] as in the RLMS analysis, and this confirmed the impact of health on

Box 4.3 The labour market impact of risk factors

Several studies have explored the impact of risk factors on labour market outcomes. The risk factors include under- and overnutrition, smoking and alcohol consumption. There is considerable literature showing the harmful effects of malnutrition or undernutrition on labour market (and broader economic) outcomes worldwide (Commission on Macroeconomics and Health 2001; Gillespie, McLachlan and Shrimpton 2003; World Bank 2006) and in the CCEE-CIS (Rokx, Galloway and Brown 2002), although typically there are no direct cost estimates for the CCEE-CIS.[a] Surprisingly few studies have examined the labour market impact of smoking. The study by Levine, Gustafson and Valenchik (1997) is a rare exception, finding that workers with otherwise typical characteristics and who smoke earn 4–8% less than non-smokers. In what appears to be a rare exception of a study on smokers in low- and middle-income countries, Lokshin and Beegle (2006) found that Albanian smokers experienced wage reductions of 21–28%.

Several studies examine simultaneous effects of smoking and drinking (Lee 1999; Lye and Hirschberg 2004; van Ours 2004; Auld 2005). One found that alcohol use in the Netherlands was associated with 10% higher wages for males while smoking reduced them by about 10% (the study found no effects of either in females) (van Ours 2004). Several other studies confirm the somewhat counter-intuitive, positive wage impact of alcohol consumption. One explanation is the beneficial health effects of moderate alcohol consumption, although it fails to consider either the very harmful health effects of excessive alcohol consumption or the absence of beneficial health effects in younger people who have little risk of cardiovascular diseases. Another explanation is alcohol is often consumed during social networking, and it is hypothesized that such consumption is associated with additional social time spent with colleagues and associates. This practice may signal to more senior staff that the individual is more motivated and committed to the firm, inducing higher wages for the individual. During such networking, workers may learn valuable information that boosts their careers and ultimately their wages (MacDonald and Shields 2001). Some refute this hypothesis, arguing that the observed results are largely a consequence of measurement problems. For instance, two studies showed that binge drinking reduced earnings among males and females in the United States (Mullahy and Sindelar 1995; Keng and Huffman 2007). Other studies also reported an adverse impact of excessive alcohol consumption on employment. Using Finnish data, one demonstrated that alcohol dependence reduced the probability that a man or woman would be in full- or part-time work by around 14 and 11 percentage points, respectively (Johansson et al. 2007; see also Johansson et al. 2006).

A relatively new but fast-growing area of research focuses on the impact of obesity on the labour market, initially in the United States (Cawley 2004; Cawley and Danziger 2004) but also in (western) Europe. In theory, being overweight should have effects similar to more-general health variables on labour market outcomes, simply because of the adverse impact of obesity on health. However, employers may also discriminate against obese job seekers or workers by offering fewer chances for employment or lower wages. Most empirical studies calculate the overall impact on labour market outcomes, without seeking to disentangle any discrimination effect from a productivity effect. Overall, considerable evidence suggests an adverse impact of obesity on labour market outcomes, but some studies conclude otherwise. If obesity has a negative impact on wages or labour participation and supply, it is clearly more pronounced among women than men. More work is needed to better explain why results vary among studies and countries, the interplay with labour market institutions and the very complex nature of the relationship between obesity and socioeconomic factors. There is some indication that some of the differences result from the imperfect measures used as a proxy for 'fatness' (Burkhauser and Cawley 2008).

An exception is the recent Global Progress Report on Vitamin and Mineral Deficiency (United Nations Children's Fund and the Micronutrient Initiative 2004), which gives some quantitative idea of the economic costs associated with micronutrient deficiencies in 80 low- and middle-income countries in central Asia and the Caucasus, including some CCEE-CIS. Those estimates do not, however, appear to be based on the kind of labour market studies described here.

wages. Men in good health earned about 30% more than those in fair, bad and very bad health, while women in good health earned 18% more than women in less good health.

Health as a determinant of labour supply

As noted above, there is more research on the impact of health on various indicators of labour supply than on wages/earnings. This may be because, given the nature of the labour market in most European countries, wages poorly reflect individual productivity. Moreover, earnings are subject to greater misreporting and non-reporting.

We have also noted how the theoretical impact of health on labour supply is ambiguous. Overall, most studies find that ill health reduces labour supply, measured by, for example, labour force participation or hours worked. Much of the research is on labour force participation by people over 50. This is particularly relevant given that low rates of labour force participation, particularly among older workers in Europe, are *one* key factor behind Europe's sluggish economic performance compared with that of the United States. This section reviews selected studies on the impact of health on labour force participation in general before dedicating a subsection to the role of health in affecting retirement decisions.

Health and labour supply in the general working age population

Many studies using panel data to examine labour supply look not only at health at one point in time but also at sudden, negative changes in health status (health shocks). To the extent that they occur unexpectedly, they are particularly good at capturing the exogenous variation in health, which is very helpful when trying to assess whether changes in health cause changes in economic variables, undisturbed by reverse causality or omitted variables.

García Gómez (2008) examined the impact that health shocks have on the probability of being employed in nine European countries. She used the ECHP and applied a matching technique combined with difference-in-differences techniques. Her results suggest that the direction of causality is indeed from health to probability of employment and then to income: individuals who suffered a health shock were significantly more likely to leave employment, and in several countries doing so was associated with a significant reduction in some types of income. As expected, the magnitude and the significance of the income declines differed across countries. Three (France, Italy and Greece) registered no significant effect, while in Denmark, the Netherlands and Ireland, which had the largest effects, a health shock reduced income by more than 7%. This difference largely relates to the fact that a health shock more than doubled the chance of being unemployed in the latter group of countries. This, in turn, may reflect different incentives created by the social security arrangements in place: in Ireland, for instance, individuals who experience deterioration in their health cannot opt to work part-time if they want to retain entitlement to disability benefits.

The Lechner and Vazquez-Alvarez study in 2004 analysed the impact of becoming disabled in Germany on the probability of being employed and found that becoming disabled reduced the probability of being employed by almost 10%. It also looked at a subsample of those in full-time work at the start of the survey. One might expect that those who become disabled would be better informed about disability policies and the labour market and, therefore, would be less at risk of unemployment than the overall sample. In fact, there was almost no difference.

Using Irish panel data covering 1995–2000, Gannon (2005) used a pooled dynamic probit model and found that disabled men whose activities were severely limited were 9 percentage points less likely to be working than non-disabled men. The corresponding figure for women was 26 percentage points. The effects of some and no limitations turn out to be less substantial.

Our study of eastern Europe and central Asia looked at, among other issues, how poor self-reported health and limited activity affected the probability of being employed in eight CIS countries. This was based on the unique (for the CIS) Living Standards, Lifestyles and Health Survey, applying an instrumental variable estimation (Suhrcke, Rocco and McKee 2007). The survey was performed only once, in 2001, but has been repeated in 2010. Table 4.3 shows how limitations in daily activities affected labour market participation. The variable was dichotomous: limited activity was either present or absent. The expected negative impact of ill health (here the proxy was activity limitations)

Table 4.3 The impact of activity limitations on labour market participation in eight countries of the Commonwealth of Independent States, 2001

Country	Change in probability of labour market participation owing to presence of activity limitation (%)
Armenia	−16.3[a]
Belarus	−25.1[a]
Georgia	−6.9[b]
Kazakhstan	−30.4[a]
Kyrgyzstan	−18.8[a]
Republic of Moldova	−22.3[a]
Russian Federation	−23.0[a]
Ukraine	−16.7[a]

Source: Suhrcke, Rocco and McKee 2007.
Notes: [a]Significant at 1%; [b]Significant at 5%.

on economic outcomes was confirmed in all surveyed countries. In Georgia, the probability that individuals whose activities were limited would participate in the labour market was at least 6.9% lower than for individuals without such limitations. This rose to 30.4% in Kazakhstan.

A similar exercise found (on the basis of a cross-sectional and panel analysis of the Bulgarian Living Standard Measurement Surveys in 1995, 1997 and 2001) that disability reduced the probability of being employed, but labour supply, in turn, had little effect on disability (Wolff 2005). The study employed a simultaneous equation model (health and employment equations) estimated separately via maximum-likelihood methods in each of the three years, as well as a simultaneous equation model on the available panel data (1995 and 1997).

Health and the labour supply of older workers: the impact of health on retirement

There is now considerable evidence that ill health plays a significant and robust role in the decision to retire. Much of the earlier research was carried out in the United States, but research from Europe is increasing.

Several reviews have concluded that the evidence is sufficient to state that poor health and negative health shocks increase the probability of retiring in high-income countries (Sammartino 1987; Currie and Madrian 1999; Deschryvere 2004; Lindeboom 2006). Health status even emerged as the main, but of course not the sole, determinant of labour supply by older workers in several studies (an important factor in the decision to retire is an individual's financial incentives, determined largely by the characteristics of the country's pension and social protection system, e.g. Gruber and Wise 1999). The review below covers some recent empirical studies on Europe but the results from different countries and time periods should be interpreted with caution as it is essential to be aware that results are sensitive to different institutional frameworks (such as pension rules, availability of disability benefits and health insurance coverage).

Hagan, Jones and Rice (2006) found that health exerted a significant and strong impact on the probability of retiring, all else being equal. They used data from nine countries (Belgium, Denmark, France, Greece, Ireland, Italy, Portugal, Spain and the United Kingdom) covered by the ECHP for 1994–2001, with a sample of individuals aged 50–64 and either employed or self-employed in 1994. They used alternative definitions of retirement (self-reported or based on the transition from activity to inactivity[9] and alternative measures of health (self-assessed health, limitations through ill health, a constructed health status measure and a measure of health shocks). They found a consistent effect of health status on retirement decisions. Acute health shocks were more important than poor health per se. Pooling data from all countries revealed that a medium health shock would, all else being equal, increase the probability of retiring by 50%, while a large one would increase it by 106% (Table 4.4).

The authors also looked at how the impact of health shocks and health stocks varied among countries, variation that may be associated with the various incentives for retirement embedded in a country's social security and tax systems. Despite this variation, the fundamental results from the pooled analysis presented above were sustained.

Kalwij and Vermeulen (2005) produced a similar cross-country analysis, using data collected in 2004 for 11 countries in the European SHARE survey. In contrast to the ECHP data used by Hagan, Jones and Rice (2006), SHARE at that time covered only one time point: panel data were not yet available. However, SHARE focused on those over 50 and had a more extensive collection of health indicators, many of them objective and not subject to the measurement bias commonly associated with the standard self-reported health variables. This makes SHARE particularly suitable for examining how health affects labour force participation by the elderly.

Kalwij and Vermeulen (2005) found that several health indicators were significantly associated with the probability that men and women aged 50–64

Table 4.4 Change in the probability of retiring resulting from a one-unit change in the health measure (pooled results)

Health measures contributing to the decision to retire	Effect on two indicators of retirement (%)	
	Self-reported retirement	Transition to inactivity
Self-assessed health	−15[a]	−18[a]
No limitation by ill health	−25[a]	−30[a]
Health stock[b]	−13[a]	−17[a]
Health shock		
Small	0	+14
Medium	+44[a]	+50[a]
Large	+47[a]	+106[a]

Source: Hagan, Jones and Rice 2006.
Notes: [a]Significance at 1% level; [b]The normalized variable 'health stock' has a mean of 0 and a standard variation of 1.

would participate in the labour force.[10] They estimated the decision of working/ not working separately for each country and for men and women. They used five health variables: maximum grip strength, whether or not the individual ever had a severe or a mild condition, whether the individual suffered from restrictions in activities of daily living and whether the individual was obese. Only in France, Greece and Switzerland did none of the health variables significantly affect the probability that men would participate in the labour force, while this was only true for women in Austria.[11] Among the statistically significant results, having ever suffered a severe condition significantly lowered the probability of women's participation in the labour force in four countries by 11–28 percentage points, while for men the range in five countries was 13–31 percentage points.

A series of country-specific analyses also confirmed that health affects retirement decisions. Most of the evidence is from western European countries, such as research by Kerkhofs, Lindeboom and Theeuws (1999) and Lindeboom and Kerkhofs (2006), who used panel data from the Netherlands. Roberts et al. (2006), using comparable longitudinal data sets for the period 1991–2002, found health to be the key determinant of whether someone would retire in Germany and the United Kingdom. Using similar British data, Disney, Emmerson and Wakefield (2006) found robust evidence that health deteriorations increased the probability that older people would transition from economic activity to inactivity. They also found that the impact of deterioration and improvement in health was asymmetrical, with a deterioration in health having a larger negative effect than the positive effect associated with a health improvement of similar magnitude. Siddiqui (1997) used longitudinal data from the Federal Republic of Germany to show that being disabled or suffering from a chronic disease significantly increased the probability of early retirement. Using Spanish survey data from 1999, Jiménez-Martin, Labeaga and Vilaplana Prieto (2005) found that (self-reported) ill health and disability shocks significantly affected the probability that older workers would continue working. Using a Danish Longitudinal Survey, Datta Gupta and Larsen (2006) found that men aged 50–69 were 8% more likely to retire two years after suffering an acute health shock (heart attack, stroke or incident cancer).

The relationship between health and retirement has been the subject of less research in the CCEE, though some work has been undertaken in the Russian Federation (Suhrcke, Rocco and McKee 2007), Albania, Bosnia and Herzegovina and Bulgaria (Favaro and Suhrcke 2006) and Estonia (Suhrcke, Võrk and Mazzuco 2006). These studies confirm that the impact of ill health on retirement is not restricted to western Europe. Ill health emerged as an important factor in anticipating the decision to retire in all these countries. In Estonia, for example, ill health increased the probability that a man would retire in the following year by 6.4% compared with a man without a chronic illness or disability. For women the corresponding figure was 5.6%.

The study on the three south-eastern European countries found a particularly strong effect in Albania, although precise cross-country comparisons cannot be made because of differences in the data. In the Russian Federation, an individual who suffers from chronic illness has a significantly higher probability of retiring in the subsequent year than the same individual free of chronic

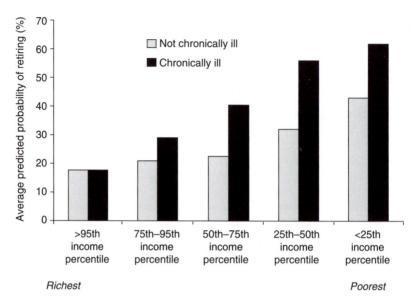

Figure 4.2 Average predicted probability of retiring in the subsequent period, based on panel logit results

Source: Suhrcke, Rocco and McKee (2007)
Note: Results refer to a hypothetical male at age 55 years.

illness (Fig. 4.2). The magnitude of effect is sizeable compared with other variables in the model. Interestingly, as the figure shows, the impact of health on retirement is particularly strong among the poor, suggesting that existing economic disadvantage may be perpetuated through ill health.

In summary, increasing research from Europe indicates that poor health and, in particular, sudden deteriorations in health, lead to earlier retirement.

Macroeconomic costs

The previous sections have shown how better health is good for the economic status of individuals. Is the same true for entire countries? This section reviews what is known, with a particular focus on research of greatest relevance to the countries of the European Region. It does not look in detail at the ways by which scourges such as human immunodeficiency virus/acquired immunodeficiency syndrome (HIV/AIDS) and malaria may impede economic growth in many low- and middle-income countries, as research on the effects of malaria (Gallup and Sachs 2001), HIV/AIDS (Bell, Devarajan and Gersbach 2006) and malnutrition (Weil 2007) are available elsewhere.

The evidence on whether better health contributes to economic growth in countries in the WHO European Region is rather mixed, and the debate is far from settled at the moment. The ultimate answer depends on at least two factors. The first is the country's economic and health status: where both are high, the scope for gains is limited, simply as a consequence of the law of diminishing returns. The second is the existing institutional setting: where retirement age is fixed and low it curbs the effect of better health on the economy. Each is considered in turn.

Does health determine economic growth?

Historical studies show that much of today's economic wealth can be attributed to historical health gains. For example, estimates indicate that about 50% of the economic growth experienced by the United Kingdom between 1780 and 1980 can be attributed to improved health and nutrition (Fogel 1994). Another study of 10 industrialized countries over periods of at least a century found improvements in health had increased the rate of economic growth by 30–40% (Arora 2001).

Findings from cross-sectional studies are less straightforward, with results differing according to whether the study looked worldwide or focused on high-income countries. Many worldwide studies consistently find that health is a robust predictor of economic growth, acting through increased savings (Silverstein, Garrison and Heinig 1995), investment in human capital (Kalemli-Ozcan, Ryder and Weil 2000), labour market participation (Commission on Macroeconomics and Health 2001), foreign direct investment (Alsan, Bloom and Canning 2004) and productivity growth (Bloom, Canning and Sevilla 2002). Although these studies cover different countries and periods and use different variables, data definitions and models, the conclusions are remarkably consistent (Levine and Renelt 1992; Sala-I-Martin, Doppelhofer and Miller 2004). Health status typically emerges as a strong predictor of subsequent economic growth in those countries, in some cases having more impact than education (Barro 1997). These findings can be used to predict the future trajectory of per capita income in a country should it achieve a defined reduction in mortality. The outcome of such an exercise in five low- and middle-income CCEE-CIS indicates potentially large income gains (Suhrcke, Rocco and McKee 2007) (Box 4.4).

However, more recently the notion that health is good for growth has come under some attack. For example, as Weil (2007: 1271) pointed out, many of the studies cited above on the growth impact of health

> suffer(s) from severe problems of endogeneity and omitted variable bias. ... More generally, the problem with the aggregate regression approach is that, at the level of countries, it is difficult to find an empirically usable source of variation in health, either in cross section or time series, that is not correlated with the error term in the equation determining income.

Endogeneity refers to the possibility that health conditions might improve as a consequence of economic development, rather than being a determinant of economic development. In their effort to overcome the endogeneity problems, Acemoglu and Johnson (2007) have succeeded in finding a suitable source of variation in health to be used as an instrument for life expectancy.[12] With life expectancy having increased exogenously, and not as a consequence of improved economic conditions, the causal contribution of good health on

Box 4.4 A calculation of the potential growth impact of reducing future adult mortality rates in five countries in central and eastern Europe and the Commonwealth of Independent States

A parsimonious cross-country growth regression for the period 1960–2000 was used initially to establish a baseline of how adult mortality, conditional on some relevant determinants of economic growth (i.e. initial per capita income, fertility rates and the economy's openness), relates to future per capita incomes (Suhrcke, Rocco and McKee 2007). It was then assumed that this relationship would also govern the relationship between adult mortality and per capita incomes in five countries: Georgia, Kazakhstan, Lithuania, Romania and the Russian Federation. In the absence of pre-existing country-specific results on the role of health in economic growth, this assumption may be a defendable first step. Three simple future scenarios for adult mortality rates from 2000 to 2025 were postulated: no change (Commission on Macroeconomics and Health 2001), a 2% per annum reduction (Suhrcke et al. 2005) and a 3% per annum reduction (Suhrcke, Rocco and McKee 2007). This provided three different scenarios for the future path of per capita incomes, as illustrated in Fig. 4.3 for the representative case of Georgia.

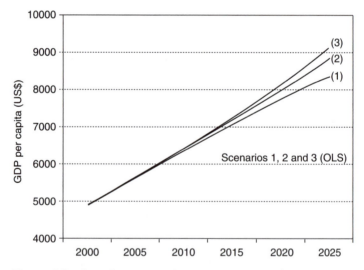

Figure 4.3 Gross domestic product (GDP) per capita forecasts based on ordinary least squares (OLS) estimates in three scenarios, Georgia

Source: Suhrcke, Rocco and McKee 2007.

The total discounted benefits of the intermediate and optimistic scenarios, compared with the benchmark scenario, can then be calculated. Table 4.5 shows the results for the five countries, using two different regression approaches: an OLS and a fixed effects regression. As expected, the fixed effects estimates produce a steeper growth path than the OLS estimates, and the 'true' effect will lie somewhere in between.

Table 4.5 Summary of discounted benefits as a share of (2000) gross domestic product (GDP) per capita in five countries

	2% per annum reduction in adult mortality rate (%)		3% per annum reduction in adult mortality rate (%		GDP per capita (US$)
	OLS	FE	OLS	FE	
Georgia	40	126	62	194	4904
Kazakhstan	26	58	40	88	7394
Lithuania	30	77	46	118	7242
Romania	40	129	61	198	4287
Russian Federation	26	62	39	95	8013

Notes: Amounts are the discounted (at 3% per year) gain from reducing adult mortality, keeping fertility rate constant at 2000 level; measured with respect to the 2000 GDP per capita in percentage terms. OLS: Ordinary least squares estimation; FE: Fixed effects model.

Even though they should be taken with great caution in light of the simplified methodology, these results suggest that the total discounted benefit, even of the relatively modest second scenario, measured by the more conservative estimation methodology (OLS), are substantial when expressed in terms of 2000 GDP. The benefits vary between 26% for the Russian Federation and Kazakhstan and 40% for Georgia and Romania.

economic development can be assessed more reliably. Surprisingly, Acemoglu and Johnson have found a negative impact of life expectancy on the growth rate of GDP per capita (but an increase in total GDP), even if they look at the income per capita of 1980 or of 2000: 40 or 60 years after the beginning of the international epidemiological transition.

This result has been interpreted in the light of Solow's model of exogenous growth: longer life expectancy causes population to rise quickly, while the stock of capital and land adjusts only slowly (Solow 1956). The resulting lower capital-to-labour ratio determines a lower productivity and an initial decline in GDP per capita. Such decline of income per capita will be subsequently compensated by higher output, through the increasing labour force, and higher capital accumulation. It can be even more than compensated if longer lives imply higher productivity, as is plausible. However, this process could take many decades, in particular in countries initially poor in capital stock – more than 60 years at least, according to Acemoglu and Johnson (2007).

Other studies that also took great care in overcoming the endogeneity problem, such as those by Ashraf, Lester and Weil (2008), Weil (2007) and Bhargava et al. (2001), found that the contribution of health to economic growth, although positive, is much smaller than that derived from the traditional growth regression studies.

Yet, the debate as to whether health affects growth, and if so how, is far from settled. Recent, more optimistic and careful assessments of the impact of health on growth, if not specifically related to chronic diseases, include those by Lorentzen, McMillan and Wacziarg (2008), Cervellati and Sunde (2009) and Aghion, Howitt and Murtin (2010).

From a European perspective, it is important to note that few of the existing studies consider whether returns from health gains diminish once a particular level of national wealth is achieved, but Bhargava et al. (2001) and Jamison, Lau and Wang (2005) have suggested that they do. Consequently, worldwide samples may not sufficiently inform thinking about high-income countries in Europe. Three studies used health expenditures as a proxy for health in OECD countries (implying that greater expenditure led to better health) and found a positive association between health expenditure and economic growth or income levels (Rivera and Currais 1999a,b; Beraldo, Montolio and Turati 2005). These results are intriguing, particularly since expenditure on health emerges as substantially more important than that on education in explaining economic growth.[13] Two studies looked at a sample of 22 developed countries between 1960 and 1985 and found that health – measured by life expectancy – had no significant impact on economic growth (Knowles and Owen 1997) or on per capita income levels (Knowles and Owen 1995). Does this mean that, above a certain level of economic development, further health gains may either have no impact or even reduce subsequent economic growth?

Closer inspection indicates that this is not necessarily the case. The most plausible explanation for these negative findings is that they may be an artefact. Life expectancies now differ relatively little among rich countries, unlike among poor countries, so the lack of explanatory power associated with life expectancy comes as no surprise (Tompa 2002). Research in rich countries necessitates the use of health indicators that can better discriminate levels of health.

This direction was taken in another recent study (Suhrcke and Urban 2009). In an analysis of 26 rich countries covering 1960–2000, cardiovascular mortality in the working-age population emerged as a robust, inverse predictor of subsequent economic growth. In one representative estimate, a 10% reduction in cardiovascular mortality was associated with a one percentage point increase in growth of per capita income, a seemingly small amount but one that has a large effect when summed over the long term.

Another explanation of why some of the earlier studies found few macroeconomic benefits from better health may be that prevailing institutional factors constrain what could be achieved. This is the case where health gains increase the proportion of a population beyond retirement age – a point taken up in the following section. If effective retirement age can be delayed in step with longevity gains, many of the negative economic consequences commonly ascribed to ageing societies could be mitigated. In other words, increasing the retirement age might allow health to finally 'deliver' its positive impact on the labour market and thus on the economy by keeping more and healthier people in the workforce as they age.

Finally, when evaluating the macroeconomic findings from these cross-country regression studies, it is important to bear in mind the general limits of this approach, whether health is included in the list of determinants or not. It is particularly important not to overstate the possibility of drawing country-specific lessons (Pritchett 2006).

Potential impact of longevity on the size of the labour force

It was hypothesized above that one reason why some studies have not found that life expectancy positively affects economic growth in high-income countries may be that the retirement age is fixed at a level far younger than average life expectancy. If so, improved population health could (at best) make only a little difference to the health and, hence, to the productivity and labour supply of the working-age population. Instead, it adds to the pool of retired people, which may be desirable from a welfare perspective, but a shrinking labour force and expanding population of elderly dependants will cause difficulties in sustaining economic growth and maintaining a fiscal balance. In 2003, OECD researchers forecast that, with unchanged labour market and immigration conditions, the labour force in the EU15 could decline by around 14% (25 million workers) by 2050 compared with the 2010 peak. This is more favourable than in Japan, where the labour force has already started this decline, but it is still far from the United States benchmark, where the labour force is projected to continue increasing, by about 26% (37 million workers), between 2005 and 2050 (Burniaux, Duval and Jaumotte 2003).

What policy implications flow from these findings in Europe? If people live longer, it may not be entirely outrageous to ask them to work longer. Increasing the effective retirement age (which has stalled or even declined in past decades) is an obvious means of averting at least part of the future labour force decline, but by how much?

A 2005 OECD study (Oliveira Martins et al. 2005) addressed this question by examining the effect of having the 'working age' – commonly assumed to range from 15 to 64 – increase along with longevity gains. The authors conservatively set an average increase of 1.2 years per decade in both longevity and retirement age over the years 2005–2050. Figure 4.4 shows what would happen to the size of the EU15 working-age population with those increases: the fairly modest adjustment would almost stabilize its size, contrasting markedly with what would happen without such adjustment.

Increasing the working-age population (thus reducing the dependency ratio) should mitigate some of the pressures on health and social expenditures. It also has the potential to contribute positively to the economy at large, although this effect will depend crucially on whether the larger working-age population also participates actively in the labour market and whether employers demand the extra labour. This illustrates the importance of complementarities in reform, some of them clearly beyond the influence of health ministries.

It is not, however, sufficient that additional older workers be in demand. It is also necessary that the additional years of life be spent in reasonably good health, enabling older people to work. None of these assumptions can be guaranteed. Nevertheless, we can at least conclude that potential exists for longevity gains to compensate for the ageing of populations in labour markets.

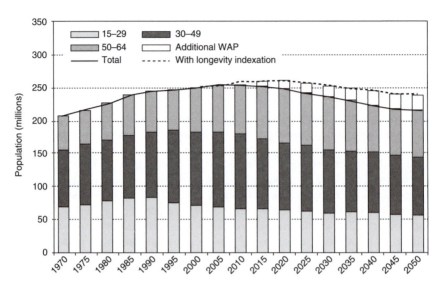

Figure 4.4   Predicted size of the EU15 working-age population with and without adjustment of upper working-age limit

Source: Oliveira Martins et al. 2005.
Notes: WAP: Working-age population.

A very limited perspective: health care costs

Upward pressure on health care spending since the mid 1980s has captured policy-makers' attention. One suggestion for containing these costs is to improve population health, which certainly sounds plausible: healthier people need less health care, which would, in turn, reduce expenditure. This idea underpinned the influential Wanless Report (2002), commissioned by the United Kingdom Treasury, but some are sceptical, suggesting that better health status may even increase future health care spending (Zweifel, Steinmann and Eugster 2005). This section sheds some light on the matter, reviewing relevant studies with a focus on the effect on health expenditures and not the effect on government expenditures in general.

Again, the question of whether investing in health will reduce future health care expenditures is not the relevant criterion when making an economic assessment of the return on investment from a welfare economic perspective, although this has not prevented use of the criterion in public policy debates.

The brief answer to the question, 'Does better health lower future health expenditures?', can only be, 'It depends'. Different studies looking at different countries with different data for different health conditions find very different results. Some of the factors that influence the results obtained are examined below, but, first, readers should be aware that many other factors also affect health expenditures, as discussed elsewhere (Oliveira Martins et al. 2005; see Chapter 3). Most of these factors, particularly technological progress, will most likely continue to contribute to sustained upward pressure on health expenditures.

Table 4.6 How different health factors may affect health care expenditures

Factor	Impact on health care expenditure
Less disease and disability at a given point in time, for a given population or at a given age	Decrease
Additional years of life	Increase
Lower *acute* health care costs of dying at older ages	Decrease
Higher *long-term* care costs of dying at older ages	Increase
Overall effect	Unknown

Therefore, in terms of health expenditures, improvements in population health can, at best, be expected only to diminish their rate of increase.

Several factors can be identified that affect health status and, acting in different directions, could affect health care expenditure:

- less disease and disability at a given point in time, for a given population or at a given age lead to lower health care expenditure at that time;
- however, the longer life that often accompanies better health increases the number of the years over which health care costs will accumulate;
- *acute* health care costs are concentrated in the period just before death, and deaths at older ages actually incur fewer costs, as treatment intensity tends to decline with the age of death;
- yet, the costs of *long-term* social care increase with age, even after controlling for proximity to death, so those costs will be higher for those dying at older ages.

Table 4.6 sets out these factors and shows their directionality more simply. The discussion below elaborates on these different factors by reviewing the relevant research findings from within and beyond Europe.

If consideration is limited to an individual at a given point in time, then clearly worse (or better) health is associated with higher (or lower) health care use and thus expenditure. For instance, Chernichovsky and Markowitz (2004), using data from Israel in 2003, found that the presence of chronic illness had a significant and strong positive impact on the number of visits to a doctor, a specialist and a nurse. In the United States, Fried et al. (2001), in a study of people aged 72 and older living in New Haven, CT in 1989, found that functional status was significantly associated with use of health care services (hospitalization, outpatient and home health care and nursing home care). The authors estimated that, compared with people living independently, stable dependence or a decline to dependence increased per capita health care expenditure by about US$ 10,000 (€6365) over two years.

Dormont, Grignon and Huber (2006) calculated that the improvement in health status of the French population between 1992 and 2000 reduced health care expenditure in 2000 by 8.6% of the country's 1992 health expenditure level (Table 4.7). However, other factors, in particular technological progress and intensity of clinical intervention among elderly people, outweighed these health expenditure savings such that the total expenditure increased by almost 50%. Also, in their model, the savings from health gains were greater than

Table 4.7 Factors causing changes in health expenditure over 1992–2000, as a percentage of total 1992 health expenditure, France

Factor	Change in aggregate health expenditures (%)
Change in population age structure	3.2
Increase in population size	3.0
Changes in practices for a given morbidity	22.1
Changes in morbidity	–8.6
Other changes	30.2
Total	*49.9*

Source: Dormont, Grignon and Huber 2006.

the costs of ageing (which increased expenditure by 3.2%). This serves as a reminder of the need, in studies at population level, to distinguish between two sets of impacts: those that result from health trends and those that result from changes in the population's age structure.

Manton et al. (2007) examined the Medicare population in the United States between 1982 and 1999. Medicare is the publicly funded health insurance programme, providing coverage to people who are aged 65 and over or meet other criteria. They calculated that reduced disability accounted for a decline in total Medicare costs of US$ 25.9 billion (€16.5 billion) in 1999 from what they would have been.

These studies looked at expenditure between two points in time; other studies try to measure whether avoiding disease and disability at earlier ages might not reduce cumulative health costs over the span of a lifetime. Living longer might exhaust the savings gained by healthier earlier years. In fact, the evidence on lifetime health costs is mixed. Some studies do suggest that better health reduces lifetime health care expenditure; others say it makes little difference; still others suggest it would lead to higher health care expenditures.

On the positive side, Liu, Daviglus and Yan (2003) found that Americans without risk factors for cardiovascular diseases in middle age had lower cumulative Medicare expenditure from age 65 until death (or advanced ages) than those with one or more adverse risk factors, even though the former lived longer. Shang and Goldman (2007) compared projections of total health care expenditure based on changes in age distribution and on changes in health (derived from life expectancy). They found that ignoring the health effect would overestimate total expenditures by 9% in 2040, by 19% in 2070 and by 22% in 2080.

On the negative side, van Baal et al. (2008) predicted that obese people and smokers in the Netherlands would incur lower health care costs over their lifetime than healthy people. They estimated lifetime costs from age 20 for three hypothetical cohorts: one of 'healthy-living' people (neither obese nor having smoked), one of obese people and one of smokers (Table 4.8). Although annual health expenditure until age 56 was highest for the obese cohort, lifetime health expenditure was highest for the healthy-living cohort, because of their longer life expectancy. However, while this may be true for the Netherlands,[14] it does

Table 4.8 Expected remaining life expectancy and lifetime health care costs for cohorts with different health-related behaviours

Outcome measure	Healthy living	Obese	Smokers
Life expectancy at age 20 (years)	64.4	59.9	57.4
Expected remaining lifetime health care costs per capita at age 20 (€)	281,000	250,000	220,000

Source: van Baal et al. 2008.

not have universal applicability. Research from the United States, where the issue has been examined more extensively, suggests that the additional lifetime medical cost associated with obesity will be substantial. According to Yang and Hall (2008), elderly men who were overweight or obese at age 65 had 6–13% more lifetime health care expenditures than the same age cohort within normal weight range at age 65. Elderly women who were overweight or obese at age 65 spent 11–17% more than those in a normal weight range. Other studies, again using data from the United States, also obtained different results from those with population in the Netherlands, finding somewhat higher lifetime medical expenditures for smokers (Sloan et al. 2004; Lakdawalla, Goldman and Shang 2005; Goldman et al. 2006). (The main reason why the United States studies found high health care costs for obesity is that it incurs high health care costs that – unlike other health behaviour-related risk factors, such as smoking – are not as highly compensated for by the expenditure-reducing effect of earlier death.) Moreover, a major United Kingdom report forecasted a significant increase in obesity-related health care expenditures in its 'business-as-usual' scenario up to the year 2050 (Butland et al. 2007).

Other studies have found that individuals in good health might have only slightly lower lifelong health care costs than those in worse health. Among them, Lubitz et al. (2003) showed that improved functional status at age 70 led to a longer total and active life expectancy, without increasing an individual's cumulative health care expenditure. For example, the estimated cumulative health care expenditure of a person with no functional limitations at age 70 would be US$ 9000 (€5729) (in 1998 dollars) lower than that of a person who experienced limitation in at least one activity of daily living, even though their life expectancy would be 2.7 years longer. Joyce et al. (2005) also found cumulative health spending to be modestly higher for those chronically ill at age 65. A 65-year-old person with a chronic condition would expect to live 0.3–3.1 years less than someone who was free of chronic conditions, but lifetime medical spending would be US$ 4000–14,000 (€2546–8912) higher. Both these studies used data from the Medicare Current Beneficiary Survey from the 1990s.

Using data from the same survey for 1992–1999 and from the 1982–1996 National Health Interview Surveys, Goldman et al. (2005) showed how an improvement in the disability status of people over 65 might substantially reduce future per capita annual health care spending, even though it would not have a great impact on overall health care spending among this age cohort.

Another predictor of health care expenditure is proximity to death (an empirical literature review is given by Raitano (2006)). However, the age at which one dies influences the health care cost of doing so, as older people tend to be treated less intensively (Seshamani and Gray 2004; Raitano 2006). Therefore, Gandjour and Lauterbach (2005) suggested that prevention (and consequently longer life) might actually decrease lifetime costs if one considers the fact that the costs of the last year of life decrease with age.

An intriguing insight in this respect was provided by Daviglus et al. (2005), who found that being healthier in earlier life reduced the cost of dying. In their study, individuals with fewer risk factors[15] for cardiovascular diseases in young adulthood or middle age (ages 33–64 years) incurred lower hospital expenditures in their last year of life. For example, the total charges (including inpatient care, skilled-nursing facility and outpatient hospital-related care) in the last year of life in the period 1984–2002 for individuals without any risk factor at younger ages were US$ 15,318 (€9750) lower than for those who had four or more risk factors. This was not solely a result of lower costs associated with cardiovascular diseases, which accounted for US$ 10,267 (€6526) of the total. The combined effects of these observations do suggest that improvements in the health of those alive today will, all else being equal, reduce costs when they die.

Balanced against this, as discussed in Chapter 3, expenditure on long-term care does seem to increase with both age and proximity to death (Spillman and Lubitz 2000; Yang, Norton and Stearns 2003; Werblow, Felder and Zweifel 2007), so the longer people live, the greater that share of overall health expenditures will be.

Finally, the Economic Policy Committee of the European Commission (2006) and the OECD (Organisation for Economic Co-operation and Development 2006) each performed projections of public health care expenditure. They calculated the potential for future savings in public health care expenditures under different health scenarios. Summarized results are presented in Table 4.9, although the numbers cannot be compared directly as they use different methodologies and assumptions in each health scenario.

These projections suggest that better health could perhaps mitigate, but not prevent entirely, projected increases in future health care expenditure. Once again, other factors influencing both the supply and demand for health care seem to have a greater impact on aggregate expenditure.

So what can be concluded from this highly condensed review of the impact of health on health care expenditure? The optimistic expectation that improved health in the future (achieved by greater efforts and investment today) will significantly mitigate or even reverse the trend of increasing health expenditures cannot be supported by the evidence presented here. Even if better health may, in some circumstances, lead to lower health care spending, other cost drivers, in particular technological advances, will more than outweigh any such expenditure-reducing effect. There is little support for the hypothesis that better health by itself is a major cost driver.

One final caution – much of the research reviewed here is from the United States, and important structural differences preclude comparison with European systems. It is essential that research of this type be given a much higher priority

Table 4.9 Projections of acute health care and long-term care expenditure, 2004–2050 and 2005–2050

Expenditure and scenarios	EPC for EU25: public expenditure (% of GDP)		OECD countries: public expenditure (% of GDP)	
	Acute health care	Long-term care	Acute health care	Long-term care
Expenditures in base year[a]	6.4	0.9	5.7	1.1
Health scenarios[b]				
Pure ageing or 'expansion of morbidity/disability' scenario (2050)	8.1	1.7	8.5	2.8
'Dynamic equilibrium' or intermediate scenario	7.3	1.3	7.7	2.3
'Compression of morbidity/disability' scenario	6.7	0.9	7.0	1.9

Sources: Economic Policy Committee of the European Commission 2006; Organisation for Economic Co-operation and Development 2006.
Notes: [a]Base year 2004 in EPC study and 2005 in OECD study; [b]Although the EPC and the OECD scenarios are summarized using the same terminology for three of their scenarios, the actual definitions and assumptions differ somewhat between the two studies. The details of these definitional differences are of secondary importance in the present context, so the reader may be referred to the original studies. The main point illustrated here is that the future course of health expenditures does differ across the different health scenarios (although it cannot prevent the overall increase); EPC: Economic Policy Committee.

in Europe, both in terms of direct support and support for the infrastructure, such as cohorts and panel surveys, that make it possible.

Conclusions and key messages

This chapter documents the evidence on some of the main dimensions of the economic costs of ill health (or the economic benefits of good health) that are relevant to the WHO European Region. Three different concepts of economic costs are presented, each policy relevant in its own way. The chapter started from the broadest and, in the view of most economists, most relevant perspective, the idea that the value of improved health (and thus the cost of ill health) is represented by the value that people individually attribute to it. Although difficult to measure in practice and not infinite, it is clearly very high. This broad or 'true' economic cost concept explicitly acknowledges the intrinsic value of health, a feature not shared by the other concepts presented here. Consequently, it demonstrates the falsity of what is all too often presented as a strict dichotomy between the 'health benefits' resulting from health investment on the one hand and the 'economic benefits' on the other. The difference lies chiefly in the measurement unit, not in the (mistaken) idea that economists would not consider the health gains by themselves as relevant.

The chapter then discussed two more-limited concepts of economic costs. The first was the economic consequences for individuals (microeconomic) and for the economy as a whole (macroeconomic). Considerable research shows that ill health negatively affects several labour market outcomes at the individual level. Evidence on the impact of health at the macroeconomic level is, in contrast, more mixed, highlighting the need for research. The second was whether improved health can save health care costs. A range of factors at play could be identified, some partly offsetting the others: the ultimate answer is a matter for empirical enquiry. Yet, even if better health will yield some savings in health care costs (which may be optimistic), such savings will likely be small and probably insignificant against the dominant cost drivers, such as technological developments.

Given limited space, it was impossible to include all the evidence or cover other important economic cost concepts, particularly the distinction between costs that justify public policy interventions from an economic perspective and those that do not, such as the distinction between external and internal costs (Suhrcke et al. 2006). As part of the microeconomic cost, the important time and labour market costs caused to household members who care for those who fall ill have not been covered.[16] Nor has the recent research on the economic cost of health inequalities, an extension of the concepts presented here, been discussed (Mackenbach, Meerding and Kunst 2007; Dow and Schoeni 2008; see Chapter 7).

The opportunity to do full justice to the enormous heterogeneity in the European Region, in terms of both economic and health measures, has also been restricted by the space available. Our earlier work attempts to situate the economic arguments in the specific socioeconomic context of the countries concerned (particularly Suhrcke, Rocco and McKee 2007), and this is clearly what is needed to provide a credible assessment of the potential macroeconomic benefits of investing in health. At a more abstract level, and at the risk of oversimplifying, it is reasonable to assume that decreasing marginal returns also apply in health: the healthier a population is, the more difficult (and costly) it will be to realize additional health gains and thus any associated economic benefits. Given the significant economic benefits that can be demonstrated even in the richer parts of the European Region, there is reason to believe that additional gains may still be possible, although may be smaller in absolute terms.

Endnotes

1. Examples include works on the EU countries (Suhrcke et al. 2005), eastern Europe and central Asia (Suhrcke, Rocco and McKee 2007) and the economic implications of noncommunicable diseases (Suhrcke et al. 2006), all available with other country- and subregion-specific studies on the WHO Regional Office for Europe web site (www. euro.who.int/socialdeterminants/develop/20050929_1, accessed 26 July 2010).

2. This analysis is restricted to a verbal description of the idea behind the calculations. Presentations and discussions of the underlying model are in Becker, Philipson and Soares (2005) and Soares (2007).

3. In general formal terms, the calculation is as follows: suppose the utility U of the hypothetical individual in the year 2003 depends on, among other factors not listed here, both life expectancy L and income Y in that year, so $U = U(L_{2003}, Y_{2003})$. The utility of the individual who has the same income but the life expectancy of 1970 would then be $U' = U(L_{1970}, Y_{2003} + a)$. To find out what the required income gain (a) is that would make the two individuals indifferent between the two situations, one just needs to equate U and U' and solve the equation for a. Of course this can only be done if a very concrete shape is assumed for the utility function with concrete numerical parameters. This very concrete shape in the concrete numerical parameters is derived and justified in Becker, Philipson and Soares (2005).

4. This chapter does not discuss 'cost-of-illness' studies, mainly for lack of space but also for reservations about how they are commonly carried out. Much like in the cost categorization here, such studies distinguish three categories for cost of illness: direct costs (mainly medical care), indirect costs (largely from foregone labour productivity) and intangible (i.e. psychological) costs, with the last rarely measured. Despite this simple categorization, cost-of-illness studies differ enormously in how and what they actually measure. A review of such studies and some critical evaluation are in Section 3.1 of Suhrcke, Võrk and Mazzuco (2006) and Section 3.2 of Suhrcke et al. (2005).

5. The authors employ single-equation fixed effects and random effects instrumental variable estimators suggested by others (Hausman and Taylor 1981; Amemiya and MaCurdy 1986; Breusch, Mizon and Schmidt 1989).

6. In an attempt to control for unobserved heterogeneity, sample selection and endogeneity, the German Socioeconomic Panel study applied estimators proposed previously (Wooldridge 1995; Semykina and Wooldridge 2006). Because of the panel structure of the data, it is possible to control for unobserved effects. A number of tests provide evidence that, for the male sample, corrections are needed, while this issue causes no problems in the female population.

7. The cross-sectional analysis was complemented with panel analysis to check the robustness of the findings. In general, the effect of health on wages continued to hold for males, although the effect was smaller: being in good health increased the wage rate by about 7.5%. Surprisingly, good health did not affect either wage rate or labour supply among female workers, unlike what appears in the cross-sectional instrumental variables estimations, where the effect on wage rates for women was even larger than it was for men.

8. While the RLMS has certain advantages, in particular the annual waves that allow comparison over time, NOBUS, so far only held once (in 2003), covered a far larger share of the population. Its health component was, however, very small compared with that in the RLMS, so a direct comparison between RLMS and NOBUS results is not possible.

9. The self-reported version was based on the self-classification of respondents as 'retired', as 1 out of 12 options for their activity status. The second, broader variable used the transition between reported activity in the labour market and inactivity as a measure of retirement. This was chosen because of doubts raised about the accuracy of the self-reported 'retired' and because transitions from activity to inactivity have been used frequently as outcome measures in analysing the effect of health on retirement. Retirement was taken as an absorbing or permanent state, so individuals were followed from work to when they first reported retirement, and any subsequent transition back to work was disregarded (Hagan, Jones and Rice 2006).

10. The countries covered were Austria, Belgium, Denmark, France, Germany, Greece, Italy, the Netherlands, Spain, Sweden and Switzerland. Data for the first wave were collected in 2004, except in Belgium and France, where they were gathered in 2004–2005.

11. The authors do not address the potential endogeneity problem but rather assume that the health indicators they employed are exogenous to labour market participation, thereby justifying the single equation probit they used, a decision further justified by the more objective nature of the health indicators available in SHARE.

12. They looked at the so-called International Epidemiological Transition, a wave of drug and chemical innovations and wide diffusion and adoption all over the world during the 1940s. Thanks to these new drugs, many communicable diseases have been successfully fought, reducing mortality, particularly among children living in the least developed countries.

13. A further – somewhat controversial – interpretation of these results warrants thought: health (and education) expenditures may be seen as proxies for the size of the welfare state. Hence, the finding that health (and/or education) expenditure enhances economic growth in high-income countries is consistent with the hypothesis that welfare expenditures more than outweigh any distortions caused by the taxation required to support them (Atkinson 1995; Lindert 2004). More work is required to validate this hypothesis.

14. Some responses to this study have expressed concern about certain underlying assumptions. Mittendorf (2008), for instance, criticized the use of average health care in the model, instead of distinguishing costs incurred by those who die versus those who survive in the respective year. With such distinction, one would see that dying later as a consequence of a healthier life reduces the costs of dying. A detailed methodological discussion would also call for scrutiny of other studies with more 'optimistic' results.

15. The authors controlled for six risk factors for cardiovascular diseases at younger ages (blood pressure, serum cholesterol, body mass index, current smoker or not, diagnosed diabetes, minor electrocardiogram abnormalities) as well as for age at death, race, sex and education.

16. Mete (2008) provided evidence on the substantial time invested by other household members in caring for chronically ill or disabled household members in Estonia, Hungary and Romania (Pardes et al. 1999), while Suhrcke et al. (2005) provide the same on impacts on the labour market).

References

Acemoglu, D. and Johnson, S. (2007) Disease and development: the effect of life expectancy on economic growth. *Journal of Political Economy*, 115(6): 925–85.

Aghion, P., Howitt, P. and Murtin, F. (2010) *The Relationship Between Health and Growth: When Lucas Meets Nelson-Phelps*, working paper no. 15813. Washington, DC: National Bureau of Economic Research.

Alsan, M., Bloom, D. and Canning, D. (2004) *The Effect of Population Health on Foreign Direct Investment*, working paper no. 10596. Cambridge, MA: National Bureau of Economic Research.

Amemiya, T. and MaCurdy, T. (1986) Instrumental variables estimation of an error components model. *Econometrica*, 54: 869–80.

Arora, S. (2001) Health, human productivity, and long-term economic growth. *Journal of Economic History*, 61(3): 699–749.

Arthur D. Little International (2000) *Public Finance Balance of Smoking in the Czech Republic.* Prague: Arthur D. Little International, http://www.tobaccofreekids.org/reports/philipmorris/pmczechstudy.pdf (accessed 7 September 2010).

Ashraf, Q.H., Lester, A. and Weil, D.N. (2008) *When Does Improving Health Raise GDP?* Providence, RI: Economics Department, Brown University.

Atkinson, A.B. (1995) The scope for a European growth initiative: is the welfare state necessarily an obstacle to economic growth? *European Economic Review,* 39: 723–30.

Auld, M.C. (2005) Smoking, drinking and income. *Journal of Human Resources,* 40(2): 505–18.

Barro, R.J. (1997) *Determinants of Economic Growth: A Cross-country Empirical Study.* Cambridge, MA: MIT Press.

Becker, G.S., Philipson, T.J. and Soares, R.R. (2005) The quantity and quality of life and the evolution of world inequality. *American Economic Review,* 95(1): 277–91.

Bell, C., Devarajan, S. and Gersbach, H. (2006) The long-run economic costs of AIDS: a model and an application to South Africa. *World Bank Economic Review,* 20: 55–89.

Beraldo, S., Montolio, D. and Turati, G. (2005) *Healthy, Educated and Wealthy: Is the Welfare State Really Harmful for Growth?* working papers in economics no. 127. Barcelona: University of Barcelona, Espai de Recerca en Economia.

Bhargava, A., Jamison, D.T., Lau, L.J. and Murray, C.J. (2001) Modelling the effects of health on economic growth. *Journal of Health Economics,* 20: 423–40.

Bloom, D., Canning, D. and Graham, B. (2003) Longevity and life cycle savings. *Scandinavian Journal of Economics,* 105(3): 319–38.

Bloom, D., Canning, D. and Sevilla, J. (2002) *Health, Worker Productivity and Economic Growth.* Pittsburgh, PA: School of Public Policy and Management, Carnegie Mellon University.

Breusch, T., Mizon, G. and Schmidt, P. (1989) Efficient estimation using panel data. *Econometrica,* 57: 695–700.

Burkhauser, R.V. and Cawley, J. (2008) Beyond BMI: the value of more accurate measures of fatness and obesity in social science research. *Journal of Health Economics,* 27(2): 519–29.

Burniaux, J.-M., Duval, R. and Jaumotte, F. (2003) *Coping with Ageing: A Dynamic Approach to Quantify the Impact of Alternative Policy Options on Future Labour Supply in OECD Countries,* working paper no. 371. Paris: Organisation for Economic Co-operation and Development.

Butland, B., Jebb, S., Kopelman, P. et al. (2007) *Tackling Obesities: Future Choices – Project Report.* London: Foresight, http://www.foresight.gov.uk/OurWork/ActiveProjects/Obesity/Obesity.asp (accessed 8 September 2010).

Cawley, J. (2004) The impact of obesity on wages. *Journal of Human Resources,* 39(2): 451–74.

Cawley, J. and Danziger, S. (2004) *Obesity as a Barrier to Employment and Earnings for Current and Former Welfare Recipients,* working paper no. 10508. Washington, DC: National Bureau of Economic Research.

Cervellati, M. and Sunde, U. (2009) *Life Expectancy and Economic Growth: The Role of the Demographic Transition,* discussion paper no. 4160. Bonn: Institut zur Zukunft der Arbeit.

Chernichovsky, D. and Markowitz, S. (2004) Aging and aggregate costs of medical care: conceptual and policy issues. *Health Economics,* 13: 543–62.

Commission on Macroeconomics and Health (2001) *Macroeconomics and Health: Investing in Health for Economic Development.* Geneva: World Health Organization Commission on Macroeconomics and Health.

Contoyannis, P. and Rice, N. (2001) The impact of health on wages: evidence from the British Household Panel Survey. *Empirical Economics,* 26: 599–622.

Costa, D.L. and Kahn, M.E. (2003) *Changes in the Value of Life, 1940–1980*. Cambridge, MA: Massachusetts Institute of Technology.

Crafts, N. (2005) *The Contribution of Increased Life Expectancy to Growth of Living Standards in the United Kingdom, 1870–2001*, working paper. London: London School of Economics, http://wpeg.group.shef.ac.uk/documents/crafts.pdf, (accessed 7 September 2010).

Currie, J. and Madrian, B.C. (1999) Health, health insurance and the labour market, in O. Ashenfelter and D. Card (eds.) *Handbook of Labour Economics*, Vol. 3. Amsterdam: Elsevier Science: 3309–415.

Cutler, D. and Richardson, E. (1997) Measuring the health of the US population. [Brookings Papers on Economic Activity.] *Microeconomics*, 29: 519–39.

Datta Gupta, N. and Larsen, M. (2006) Do health shocks increase retirement more when workers are universally insured? in *Proceedings of an Institute for the Study of Labor Conference: The Well-Being of the Elderly: Income, Consumption, and Health – Cross-Country Perspectives*, Bonn, 22–23 May, http://www.iza.org/conference_files/eld2006/datta%20gupta_n349.pdf (accessed 7 September 2010).

Daviglus, M.L., Liu, K., Pirzada, A. et al. (2005) Cardiovascular risk profile earlier in life and medicare costs in the last year of life. *Archives of Internal Medicine*, 165: 1028–34.

Deschryvere, M. (2004) *Health and Retirement Decisions: An Update of the Literature*, discussion papers no. 932. Helsinki: Elinkeinoelämän Tutkimuslaitos.

Disney, R., Emmerson, C. and Wakefield, M. (2006) *Ill Health and Retirement in Britain: A Panel Data-based Analysis*, working paper no. 03/02. London: Institute for Fiscal Studies.

Dormont, H., Grignon, M. and Huber, H. (2006) Health expenditure growth: reassessing the threat of ageing, *Health Economics*, 15: 947–63.

Dow, W. and Schoeni, R.F. (2008) Economic value of improving the health of disadvantaged Americans. Technical report for *Overcoming Obstacles to Health*, a report from the Robert Wood Johnson Foundation to the Commission to Build a Healthier America. http://www.commissiononhealth.org/PDF/7626470d-e944-4dfe-9f8c-3fd2dad98472/Technical%20Report-Economic%20Value%20of%20Improving%20Health.pdf (accessed 8 September 2010).

Economic Policy Committee of the European Commission (2006) *The Impact of Ageing on Public Expenditure: Projections for the EU25 Member States on Pensions, Health Care, Long-term Care, Education and Unemployment Transfers (2004–2050)*, special report no. 1. Brussels: Directorate-General for Economic and Financial Affairs of the European Commission.

Eurostat (2008) Online database. Brussels: European Commission, http://europa.ec/eurostat/ (accessed 7 September 2010).

Favaro, D. and Suhrcke, M. (2006) Health as a driver of economic development: conceptual framework and related evidence for south-eastern Europe, in WHO Regional Office for Europe and Council of Europe Development Bank (eds.) *Health and Economic Development in South-eastern Europe*. Copenhagen: WHO Regional Office for Europe and Council of Europe Development Bank: 71–85.

Fogel, R.W. (1994) Economic growth, population theory and physiology: the bearing of long-term process on the making of economic policy. *American Economic Review*, 84(3): 369–95.

Fried, T.R., Bradley, E.H., Williams, C.S. and Tinetti, M.E. (2001) Functional disability and health care expenditures for older persons. *Archives of Internal Medicine*, 161(21): 2602–7.

Gallup, J.L. and Sachs, J.D. (2001) The economic burden of malaria. *American Journal of Tropical Medicine and Hygiene*, 64: 85–96.

Gambin, L.M. (2005) *The Impact of Health on Wages in Europe: Does Gender Matter?* working paper no. 05/03. York: Department of Economics University of York.

Gandjour, A. and Lauterbach, K.W. (2005) Does prevention save costs? Considering deferral of the expensive last year of life. *Journal of Health Economics,* 24: 715–24.

Gannon, B. (2005) A dynamic analysis of disability and labour force participation in Ireland. *Health Economics,* 14: 925–38.

García Gómez, P. (2008) *Institutions, Health Shocks and Labour Outcomes Across Europe,* working paper no. 2008–01. Madrid: Fundación de Estudios de Economia Aplicada, http://www.fedea.es/pub/Papers/2008/dt2008-01.pdf (accessed 7 September 2010).

Gillespie, S., McLachlan, M. and Shrimpton, R. (2003) *Combating Malnutrition: Time to Act.* Washington, DC: World Bank.

Goldman, D.P., Cutler, D.M., Shang, B. and Joyce, G.F. (2006) The value of elderly disease prevention. *Forum for Health Economics & Policy,* 9(2): article 1, http://www.bepress.com/fhep/biomedical_research/1 (accessed 8 September 2010).

Goldman, D.P., Shang, B., Bhattacharya, J. et al. (2005) Consequences of health trends and medical innovation for the future elderly. *Health Affairs,* 24(Suppl. 2): W5R5–17.

Griliches, Z. (1992) The search for R&D spillovers. *Scandinavian Journal of Economics,* 94: 29–47.

Gruber, J. and Wise, D.A. (1999) *Social Security and Retirement Around the World.* Chicago, IL: University of Chicago Press for National Bureau of Economic Research.

Haacker, M. (2004) *The Macroeconomics of HIV/AIDS.* Washington, DC: International Monetary Fund.

Hagan, R., Jones, A.M. and Rice, N. (2006) *Health and Retirement in Europe,* working paper no. 06/10. York: Department of Economics University of York.

Hausman, J.A. and Taylor, W.E. (1981) Panel data and unobservable individual effect. *Econometrica,* 49: 1377–98.

Jäckle, R. (2007) *Health and Wages: Panel Data Estimates Considering Selection and Endogeneity,* working paper no. 43. Munich: Institute for Economic Research, University of Munich.

Jamison, D., Lau, L. and Wang, J. (2005) Health's contribution to economic growth in an environment of partially endogenous technical progress, in G. Lopez-Casasnovas, B. Rivera and L. Currais (eds.), *Health and Economic Growth: Findings and Policy Implications.* Cambridge, MA: MIT Press: 67–91.

Jiménez-Martín, S., Labeaga, J.M. and Vilaplana Prieto, C. (2005) *A Sequential Model for Older Workers' Labor Transitions After a Health Shock.* Rochester, NY: Social Science Research Network, http://ssrn.com/abstract=1001630 (accessed 7 September 2010).

Johansson, E., Alho, H., Kiiskinen, U. and Poikolainen, K. (2006) Abstaining from alcohol and labour market underperformance: have we forgotten the 'dry' alcoholics? *Alcohol and Alcoholism,* 41(5): 574–79.

Johansson, E., Alho, H., Kiiskinen, U. and Poikolainen, K. (2007) The association of alcohol dependency with employment probability: evidence from the population survey 'Health 2000 in Finland'. *Health Economics,* 16(7): 739–54.

Jones, A. (2007) *Applied Econometrics for Health Economists: A Practical Guide,* 2nd edn. Oxford: Radcliffe Publishing for the Office of Health Economics.

Joyce, G.F., Keeler, E.B., Shang, B. and Goldman, D.P. (2005) The lifetime burden of chronic disease among the elderly. *Health Affairs,* 24(Suppl. 2): W5R18–29.

Kalemli-Ozcan, S., Ryder, H.E. and Weil, D.N. (2000) Mortality decline, human capital investment and economic growth. *Journal of Development Economics,* 62: 1–23.

Kalwij, A. and Vermeulen, F. (2005) *Labour Force Participation of the Elderly in Europe: the Importance of being Healthy,* discussion paper no. 1887. Bonn: Institute for the Study of Labor.

Keng, S.-H. and Huffman, W.E. (2007) Binge drinking and labor market success: a longitudinal study on young people. *Journal of Population Economics,* 20(1): 35–54.

Kerkhofs, M., Lindeboom, M. and Theeuws, J. (1999) Retirement, financial incentives and health. *Labour Economics*, 6: 203–27.

Knowles, S. and Owen, P. (1995) Health capital in cross-country variation in income per capita in the Mankiw–Romer–Weil model. *Economic Letters*, 48: 99–106.

Knowles, S. and Owen, P.D. (1997) Education and health in an effective-labour empirical growth model. *Economic Record*, 73(223): 314–28.

Lakdawalla, D.N., Goldman, D.P. and Shang, B. (2005) The health and cost consequences of obesity among the future elderly. *Health Affairs*, 24(Suppl. 2): W5R30–41.

Laxminarayan, R., Klein, E., Dye, C., Floyd, K., Darley, S. and Adeyi, O. (2007) *Economic Benefit of Tuberculosis Control*, policy research working paper no. 4295. Washington, DC: World Bank.

Lechner, M. and Vazquez-Alvarez, R. (2004) *The Effect of Disability on Labour Market Outcomes in Germany: Evidence from Matching*, discussion paper no. 4223. London: Centre for Economic Policy Research.

Lee, Y. (1999) *Wage Effects of Drinking and Smoking: An Analysis Using Australian Twins Data*, working paper no. 99–22. Perth: University of Western Australia.

Leonhardt, D. (2007) Free lunch on health? Think again. *New York Times*, 8 August, http://www.nytimes.com/2007/08/08/business/08leonhardt.html (accessed 7 September 2010).

Levine, P.B., Gustafson, T.A. and Valenchik, A.D. (1997) More bad news for smokers? The effects of cigarette smoking on wages. *Industrial and Labor Relations Review*, 50: 493–509.

Levine, R. and Renelt, D. (1992) A sensitivity analysis of cross-country growth regressions. *American Economic Review*, 82: 942–63.

Lindeboom, M. (2006) Health and work of older workers, in A.M. Jones (ed.) *The Elgar Companion to Health Economics*. Cheltenham: Edward Elgar: 26–35.

Lindeboom, M. and Kerkhofs, M. (2006) *Subjective Health Measures, Reporting Errors and Endogeneity in the Relationship between Health and Work*, research paper series 16–46. Rome: Centre for Economic and International Studies, University of Rome Tor Vergata.

Lindert, P. (2004) *Growing Public: Social Spending and Economics Growth Since the Eighteenth Century*. Cambridge: Cambridge University Press.

Liu, K., Daviglus, M.L. and Yan, L. (2003) Cardiovascular disease (CVD) risk factor status earlier in adulthood and cumulative health care costs from age 65 to the point of death. *Circulation*, 108: IV-722.

Lokshin, M. and Beegle, K. (2006) *Forgone Earnings from Smoking: Evidence for a Developing Country*, policy research working paper no. 4018. Washington, DC: World Bank.

Lorentzen, P., McMillan, J. and Wacziarg, R. (2008) Death and development. *Journal of Economic Growth*, 13: 81–124.

Lubitz, J., Cai, L., Kramarow, E. and Lentzner, H. (2003) Health, life expectancy, and health care spending among the elderly. *New England Journal of Medicine*, 349: 1048–55.

Lye, J.N. and Hirschberg, J. (2004) Alcohol consumption, smoking and wages. *Applied Economics*, 36: 1807–17.

MacDonald, Z. and Shields, M.A. (2001) The impact of alcohol consumption on occupational attainment in England. *Economica*, 68(271): 427–53.

Mackenbach, J.P., Meerding, W.J. and Kunst, A.E. (2007) *Economic Implications of Socioeconomic Inequalities in Health in the European Union*. Luxembourg: Directorate-General for Health and Consumer Protection of the European Commission.

Mankiw, N., Gregory, D.R. and Weil, D.N. (1992) A contribution to the empirics of economic growth. *Quarterly Journal of Economics*, 107(2): 407–37.

Manton, K.G., Lowrimore, G.R., Ullian, A.D., Gu, X. and Tolley, H.D. (2007) Labor force participation and human capital increases in an aging population and implications for US research investment. *Proceedings of the National Academy of Sciences of the USA*, 104(26): 10802–7.

McCain, M.N. and Mustard, J.F. (1999) *Reversing the Real Brain Drain: Early Years Study, Final Report*. Toronto, Ontario Children's Secretariat.

Mete, C. (2008) *Economic Implications of Chronic Illness and Disability in Eastern Europe and the former Soviet Union*. Washington, DC: World Bank.

Miller, T.R. (2000) Variations between countries in values of statistical life. *Journal of Transport Economics and Policy*, 34(2): 169–88.

Mittendorf, T. (2008) Are average cost figures correct in this context? Response to van Baal *et al. PLoS Medicine*, http://www.plosmedicine.org/annotation/listThread.action; jsessionid=43CF3A202803DC41D351B293108C180D?inReplyTo=info%3Adoi%2F1 0.1371%2Fannotation%2Ffd383a37-78af-4ef9-83b3-21ae90edba69&root=info%3Ad oi%2F10.1371%2Fannotation%2Ffd383a37-78af-4ef9-83b3-21ae90edba69 (accessed 16 September 2010).

Mullahy, J. and Sindelar, J.L. (1995) Health, income, and risk aversion: assessing some welfare costs of alcoholism and poor health. *Journal of Human Resources*, 30(3): 439–59.

Nadiri, M.I. (1993) *Innovations and Technological Spillovers*, economic research report no. 93–31. New York: CV Starr Center for Applied Economics, New York University.

Nordhaus, W. (2003) The health of nations: the contribution of improved health to living standards, in K.M. Murphy and R.H. Topel (eds.) *Exceptional Returns: The Value of Medical Research*. Chicago, IL: University of Chicago Press: 9–40.

Oliveira Martins, J., Frédéric, Gonand, F., Antolín, P., de la Maisonneuve, C. and Yoo, K.-Y. (2005) *The Impact of Ageing on Demand, Factor Markets and Growth*, economics working paper no. 420. Paris: Organisation for Economic Co-operation and Development.

Organisation for Economic Co-operation and Development (2006) *Projecting OECD Health and Long-term Care Expenditures: What are the Main Drivers?* economics working paper, no. 477. Paris: Organisation for Economic Co-operation and Development.

Pardes, H., Manton, K.G., Lander, E.S., Tolley, H.D., Ullian, A.D. and Palmer, H. (1999) Effects of medical research on health care and the economy. *Science*, 283: 36–7.

Pritchett, L. (2006) The quest continues. *Finance and Development*, 43: 18–22.

Raitano, M. (2006) *The Impact of Death-related Costs on Health-care Expenditure: A Survey*, research report no. 17. Brussels: European Network of Economic Policy Research Institutes, http://www.enepri.org/files/Publications/RR17.pdf (accessed 8 September 2010).

Rivera, B. and Currais, L. (1999a) Economic growth and health: direct impact or reverse causation? *Applied Economics Letters*, 6: 761–4.

Rivera, B. and Currais, L. (1999b) Income variation and health expenditure: evidence for OECD countries. *Review of Development Economics*, 3(3): 258–67.

Roberts, J., Rice, N., Schellhorn, M. and Jones, A.M. (2006) *Health, Retirement and Inequality: Can Germany and the United Kingdom Learn From Each Other?* London: Anglo German Foundation.

Rokx, C., Galloway, R. and Brown, L. (2002) *Prospects for Improving Nutrition in Eastern Europe and Central Asia*. Washington, DC: World Bank.

Sala-I-Martin, X., Doppelhofer, G. and Miller, R.I. (2004) Determinants of long-term growth: a Bayesian averaging of classical estimates (BACE) approach. *American Economic Review*, 94(4): 813–35.

Sammartino, F.J. (1987) The effect of health on retirement. *Social Security Bulletin*, 50(2): 31–47.

Semykina, A. and Wooldridge, J.M. (2006) *Estimating Panel Data Models in the Presence of Endogeneity and Selection: Theory and Application*. Tallahassee, FL: Florida State University.

Seshamani, M. and Gray, A. (2004) Ageing and health-care expenditure: the red herring argument revisited. *Health Economics*, 13: 303–14.

Shang, B. and Goldman, D. (2007) Does age or life expectancy better predict health care expenditures? *Health Economics*, 17(4): 487–501.

Siddiqui, S. (1997) The impact of health on retirement behaviour: empirical evidence from West Germany. *Econometrics and Health Economics*, 6: 425–38.

Silverstein, S.C., Garrison, H.H. and Heinig, S.J. (1995) A few basic economic facts about research in the medical and related life sciences. *FASEB Journal*, 9: 833–40.

Sloan, F., Ostermann, J., Conover, C., Donald, H., Taylor. J. and Picone, G. (2004) *The price of smoking*. Cambridge, MA: MIT Press.

Soares, R.R. (2007) Health and the evolution of welfare across Brazilian municipalities. *Journal of Development Economics*, 84(2): 590–608.

Solow, R.M. (1956) A contribution to the theory of economic growth. *Quarterly Journal of Economics*, 70(1): 65–94.

Spillman, B.C. and Lubitz, J. (2000) The effect of longevity on spending for acute and long-term care. *New England Journal of Medicine*, 342(19): 1409–15.

Strauss, J. and Thomas, D. (1998) Health, nutrition and economic development. *Journal of Economic Literature*, 36: 766–817.

Suhrcke, M. and Urban, D. (2009) Are cardiovascular diseases bad for economic growth? *Health Economics*, ePub doi: 10.1002/hec.1565 8.

Suhrcke, M., Rocco, L. and McKee, M. (eds.) (2007) *Health: A Vital Investment for Economic Development in Eastern Europe and Central Asia*. Copenhagen: WHO Regional Office for Europe on behalf of the European Observatory on Health Systems and Policies, http://www.euro.who.int/__data/assets/pdf_file/0003/74739/E90569.pdf (accessed 2 September 2010).

Suhrcke, M., Võrk, A. and Mazzuco, S. (2006) *The Economic Consequences of Ill Health in Estonia*. Copenhagen: WHO Regional Office for Europe.

Suhrcke, M., Nugent, R.A., Stuckler, D. and Rocco, L. (2006) *Chronic Disease: An Economic Perspective*. London: Oxford Health Alliance.

Suhrcke, M., McKee, M., Sauto Arce, R., Tsolova, S. and Mortensen, J. (2005) *The Contribution of Health to the Economy in the European Union*. Brussels: European Commission.

Tompa, E. (2002) *The Impact of Health on Productivity: Empirical Evidence and Policy Implications*. Ontario: Centre for the Study of Living Standards, http://www.csls.ca/repsp/2/emiletompa.pdf (accessed 8 September 2010).

United Nations Children's Fund and the Micronutrient Initiative (2004) *The Micronutrient Initiative: Vitamin and Mineral Deficiency – A Global Assessment*. Ottawa: United Nations Children's Fund and Micronutrient Initiative.

Usher, D. (1973) An imputation to the measure of economic growth for changes in life expectancy, in M. Moss (ed.) *The Measurement of Economic and Social Performance*. New York: Columbia University Press for the National Bureau of Economic Research: 193–226.

van Baal, P.H.M., Polder, J.J., de Wit, G.A. et al. (2008) Lifetime medical costs of obesity: prevention no cure for increasing health expenditure. *PLoS Medicine*, 5(2): e29.

van Ours, J.C. (2004) A pint a day raises a man's pay; but smoking blows that gain away. *Journal of Health Economics*, 23: 863–86.

Viscusi, W.K. and Aldy, J.E. (2003) *The Value of a Statistical Life: A Critical Review of Market Estimates Throughout the World*, working paper no. 9487. Washington, DC: National Bureau of Economic Research.

Wanless, D. (2002) *Securing Our Future Health: Taking a Long-term View: Final Report*. London: The Stationery Office.

Weil, D.N. (2007) Accounting for the effect of health on economic growth. *Quarterly Journal of Economics*, 122: 1265–1306.

Werblow, A., Felder, S. and Zweifel, P. (2007) Population ageing and health care expenditure: a school of 'red herrings'? *Health Economics*, 16(10): 1109–26.

Wolff, F.C. (2005) Disability and labour supply during economic transition: evidence from Bulgaria. *Labour*, 19(2): 303–41.

Wooldridge, J.M. (1995) Selection corrections for panel data models under conditional mean independence assumptions. *Journal of Econometrics*, 68: 115–32.

World Bank (2006) *Repositioning Nutrition as Central to Development: A Strategy for Large-scale Action*. Washington, DC: World Bank.

WHO Regional Office for Europe (2007) *Health For All Database*. Copenhagen: WHO Regional Office for Europe.

Yang, Z. and Hall, A.G. (2008) The financial burden of overweight and obesity among elderly Americans: the dynamics of weight, longevity, and health care cost. *Health Services Research*, 43: 849–68.

Yang, Z., Norton, E.C. and Stearns, S.C. (2003) Longevity and health care expenditures: the real reasons older people spend more. *Journals of Gerontology Series B: Psychological Sciences and Social Sciences*, 58(1): S2–10.

Zweifel, P., Steinmann, L. and Eugster, P. (2005) The Sisyphus syndrome in health revisited. *International Journal of Health Care Finance and Economics*, 5: 127–45.

chapter five

Saving lives? The contribution of health care to population health

Ellen Nolte, Martin McKee, David Evans and Marina Karanikolos

Introduction

The question of whether health services make a meaningful contribution to population health has long been debated (McKee 1999). Writing from a historical perspective in the late 1970s, several authors argued persuasively that health care had contributed little to the observed decline in mortality that had occurred in industrialized countries between the mid-nineteenth and mid-twentieth century. For example, Thomas McKeown (1979) showed how the largest part of the decline in mortality from tuberculosis in England and Wales between 1848/1854 and 1971 predated the introduction of immunization or effective chemotherapy. Factors outside the health care sector (particularly nutrition), as well as improvements in the environment, were seen as the most likely explanation of these declines (McKinley and McKinley 1977; Cochrane, St Leger and Moore 1978; McKeown 1979). Others, such as Ivan Illich (1976), have argued that developments in health care in the 1950s and 1960s were actually damaging health, introducing the term iatrogenesis or physician-produced disease.

Recent reassessments of the impact of health care on population health have challenged whether these arguments are applicable now (Nolte, Bain and McKee 2009), although there is a consensus that McKeown and others were correct in concluding that 'curative medical measures played little role in mortality decline prior to mid-twentieth century' (Colgrove 2002).

However, the scope of health care has changed substantially, particularly in the second half of the twentieth century. Many conditions that would once have been fatal can now be cured, such as common childhood infections. The discovery of insulin has transformed juvenile-onset diabetes (type 1) from what was once an acute, rapidly fatal disease of childhood into one that is compatible with a normal lifespan. The recent development of antiretroviral drugs is bringing about a similar change with HIV/AIDS. There are changes not only in the more obvious areas (such as new pharmaceuticals and technology) but also through new and more effective ways of organizing care (such as the introduction of multidisciplinary stroke units or integrated screening programmes) and the development of evidence-based care. The last enables traditional but ineffective treatments to be discarded while those that are innovative and effective are adopted and diffused more rapidly.

Consequently, the question is no longer whether health care contributes to population health but by how much? This chapter seeks to answer this question. It begins by describing a range of approaches to quantifying this impact and then summarizes the evidence on quantitative estimates of the contribution of health care to population health. It also includes a description of a new WHO approach developed to help policy-makers to choose which interventions to support in order to achieve the greatest health benefits within available resources.

Measuring the impact of health care on population health

Approaches that have been developed in an attempt to quantify the contribution of health care to population health include the inventory approach, the production function approach (Buck, Eastwood and Smith 1999), the concept of avoidable mortality and the tracer concept (Kessner, Kalk and Singer 1973). This section summarizes and updates our earlier review of these approaches (Nolte and McKee 2004).

The inventory approach

The inventory approach examines individual health services, identifies the target population for each service and quantifies their effect on the burden of disease. Examples include early work by McKinley and McKinley (1977), who estimated that 3.5% of the observed decline in infectious disease mortality in the United States since 1900 could be attributed to the introduction of chemotherapeutical and prophylactic interventions in the early twentieth century. Similarly, Mackenbach (1996) calculated that up to 4.8% of the total decline in infectious disease mortality in the Netherlands between 1875/1879 and 1970 could be linked to the introduction of antibiotics in the mid-1940s.

Others used published evidence on the effectiveness of individual health service interventions to estimate the potential gain in life expectancy attributable to their introduction. Thus, Bunker, Frazier and Mosteller (1994) examined the impact of 13 (clinical) preventive services, such as cervical cancer screening, and 13 curative services, such as treatment of cervical cancer, in the United States. They estimated that preventive services had achieved a gain in life expectancy of 1.5 years; curative services gained an estimated 3.5 to 4 years. Taken together, these calculations suggest that about half of the total gain in life expectancy (between 7 and 7.5 years in the United States since 1950) may be attributed to preventive and curative clinical services (Bunker 1995).

Cutler and McClellan (2001) examined the impact of technological advances in medical care on selected conditions. Looking specifically at survival from heart attacks among Medicare beneficiaries in the United States between 1984 and 1998, and linking this to changes in treatment and associated costs, they estimate that every US$ 1 spent on treatment had produced a health gain of US$ 7. They concluded that 'technology increases spending, but the health benefits more than justify the added costs'. Improved treatment of depression and cataract was also found to achieve net benefits when monetary values were applied to improvements in quality of life (i.e. reduction in time spent depressed or an improvement in vision).

One limitation of the type of analysis undertaken by Bunker, Frazier and Mosteller (1994) is that they rest on the assumption that health gains reported in clinical trials will translate directly into health gains at the population level. This is not necessarily the case as trial participants are often a highly selected subset of the population – some recent trial participants had characteristics found in less than 5% of those who will eventually receive the treatment (Britton et al. 1999). Also, the analysis undertaken by Cutler and McClellan only provides information about the potential health gain for those who have access to care. A further concern is that the intrinsically selective nature of the inventory approach, limited to certain specific services, fails to capture the combined effects of individual and integrated packages of care (Buck, Eastwood and Smith 1999). Hence, it may be more effective to offer a package of measures rather than single interventions to detect a range of diseases at an early stage. It also fails to consider how services are organized. For example, the impact of a screening service for detecting the precursors of cervical cancer will largely depend on how the actual screening programme is organized: a proactive approach invites a defined population (e.g. community) to attend screening, whereas an opportunistic approach is restricted to patients who consult a health practitioner usually for reasons other than screening.

The production function approach

The production function approach describes 'the production of health in terms of a function of possible explanatory variables' (Buck, Eastwood and Smith 1999). Studies adopting this approach usually examine how health care inputs and other potentially explanatory variables impact on some health measure (health care output), using regression analysis.

The findings of such analyses have been mixed, often identifying relationships that run counter to what would have been expected. For example, in a cross-sectional analysis of 18 developed countries, Cochrane, St Leger and Moore (1978) found that a higher number of doctors per capita correlated with *increased* mortality at young ages. In contrast, GNP per capita showed a strong and consistent negative association with mortality. Others have also failed to identify strong and consistent relationships between health care indicators such as health care expenditure and health outcomes (usually infant mortality or life expectancy) after controlling for other factors, whereas socioeconomic factors were found to be powerful determinants of health outcomes (Martini et al. 1977; Kim and Moody 1992; Babazono and Hillman 1994).

More recent work has provided more consistent evidence. Cremieux, Ouellette and Pilon (1999) showed that a 10% reduction in health care spending in Canadian provinces was associated with an increased infant mortality of about 0.5%, and a life expectancy that was 6 months lower in men and 3 months lower in women. This relationship was independent of a number of (socio) economic and lifestyle variables. In a cross-country analysis that examined the determinants of health outcomes in 21 OECD countries, Or (2000) found a significant negative relationship between health expenditure and premature mortality among women as measured in potential years of life lost. In a subsequent analysis of the same OECD countries, Or (2001) also found a strong and significant negative association between the number of doctors and premature and infant mortality, as well as life expectancy at age 65, suggesting that, all else being equal, a 10% increase in doctors would reduce premature mortality by almost 4% in women and 3% in men. There was also evidence that a larger share of public financing of health care was associated with lower rates of premature and infant mortality.

A branch of this work has extended the approach to measure the efficiency with which inputs are used to produce health, using both parametric and non-parametric techniques (Hollingsworth 2003). Inefficiency is taken to be the gap between the level of health that could have been achieved with the observed inputs and what is actually achieved. This type of analysis had been used extensively for measuring hospital efficiency over the years, but since *The World Health Report 2000* (World Health Organization 2000) it has also been applied widely to measuring the comparative efficiency of health systems, often using panel data (Evans et al. 2001; Greene 2004; Jacobs, Smith and Street 2006).

However, production function studies have some important limitations. The contribution of health care to population health is likely to operate over a period of time, with potentially considerable time lags between intervention and outcome. Yet, data availability means that the usual approach is to associate current outcomes with contemporary (or recent) inputs although it is possible that inputs in earlier periods would also have impacted on population health at the current time (Gravelle and Blackhouse 1987). It can also be difficult to interpret efficiency from these models because they do not incorporate variations in input prices across countries, nor do they generally allow for multiple objectives of health policy (Ravallion 2005). What appears to be inefficiency could simply reflect the fact that a country is pursuing other objectives in addition to improving population health, for example reducing inequalities. What is important is that the vast majority of recent studies show a significant and positive correlation between health spending and health outcomes even after controlling for measurable confounders.

Avoidable mortality

The concept of avoidable mortality, as used over the last three decades, originates from the Working Group on Preventable and Manageable Diseases led by David

Rutstein of Harvard Medical School in the United States in the 1970s (Rutstein et al. 1976). This introduced the notion of 'unnecessary untimely deaths' by proposing a list of conditions from which death should not occur in the presence of timely and effective medical care. These 'sentinel health events' were to serve as an index of the quality of care. These were of two types: (i) those where each death justifies an immediate enquiry into the question of why it happened (e.g. death from cervical cancer), and (ii) those where not every single case is considered preventable or manageable but appropriate medical care should be associated with fewer deaths (e.g. the vascular consequences of treated or untreated hypertension).

Charlton et al. (1983) were the first to apply this concept at the population level to analyse regional variation in mortality in England and Wales in 1974–1978. They also introduced the terms 'avoidable deaths' and '[conditions] amenable to medical intervention'. Based on the list presented by Rutstein et al. (1976), they selected 14 disease groups to reflect different aspects of health care (including primary care, general practice referrals to hospitals and hospital care) with age limits for each cause, usually 5–64 years (Charlton, Bauer and Lakhani 1984). This concept was adopted widely, particularly in Europe, and applied to routinely collected mortality data. It gained momentum with the European Commission Concerted Action Project on Health Services and 'Avoidable death', established in the early 1980s. This project built on the work by Charlton et al. (1983) and led to the publication of the *European Community Atlas of 'Avoidable Death'* in 1988 (Holland 1986, 1988). This major work has been updated twice (Holland 1991, 1993, 1997).

Much of this work dates back to the 1980s and early 1990s, but recently the concept has been revitalized as a potentially useful tool to assess the quality and performance of health systems. Thus, reviewing the work on avoidable mortality that had been published until 2003, Nolte and McKee (2004) demonstrated how improvements in access to effective health care have had a measurable impact in many countries during the 1980s and 1990s. The findings of this review are discussed, along with the limitations of the concept of avoidable mortality, in more detail below.

The tracer concept

The concept of tracer conditions was proposed by the Institute of Medicine in the United States in the late 1960s as a means to evaluate health policies (Kessner, Kalk and Singer 1973). Borrowing from natural sciences, it is based on the premise that tracking a few carefully selected health problems can provide a means to identify the strengths and weaknesses of the health care system and so assess its quality. It defined a set of criteria to be met by a potential tracer condition, the core elements being a clear case definition and ease of diagnosis, sufficiently common, evidence that (an) effective well-defined health care intervention(s) exists and measurable outcomes that reflect the use of effective health care.

The original concept envisaged the use of tracers as a means to evaluate discrete health service organizations or individual health care providers. However, the concept may also be applied at the system level in order to provide insights into its strengths and weaknesses. Here, the selection of tracer conditions will depend on the elements of the system being studied. For example, diabetes outcomes might be used as a measure of the performance of health systems in relation to chronic illness (Nolte, Bain and McKee 2006). Deaths from diabetes among young people have been interpreted as sentinel health events that should raise questions about the quality of health care delivery (McColl and Gulliford 1993). The optimal management of diabetes requires coordinated inputs from a wide range of health professionals, access to essential medicines and monitoring and, ideally, a system that promotes patient empowerment. Measures of diabetes outcome may, therefore, provide important insights into primary and specialist care, and into systems for communicating among them.

The use of this concept is described in more detail elsewhere (McKee and Nolte 2009; Nolte, Bain and McKee 2009). In brief, it involves selecting a condition that can capture a range of aspects of health system performance and then undertaking a rapid appraisal to understand in what ways the system is succeeding or failing to deliver optimal care. Diabetes is one of the more commonly used conditions as individuals with this condition (at least those requiring insulin) are usually easily identifiable and the principles of good management are agreed. The process involves collection of data from a variety of sources, including written material such as official policy documents and guidelines, surveys (if they exist) and interviews and focus groups with patients, providers and policy-makers. Analysis focuses on the inputs to care (physical, such as facilities and pharmaceuticals; human, such as trained health workers and empowered patients; knowledge, such as evidence-based guidelines; and social, such as social support and communication systems), as well as the integration of these elements.

Research using this approach in Kyrgyzstan (Hopkinson et al. 2004) and Georgia (Balabanova et al. 2009) has shown how, while many of the inputs are in place, critical gaps and a failure to integrate the inputs often result in patients receiving treatment that is far from ideal.

Although such studies focus on a single tracer, the problems they identify are often generic. Therefore, diabetes can be seen as an example of a much larger group of complex chronic diseases requiring long-term treatment by multiprofessional teams with the active involvement of informed and empowered patients.

By how much does health care contribute to population health?

Given the premise that health care can indeed contribute to population health, how much of a difference does it actually make? This section uses the concept of avoidable mortality to estimate the impact of health services on population health as measured by mortality. The notion of amenable conditions (amenable mortality) is used to refer specifically to death that may be averted through health care interventions (Nolte and McKee 2004). Health care interventions in this context generally include primary care, hospital care, collective health services (such as screening) and public health programmes (such as immunization) (Holland 1986). The interpretation of this concept will be discussed in more detail below.

Amenable deaths: contribution to total mortality

Table 5.1 presents an overview of selected studies that have analysed trends in amenable mortality over time. It shows that its importance as a proportion of total mortality has varied between countries and over time, ranging from a low of 4.4% of total mortality among men in Belgium in 1990–1994 to 45% among women in Romania in 2000–2002. This variation is largely attributable to differences in the classification of the causes of death and the age limit up to which death is considered amenable to health care. In particular, studies examining trends in the 1960s and 1970s used a rather limited range of 10–13 conditions that were considered amenable to health care, along with an upper age limit of 65 years (Charlton and Velez 1986; Poikolainen and Eskola 1986; Berneat Gil and Rathwell 1989; Gaižauskienė and Gurevičius 1995; Simonato et al. 1998; Humblet, Lagasse and Levêque 2000; Logminiene et al. 2004; James, Manuel and Mao 2006), reflecting the scope of health care and life expectancies at that time.

However, the choice of 65 years as an upper cut-off point for amenable deaths seems inconsistent with life expectancies at birth, which that are now in the late 70s or early 80s in many industrialized countries. Also, the scope of health care has changed immensely over the past decades, particularly since the 1980s. More recent analyses have, therefore, expanded the list of conditions considered amenable in order to reflect the changing scope of health care and have extended the age limit to 75 years to better reflect increasing expectation of life in industrialized countries (Mackenbach et al. 1988; Nolte et al. 2002; Newey et al. 2004; Stirbu et al. 2006; Weisz et al. 2007; Nolte and McKee 2008). Consequently, the impact of health care as measured by amenable mortality in more recent analyses tends to be higher than in earlier studies, accounting for between 20% of total mortality among men and over 40% among women (Table 5.1).

Variation over time

Another way of looking at the impact of health care on population health using amenable mortality is to examine trends over time. An early review of aggregate studies found considerable declines in recent decades in mortality for most or all conditions considered amenable to medical intervention (Mackenbach, Bouvier-Colle and Jougla 1990).

To account for the likely confounding effects of improving socioeconomic conditions and spontaneous declines in the incidence of a number of amenable causes, the authors compared trends in amenable mortality with trends in mortality from other conditions. This generally demonstrated that mortality from amenable causes declined much more rapidly than mortality from other (not amenable) causes. Thus, in the Netherlands, amenable mortality declined,

Table 5.1 Amenable mortality as a proportion of total mortality as reported in selected studies

Time period	Region/country	Conditions amenable to health care		Source
		No. conditions (age range, years)	Percentage of all deaths[a]	
1956–1978	England & Wales, France, Italy, Japan, Sweden, United States	10 (5–64)	1956: 15.8 (Sweden), 33.3 (Japan) 1978: 6.3 (United States), 19.6 (Japan)	Charlton and Velez 1986
1955/59–1990/94	21 European countries	12 (5–64)	1955/59: 22 (m+f) 1990/94: 7.6 (m), 8.9 (f)	Simonato et al. 1998
1960–1984	Spain	13 (5–64)	1960: 19.0 1984: 8.9	Bernat Gil and Rathwell 1989
1969–1981	Finland	21 (0–64)	1969: 8.2 (m), 13.4 (f) 1981: n/a	Poikolainen and Eskola 1986
1969–1984	Netherlands	13 (0–75)	1969: 18.4 1984: 11.8	Mackenbach et al. 1988
1970–1990, 1991–1999	Lithuania	11 (0–64)	1970–1990: 11.8 (m), 21.0 (f) 1991–1999: 10.8 (m), 21.0 (f)	Gaižauskienė and Gurevičius 1995; Logminiene et al. 2004
1974/78–1990/94	Belgium	13 (1–64)	1974/78: 7.3 (m), 20.8 (f) 1990/94: 4.4 (m), 20.0 (f)	Humblet, Lagasse and Levêque 2000

1975/79–1995/99	Canada	13[b] (0–64)	1975/79: 7.3 (m), 21.9 (f) 1995/99: 5.0 (m), 19.8 (f)	James, Manuel and Mao 2006
1980–1996/97	East and west Germany,[c] Poland	29[b] (<75)	1980: 14.9 (m, West Germany), 30.0 (f, Poland) 1996/97: 10.6 (m, West Germany), 27.9 (f, Poland)	Nolte et al. 2002
1988/90–1998/2000	England & Wales, France, United States	21[b] (<75)	1988/90: 19 (France), 22 (United States) 1998/2000: 20 (France), 24 (United States)	Weisz et al. 2007
1988/90–1998/2000	Inner London (United Kingdom), Manhattan (United States), Paris (France)	21[b] (<75)	1988/90: 18 (Paris), 23 (Manhattan) 1998/2000: 20 (Paris), 25 (Inner London, Manhattan)	Weisz et al. 2007
1990/91–2000/02	EU27	33 (<75)	1990/91: 13 (m, Netherlands), 44 (f, Romania) 2000/02: 12 (m, France), 45 (f, Romania)	Newey et al. 2004
1995/2000	Netherlands	25[b] (<75)	1995/2000: 23 (m), 32 (f)	Stirbu et al. 2006
1997/98–2002/03	19 OECD countries	33[d] (<75)	2002/03: 15 (m, France), 36 (f, Greece, Portugal)	Nolte and McKee 2008

Note: [a]Both sexes combined if not stated, otherwise male (m) and female (f) given; [b]Excluding ischaemic heart disease; [c]East and west Germany refers, respectively, to the German Democratic Republic and the Federal Republic of Germany until 1989 and the eastern and western parts of Germany thereafter; [d]Including 50% of deaths from ischaemic heart disease; n/a: not available.

on average, by 6% per year between 1950 and 1984 in both men and women. Among women, mortality from other conditions fell by only a mere 2% per year; among men, there was no change. These findings indicate that health care did indeed contribute to improving population health as measured by mortality.

These conclusions receive support from other studies of changes in amenable mortality, which have been reviewed by Nolte and McKee (2004). In brief, mortality from amenable conditions in a range of industrialized countries was found to decline more rapidly between the 1960s/1970s and 1980s/1990s than mortality from other causes not considered amenable to health care. However, the pace of change has varied between countries, with some indication of an acceleration of observed declines in the 1980s in particular (Box 5.1) (Charlton and Velez 1986; Boys, Forster and Jōzan 1991; Simonato et al. 1998; Nolte et al. 2002).

More recent analyses of changes in amenable mortality in 12 Member States of the EU between 1980 and 1998 confirm these observations. They demonstrate how reductions in amenable deaths contributed substantially to an overall improvement in life expectancy between birth and age 75 (life expectancy 0–75) in all 12 countries (Fig. 5.1).

During the 1980s, male life expectancy (0–75) increased by between 0.37 years in Spain and 2.14 years in Portugal (women: 0.31 years in Denmark to 1.42 years in Portugal). Among men, between 17% (Denmark) and 80% (Greece) of this increase was attributable to falling mortality from amenable conditions (women: 8% in the Netherlands to 67% in Greece). The largest contribution came from declining deaths in infancy but reductions in deaths among the middle aged was equally or even more important in some countries: Denmark, the Netherlands, the United Kingdom, France (for men) and Sweden (for women).

During the 1990s, the overall increase in life expectancy (0–75) was somewhat smaller, ranging between 0.31 years (Greece) and 1.61 years (Finland) among

Box 5.1 Comparing trends over time

An historical comparison of the former Soviet Union (the Russian Federation after 1991) and the United Kingdom showed that both countries had similar levels of amenable mortality in the mid-1960s, at a time when effective, safe and acceptable treatments for many of the most common conditions (particularly hypertension) were just becoming available (Andreev et al. 2003). Death rates in the United Kingdom then began to decline steadily, but they remained almost unchanged in the Soviet Union. This can be explained by the United Kingdom's ability to purchase and distribute these new treatments to those in need. The Soviet authorities lacked the domestic manufacturing capacity, funds for imports and the distribution systems that would have made this possible. The widening gap was exacerbated by the growing acceptance of evidence-based practice outside the Soviet Union but not within it (McKee 2007).

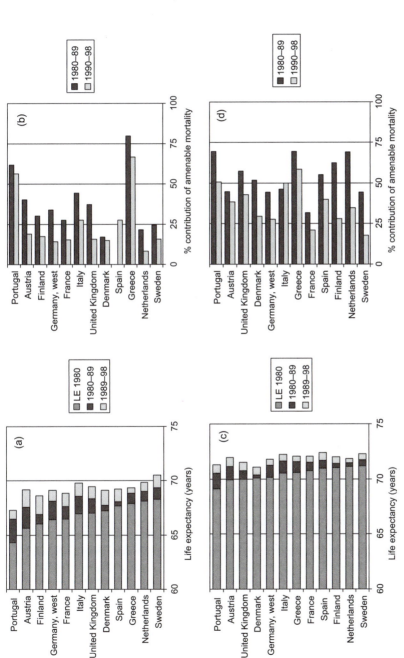

Figure 5.1 The contribution of amenable mortality to changing life expectancy (0–75 years) among men and women in 12 European countries.

Notes: (a,c) Changes in life expectancy (0–75) for men (a) and women (c); (b,d) percentage contribution of amenable mortality to changing life expectancy in 12 EU countries, 1980–1998, for men (b) and women (d).

Source: Adapted from Nolte and McKee 2004.

men and 0.31 (the Netherlands) and 0.78 years (Portugal) among women (Fig. 5.1). Reductions in amenable mortality also made a somewhat smaller contribution to improvements in life expectancy. Among men, falling amenable mortality now accounted for only 8% in the Netherlands and around 15% in France, Federal Republic of Germany, Sweden and the United Kingdom. However, it remained an important contributor in southern Europe, particularly in Portugal and Greece, accounting for 56% and 67%, respectively, of the total improvement in life expectancy (0–75). Among women, the impact of amenable mortality on changing life expectancy (0–75) also declined somewhat in the 1990s but still accounted for at least 20% of the total improvement in Sweden, and up to 59% in Greece. As in the 1980s, the impact of amenable mortality among men was largely attributable to a continuous decline in infant mortality in most countries. However, among women, declining amenable mortality among the middle aged was more important in all countries except those in southern Europe.

Although the rate of decline in amenable deaths began to slow in many countries in the 1990s, it is important to note that rates continue to fall, even in those countries that had already achieved low levels. This can be seen in a comparison of 19 industrialized countries between 1997/1998 and 2007/2008, although the scale and pace of change varied (Nolte and McKee 2008). The largest reductions were seen not only in countries with the highest initial levels (including Finland, Ireland and the United Kingdom) but also in some countries that had been performing better initially (such as Austria, Australia, the Netherlands and Norway). In contrast, the United States started from a relatively high level of avoidable mortality but experienced much smaller reductions (Fig. 5.2).

In summary, analysis of changes in amenable mortality published so far paint a rather consistent pattern of substantial declines that have generally been much more rapid than declines in mortality from other causes. These findings confirm Mackenbach's earlier conclusions that: 'at least part of the mortality decline from amenable conditions is due to improvements in health care' (Mackenbach, Bouvier-Colle and Jougla 1990: 109).

Selection of 'avoidable' conditions and the attribution of health outcomes

One of the key challenges involved in applying the concept of avoidable mortality is to define the list of conditions to be included. A death from any cause is typically the final event in a complex chain of processes that include underlying social and economic factors and lifestyles, as well as preventive and curative health care. The previous section used the term 'amenable' specifically to refer to deaths from causes that can be averted through health care interventions. These interventions encompass primary and hospital care as well as preventive services such as screening and immunization. Others have offered different interpretations of this concept, distinguishing three tiers – primary, secondary and tertiary avoidability (analogous to primary, secondary and tertiary prevention) – without specifying what part of the health system should

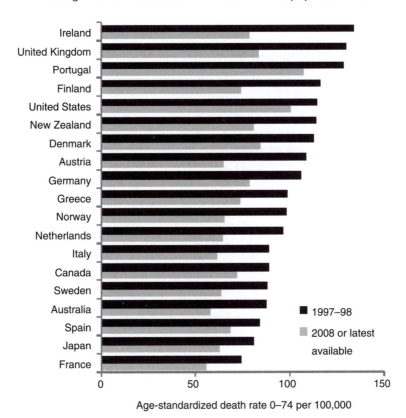

Figure 5.2 Mortality from amenable conditions (men and women combined), aged 0–74 years, in 19 OECD countries, 1997–1998 and 2007–2008

Source: Adapted and updated from Nolte and McKee 2008.
Notes: The data used are from 2008 where possible and otherwise the latest available: Australia (2006), Austria (2007/08), Canada (2004), Denmark (2005/06), Finland (2007/08), France (2007), Germany (2006), Greece (2007/08), Ireland (2007/08), Italy (2007), Japan (2008), Netherlands (2008), New Zealand (2005/06), Norway (2006/07), Portugal (2002/03), Spain (2005), Sweden (2006/07), United Kingdom (2007), United States (2005). Two-year averages were used for countries with populations of 10 million and less.

undertake these roles (Box 5.2). Yet others have sought to distinguish between wider public health measures (primary prevention) and more specific health care measures (secondary prevention and treatment), defining preventable conditions as the former and treatable (or amenable) conditions as the latter (Rutstein et al. 1976; Holland 1988; Nolte and McKee 2004).

Some clarification is required as these differences in interpretation of the underlying concept and consequent terminology can be confusing. *Amenable* conditions are defined as those from which it is reasonable to expect death to be averted even after the condition has developed. This includes conditions such as appendicitis and hypertension, where the medical nature of the intervention required is apparent. It also includes causes of death susceptible

Box 5.2 Primary, secondary and tertiary avoidable mortality

Simonato et al. (1998) have differentiated avoidable causes of death into (i) causes amenable to primary prevention (i.e. health and wider societal policies, such as lung cancer, liver cancer, or injury and poisoning), (ii) causes/conditions amenable to early detection and treatment (e.g. skin, breast or cervical cancer), and (iii) causes amenable to improved treatment and medical care (e.g. leukaemia, hypertension, peptic ulcer, hernia). Tobias and Jackson (2001) refined this approach further by classifying each condition not as entirely 'avoidable' by either primary *or* secondary *or* tertiary actions but by partitioning causes among these three categories, using an expert consensus method. Thus each condition considered avoidable was assigned relative weights reflecting the scope of its potential avoidability within each category. For example, deaths from hypertensive disease could be avoided by primary, secondary and tertiary actions, contributing in the proportions 0.3, 0.65 and 0.05, respectively. The final list compiled by Tobias and Jackson (2001) included 56 conditions or groups of conditions, 24 of which were considered to be avoidable largely through primary prevention (preventing the condition from developing), 16 mainly through secondary prevention (early detection and intervention intended to delay progression of disease or recurrence of events) and 16 mainly through tertiary prevention (reducing case-fatality by medical or surgical treatment).

to secondary prevention through early detection and effective treatment, such as cancer of the cervix uteri (for which effective screening programmes exist) and tuberculosis where (although the acquisition of disease is largely driven by socioeconomic conditions) timely treatment is effective in preventing death.

In contrast, *preventable* conditions include causes where the etiology is, to a considerable extent, related to lifestyle factors, most importantly the use of alcohol and tobacco (e.g. liver cirrhosis, lung cancer). This group also includes deaths responsive to legal measures such as traffic safety (speed limits, use of seat-belts and motorcycle helmets). This refinement of the concept of avoidable mortality makes it possible to distinguish improvements in health care from the impact of policies outside the health sector that also impact on the public's health.

These definitions are not clear cut, however, and clearly some conditions have features that place them on an interface between the amenable and preventable categories. For example, declining mortality from cardiovascular and cerebrovascular diseases may substantially reflect changes in diet and so be considered preventable, whereas reductions in mortality from traffic injuries may also be a result of improvements in emergency care, and thus considered to be amenable. As a consequence, these findings should be interpreted with judgement informed by an understanding of the natural history and scope for prevention and treatment of the condition in question. However, by differentiating avoidable mortality into causes that are amenable to health care and those considered preventable it is possible to distinguish improvements in health care from the impact of policies outside the health sector that also impact on the public's health, such as tobacco and alcohol policies (Westerling 1992; Albert et al. 1996).

This refined approach has previously been applied to 20 Member States of the EU for which data were available, examining the period 1990/1991 to 2000/2002 (Newey et al. 2004), an exercise updated here with the latest available data for these countries. Amenable conditions (including causes that are responsive to health care as defined above, e.g. cervical cancer, hypertension, appendicitis) were separated from preventable causes that are considered responsive to interventions that are usually outside the direct control of the health services (e.g. lung cancer, preventable by policies that reduce smoking; and cirrhosis, preventable by policies that reduce hazardous drinking).

This analysis showed that levels of amenable mortality in 1990/1991 and 2007/2008 were highest in central and eastern European countries (particularly Romania, Bulgaria, Latvia and Hungary). Portugal was the only former EU15 country displaying similarly high levels in 1990/1991 (Fig. 5.3). Levels were lowest in France (women) and Sweden (men). All countries experienced substantial declines of about one-third in amenable mortality during the examined period. The largest gains were seen in Slovenia, Austria, Finland and the Czech Republic; the exception was Lithuania (men), where amenable mortality actually increased.

Rates of preventable mortality were also highest in the eastern part of the WHO European Region in 1990/1991, particularly in Hungary. Among women, high rates were also seen in the United Kingdom. Unlike the situation with amenable causes, there have been consistent declines in preventable mortality among men (except in Romania, Bulgaria and Lithuania) but not among women (Fig. 5.4). The declines among men were most prominent in Italy, Austria, the Netherlands, Czech Republic, Germany, the United Kingdom and Slovenia – at over 20%. Preventable mortality rose among women in several Member States, particularly Lithuania, Poland, Romania, Czech Republic, Finland, Sweden and the Netherlands (the last reflects rising levels of smoking-related disease).

This refined definition of avoidable mortality makes possible a more detailed diagnosis of successes in health care and wider societal policies that impact on population health. Thus, in terms of amenable mortality, this analysis suggests that both Romania and Bulgaria have a considerable way to go to achieve the health outcomes seen in their neighbours to the west. In contrast, most countries that joined the EU in 2004 have made considerable progress in modernizing their health systems. This is reflected by the improvements in amenable mortality, although further sizeable improvements are possible. Patterns of preventable mortality call for strengthening of policies and their implementation, particularly for women in the countries of central and eastern Europe where rates of lung cancer mortality increased substantially. However, almost everywhere there is a need for the continued development of both tobacco and alcohol policies.

Taken together, these findings are consistent with the interpretation that the effect of the widespread use of modern treatment became apparent first in northern Europe (beginning in the late 1970s), spread to southern Europe in the early 1990s and began to be seen in parts of central Europe by the late 1990s.

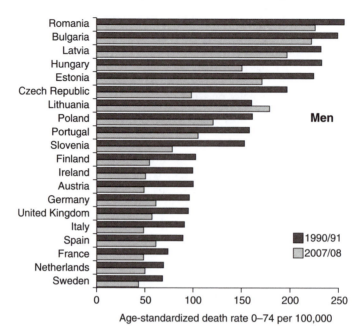

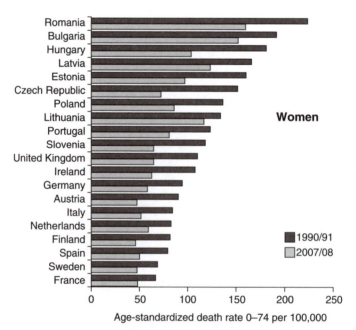

Figure 5.3 Mortality from amenable conditions, aged 0–74 years, in 20 European Union countries, 1990/91 and 2007/08

Source: Adapted and updated from Newey et al. 2004.

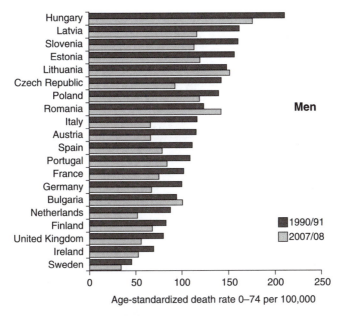

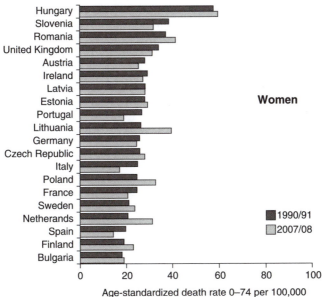

Figure 5.4   Mortality from preventable conditions, age 0–74 years, in 20 European Union countries, 1990/91 and 2007/08

Source: Adapted and updated from Newey et al. 2004.
Notes: The latest data available for each country was as follows: Austria (2007/08), Bulgaria (2007/08), Czech Republic (2007/08), Estonia (2007/08), Finland (2007/08), France (2007), Germany (2006), Hungary (2007/08), Ireland (2007/08), Italy (2007), Latvia (2007/08), Lithuania (2007/08), Netherlands (2008), Poland (2008), Portugal (2002/03), Romania (2008), Slovenia (2007/08), Spain (2005), Sweden (2006/07), United Kingdom (2007). Two-year averages were used for countries with populations of 10 million and less.

Assessing morbidity

The approaches to measuring the impact of health care on population health described here have one obvious limitation – their focus on mortality. Mortality is (at best) an incomplete measure of health care performance and is irrelevant for those services that are focused primarily on relieving pain and improving quality of life.

Bunker and colleagues tried to overcome this limitation by further assessing the potential impact of medical care on the quality of life (Bunker, Frazier and Mosteller 1994). Using published evidence on the effects of specific treatments for a certain illness or condition, they examined 'magnitude of relief in treated patients', subsequently translated into 'potential years of relief per 100 population' (Bunker 1995). Looking at 19 conditions as diverse as unipolar depression, terminal cancer (severe pain) and cataract, they estimated that an individual has, on average, been relieved (from pain, by restoring function, by preventing complications) from about five years of poor quality life as a result of medical care. Although providing different and potentially useful results, it uses the inventory approach described previously for mortality and, therefore, is subject to the same methodological problems.

Reliable data on morbidity remain scarce. Some progress has been made by setting up registries of diseases for conditions such as diabetes, myocardial infarction or stroke. These supplement the more widely established cancer registries but often cover only very small parts of the population in any country. In contrast, routinely collected health service utilization data such as inpatient data or consultations of general practitioners and/or specialists usually cover an entire region or country. However, such data ignore those who need care but fail to seek it and also are highly susceptible to changes in the accessibility of services.

Buck, Eastwood and Smith (1999) have also pointed to the importance of non-health outcomes of health care. These would include, among others, the potential impact on the general well-being (of society) of the redistributional effects of health care. Another issue is the intrinsic value of the health care process itself (process utility). This is the potential benefit to patients of being able to transfer responsibility for decision-making – and any potential risks related to those decisions – to their agents (i.e. doctors), thereby relieving themselves of responsibility for difficult decisions and gaining the reassurance that results from the transfer of expert information. A related benefit of organized health care, where this involves an element of redistribution, is alleviation of the risk of impoverishment as a consequence of disease.

Effective health service interventions

Policy-makers fortunate to obtain additional resources may ask what they should do to maximize health gain. Their considerations can be informed by cost-effectiveness analyses. The means of doing so are now institutionalized in several countries, typically to guide decisions about funding pharmaceuticals (Hoffmann and von der Schulenburg 2000) but, in a few cases, to examine other types of intervention also. A widely studied example is the National Institute for Health and Clinical Excellence (NICE) in the United Kingdom (Appleby, Devlin and Parkin 2007). Such organizations assess the costs and effects of new options, arguing – sometimes implicitly – that they are cost-effective if the costs per unit of health outcome are lower than some specified threshold. Patient health outcomes are frequently measured in terms of mortality rates or intermediate indicators such as life-years saved or gained, disability-adjusted life-years averted (DALYs) or quality-adjusted life-years (QALYs) gained. For example, NICE usually measures health outcomes in terms of QALYs and has used a threshold of between €26,000 and €39,000 per QALY gained to determine acceptability. However, certain additional questions are necessary. Where might the funds required for cost-effective innovations come from? There are rarely mechanisms to disinvest in interventions that are discovered to be ineffective. What is the potential impact at a population level? In aggregate, more may be gained by an inexpensive intervention that yields a small gain among large numbers of people than by a more expensive intervention that yields a large benefit in a few. Examples might be treatment of mild and severe hypertension, respectively. Furthermore, it is important not to consider interventions in isolation; there may be economies of scale from creating a package of blood pressure reduction, nicotine replacement therapy and advice on exercise and diet that would not be achieved by the implementation of each in isolation.

To address these challenges, WHO has developed the *CHO*osing *I*nterventions that are *Cost-E*ffective (WHO-CHOICE) project (World Health Organization 2005). Recognizing that the information needed to evaluate all possible interventions, at different levels of coverage, and with different types of interaction, was beyond the capacity of many countries, it sought to provide a set of 'priors' that countries could use. It has undertaken the analysis of over 800 interventions so far, taking account of scale and interactions. It has also sought to assess whether the most cost-effective mix of interventions is currently being undertaken, at the same time as assessing what would be appropriate if more resources became available. Calculations were made for 14 different subregions, broadly following WHO geographical boundaries but taking account of different levels of child and adult mortality. Tools have been developed that allow countries to modify and adjust the subregional estimates to their own epidemiological and cost structures.

Table 5.2 provides an example, which shows combinations of interventions that could be used in the management of breast cancer, in this case using data from WHO EUR A Region, which covers western Europe. Column one contains a code for the intervention package, which is described in column two. Columns three and four show total costs and total health benefits in terms of DALYs averted, for a population of 1 million. The last column illustrates how the cost per DALY averted would change as different combinations are implemented.

This type of information, adjusted to country costs and epidemiology, can help policy-makers to choose the most appropriate combination of interventions for any given availability of resources, taking account of many other factors that must influence decisions about priorities – issues of equity and acceptability, for example. The findings from this exercise can also be used to compare the

Table 5.2 Cost-effectiveness analysis of treatments for breast cancer in EUR A Region

Intervention package (1)	Interventions (2)	Cost per 1 million population per year (international dollars) (3)	DALYs per 1 million population per year (4)	Average cost per DALY (5)
BRC1	Partial mastectomy + axillary dissection + radiotherapy	758,464	1010	751
BRC2	BRC1 intervention + endocrine therapy	856,525	406	2111
BRC3	BRC1 intervention endocrine therapy + chemotherapy	1,912,371	451	4241
BRC4	Chemotherapy + endocrine therapy + palliative treatment	725,996	21	35,148
BRC5	BRC1 + BRC4 intervention	2,699,960	1913	1411
BRC6	BRC1 + BRC4 intervention + biennial screening	4,458,312	5630	792

Source: World Health Organization 2005.
Notes: Eur A: Andorra, Austria, Belgium, Croatia, Cyprus, Czech Republic, Denmark, Finland, France, Germany, Greece, Iceland, Ireland, Israel, Italy, Luxembourg, Malta, Monaco, Netherlands, Norway, Portugal, San Marino, Slovenia, Spain, Sweden, Switzerland, United Kingdom; DALYs: Disability-adjusted life-years; *BRAC*: Breast cancer gene.

incremental benefit (measured in terms of the cost of gaining an additional DALY) of interventions aimed at very different health problems as an aid to broader types of priority setting (Evans et al. 2005).

Conclusions

The evidence reviewed in this chapter demonstrates that health systems have varying success in achieving a key component of performance – saving lives. This matters. If the United States had achieved levels of amenable mortality comparable to those seen in the best performing European countries, over 100,000 fewer American citizens would have died in 2002. Today, it is apparent that countries at similar levels of economic development differ in their ability to protect their citizens from avoidable death.

Differences in performance can be identified by applying the concept of amenable mortality to existing mortality data in order to make an initial diagnosis at health system level. However, it is essential to go beyond the broad comparisons to understand why differences are seen. This will involve looking in detail at the causes of death responsible for these differences, although this can be methodologically challenging in small countries where there may be few deaths in certain categories. The tracer concept is one way of looking at any conditions identified as problematic but there are others (such as confidential enquiries into perioperative or maternal deaths). The choice will depend on the potential problem identified. Of course, this highlights the importance of investment in capacity to undertake such studies, which is lacking in many countries.

The next question concerns what to do. Obviously, this will depend on the probe, but again it highlights the importance of having an established health service research infrastructure that can guide policy.

One question is often asked: if additional funds suddenly became available, how might they be invested to achieve the optimal benefit? Clearly, it is impossible to provide a single list of the most effective health service interventions. Any selection must take account of contextual factors such as underlying health status, the value attached to different health states and the level of existing infrastructure. The WHO-CHOICE initiative, described above, offers a framework that can be adapted to help each country decide.

References

Albert, X., Bayo, A., Alfonso, J.L., Cortina, P. and Corella, D. (1996) The effectiveness of health systems in influencing avoidable mortality: a study in Valencia, Spain, 1975–90. *Journal of Epidemiology and Community Health*, 50: 320–5.

Andreev, E.M., Nolte, E., Shkolnikov, V.M., Varavikova, E. and McKee, M. (2003) The evolving pattern of avoidable mortality in Russia. *International Journal of Epidemiology*, 32: 437–46.

Appleby, J., Devlin, N. and Parkin, D. (2007) NICE's cost effectiveness threshold. *British Medical Journal*, 335: 358–9.

Babazono, A. and Hillman, A.L. (1994) A comparison of international health outcomes and health care spending. *International Journal of Technical Assessment of Health Care*, 10: 376–81.

Balabanova, D., McKee, M., Pomerleau, J., Rose, R. and Haerpfer, C. (2009) Navigating the health system: diabetes care in Georgia. *Health Policy and Planning*, 24(1): 46–54.

Bernat Gil, L.M. and Rathwell, T. (1989) The effect of health services on mortality: amenable and non-amenable causes in Spain. *International Journal of Epidemiology*, 18: 652–7.

Boys, R.M., Forster, D.P. and Jõzan, P. (1991) Mortality from causes amenable and non-amenable to medical care: the experience of eastern Europe. *British Medical Journal*, 303: 879–83.

Britton, A., McKee, M., Black, N., McPherson, K., Sanderson, C. and Bain, C. (1999) Threats to applicability of randomised trials: exclusions and selective participation. *Journal of Health Service Research Policy*, 4: 112–21.

Buck, D., Eastwood, A. and Smith, P.C. (1999) Can we measure the social importance of health care? *International Journal of Technical Assessment of Health Care*, 15: 89–107.

Bunker, J.P. (1995) Medicine matters after all. *Journal of the Royal Society of Medicine*, 29: 105–12.

Bunker, J.P., Frazier, H.S. and Mosteller, F.L. (1994) Improving health: measuring effects of medical care. *Milbank Quarterly*, 72: 225–58.

Charlton, J.R.H. and Velez, R. (1986) Some international comparisons of mortality amenable to medical intervention. *British Medical Journal*, 292: 295–301.

Charlton, J.R.H., Bauer, R. and Lakhani, A. (1984) Outcome measures for district and regional health care planners. *Commun Medicine*, 6: 306–15.

Charlton, J.R.H., Hartley, R.M., Silver, R. and Holland, W.W. (1983) Geographical variation in mortality from conditions amenable to medical intervention in England and Wales. *Lancet*, i: 691–6.

Cochrane, A.L., St, Leger, A.S. and Moore, F. (1978) Health service 'input' and mortality 'output' in developed countries. *Journal of Epidemiology and Community Health,* 32: 200–5.

Colgrove, J. (2002) The McKeown thesis: a historical controversy and its enduring influence. *American Journal of Public Health,* 92: 725–9.

Cremieux, P.-Y., Ouellette, P. and Pilon, C. (1999) Health care spending as determinants of health outcomes. *Health Economics;* 8: 627–39.

Cutler, D.M. and McClellan, M. (2001) Is technological change in medicine worth it? *Health Affairs,* 20(5): 11–29.

Evans, D.B., Tandon, A., Murray, C.J. and Lauer, J.A. (2001) The comparative efficiency of national health systems in producing health. *British Medical Journal,* 323: 307–10.

Evans, D.B., Lim, S.S., Adam, T. and Tan-Torres Edejer, T. for the WHO-CHOICE MDG Team (2005) Achieving the Millennium Development Goals for health: evaluation of current strategies and future priorities for improving health in developing countries. *British Medical Journal,* 331: 1457–61.

Gaižauskienė, A. and Gurevičius, R. (1995) Avoidable mortality in Lithuania. *Journal of Epidemiology and Community Health,* 49: 281–4.

Gravelle, H.S.E. and Blackhouse, M.E. (1987) International cross-section analysis of the determination of mortality. *Social Science and Medicine,* 25: 427–41.

Greene, W.H. (2004) Distinguishing between heterogeneity and inefficiency: stochastic frontier analysis of the World Health Organization's panel data on national health care systems. *Health Economics,* 13: 959–80.

Hoffmann, C. and von der Schulenburg, J.M. (2000) The influence of economic evaluation studies on decision making. A European survey. The EUROMET group. *Health Policy,* 52: 179–92.

Holland, W.W. (1986) The 'avoidable death' guide to Europe. *Health Policy,* 6: 115–17.

Holland, W.W. (ed.) (1988) *Commission of the European Communities Health Services Research Series No. 3: European Community Atlas of 'Avoidable Death'.* Oxford: Oxford University Press.

Holland, W.W. (ed.) (1991) *Commission of the European Communities Health Services Research Series No. 6: European Community Atlas of 'Avoidable Death',* 2nd edn, Vol. I. Oxford: Oxford University Press.

Holland, W.W. (ed.) (1993) *Commission of the European Communities Health Services Research Series No. 9: European Community Atlas of 'Avoidable Death'. European Community atlas of 'avoidable death',* 2nd edn, Vol. II. Oxford: Oxford University Press.

Holland, W.W. (ed.) (1997) *European Community Atlas of 'Avoidable Death' 1985–89.* Oxford: Oxford University Press.

Hollingsworth, B. (2003) Non-parametric and parametric applications measuring efficiency in health care. *Health Care Management Science,* 6: 203–18.

Hopkinson, B., Balabanova, D., McKee, M. and Kutzin, J. (2004) The human perspective on health care reform: coping with diabetes in Kyrgyzstan. *International Journal of Health Planning Management,* 19: 43–61.

Humblet, P.C., Lagasse, R. and Levêque, A. (2000) Trends in Belgian premature avoidable deaths over a 20 year period. *Journal of Epidemiology and Community Health,* 54: 687–91.

Illich, I. (1976) *Limits to Medicine.* London: Marion Boyars.

Jacobs, R., Smith, P.C. and Street, A. (2006) *Measuring Efficiency in Health Care: Analytical Techniques and Health Policy.* Cambridge: Cambridge University Press.

James, P.D., Manuel, D.G. and Mao, Y. (2006) Avoidable mortality across Canada from 1975 to 1999. *BMC Public Health,* 6: 173.

Kessner, D.M., Kalk, C.E. and Singer, J. (1973) Assessing health quality: the case of tracers. *New England Journal of Medicine,* 288: 189–94.

Kim, K. and Moody, P.M. (1992) More resources better health? A cross-sectional perspective. *Social Science and Medicine,* 34: 937–42.

Logminiene, Z., Nolte, E., McKee, M., Valius, L. and Gaizauskiene, A. (2004) Avoidable mortality in Lithuania: 1991–1999 compared with 1970–1990. *Public Health,* 118: 201–10.

Mackenbach, J.P. (1996) The contribution of medical care to mortality decline: McKeown revisited. *Journal of Clincial Epidemiology,* 49: 1207–13.

Mackenbach, J.P., Bouvier-Colle, M.H. and Jougla, E. (1990) 'Avoidable' mortality and health services: a review of aggregate data studies. *Journal of Epidemiology and Community Health,* 44: 106–11.

Mackenbach, J.P., Looman, C.W., Kunst, A.E., Habbemam, J.D. and van der Maas, P.J. (1988) Regional differences in decline of mortality from selected conditions: the Netherlands, 1969–1984. *International Journal of Epidemiology,* 17: 821–9.

Martini, C.J.M., Allan, G.J.B., Davison, J. and Backett, E.M. (1977) Health indexes sensitive to medical care variation. *International Journal of Health Services,* 7: 293–309.

McColl, A.J. and Gulliford, M.C. (1993) *Population Health Outcome Indicators for the NHS. A Feasibility Study.* London: Faculty of Public Health Medicine of the Royal Colleges of Physicians.

McKee, M. (1999) For debate: does health care save lives? *Croatian Medical Journal,* 40: 123–8.

McKee, M. (2007) Cochrane on Communism: the influence of ideology on the search for evidence. *International Journal of Epidemiology,* 36: 269–73.

McKee, M. and Nolte, E. (2009) Chronic care, in P.C. Smith, E. Mossialos, I. Papanicolas and S. Leatherman (eds.) *Performance Measurement for Health System Improvement: Experiences and Prospects.* Cambridge: Cambridge University Press: 406–25.

McKeown, T. (1979) *The Role of Medicine: Dream, Mirage or Nemesis?* Oxford: Blackwell.

McKinley, J.B. and McKinley, S.M. (1977) The questionable contribution of medical measures to the decline of mortality in the United States in the twentieth century. *Milbank Quarterly,* 55: 405–28.

Newey, C., Nolte, E., Mossialos, E. and McKee, M. (2004) *Avoidable Mortality in the Enlarged European Union.* Paris: Institut des Sciences de la Santé.

Nolte, E. and McKee, M. (2004) *Does Healthcare Save Lives? Avoidable Mortality Revisited.* London: Nuffield Trust.

Nolte, E. and McKee, M. (2008) Measuring the health of nations: updating an earlier analysis. *Health Affairs,* 27: 58–71.

Nolte, E., Bain, C. and McKee, M. (2006) Chronic diseases as tracer conditions in international benchmarking of health systems: the example of diabetes. *Diabetes Care,* 29: 1007–11.

Nolte, E., Bain, C. and McKee, M. (2009) Population health, in P.C. Smith, E. Mossialos, I. Papanicolas and S. Leatherman (eds.) *Performance Measurement for Health System Improvement: Experiences and Prospects.* Cambridge: Cambridge University Press: 27–62.

Nolte, E., Scholz, R., Shkolnikov, V. and McKee, M. (2002) The contribution of medical care to changing life expectancy in Germany and Poland. *Social Science and Medicine,* 55: 1907–23.

Or, Z. (2000) Determinants of health outcomes in industrialised countries: a pooled, cross-country, time-series analysis. *OECD Economic Studies,* 30: 53–77.

Or, Z. (2001) *Labour Market and Social Policy Occasional Papers no. 46: Exploring the Effects of Health Care on Mortality across OECD Countries.* Paris: Organisation for Economic Co-operation and Development.

Poikolainen, K. and Eskola, J. (1986) The effect of health services on mortality: decline in death rates from amenable and non-amenable causes in Finland, 1969–1981. *Lancet,* i: 199–202.

Ravallion, M. (2005) On measuring aggregate social efficiency. *Economic Development and Cultural Change*, 53: 273–92.

Rutstein, D.D., Berenberg, W., Chalmers, T.C., Child, C.G., Fishman, A.P. and Perrin, E.B. (1976) Measuring the quality of medical care. *New England Journal of Medicine*, 294: 582–8.

Simonato, L., Ballard, T., Bellini, P. and Winkelmann, R. (1998) Avoidable mortality in Europe 1955–1994: a plea for prevention. *Journal of Epidemiology and Community Health*, 52: 624–30.

Stirbu, I., Kunst, A.E., Bos, V. and Mackenbach, J.P. (2006) Differences in avoidable mortality between migrants and the native Dutch in the Netherlands. *BMC Public Health*, 6: 78.

Tobias, M. and Jackson, G. (2001) Avoidable mortality in New Zealand, 1981–97. *Australian and New Zealand Journal of Public Health*, 25: 12–20.

Weisz, D., Gusmano, M.K., Rodwin, V.G. and Neuberg, L.G. (2007) Population health and the health system: a comparative analysis of avoidable mortality in three nations and their world cities. *European Journal of Public Health*, 18: 166–72.

Westerling, R. (1992) 'Avoidable' causes of death in Sweden 1974–85. *Quality Assurance and Health Care*, 4: 319–28.

World Health Organization (2000) *The World Health Report 2000. Health Systems: Improving Performance*. Geneva: World Health Organization. http://www.who.int/whr/2000/en/ (accessed 1 September 2010).

World Health Organization (2005) *CHOICE: CHOosing Interventions that are Cost Effective*. Geneva: World Health Organization, http://www.who.int/choice (accessed 8 September 2010).

chapter SIX

The contribution of public health interventions: an economic perspective

David McDaid and Marc Suhrcke

Introduction

This chapter provides an overview of the economic argument for investment in public health and health-promoting interventions. It begins by highlighting briefly the nature of health problems in the WHO European Region and illustrates that, at least in principle, a large share of the existing disease burden is preventable through early intervention – within and outside the health care system. The chapter highlights the case for the use of economic evaluation as a tool in the policy-making process. This is followed by a discussion of the state of the evidence-base on cost-effectiveness (providing examples from different areas of public health and health promotion) and focusing particularly on interventions delivered outside the health system. The chapter concludes with a discussion of the challenges and future opportunities in the field.

Nature of health problems in Europe

Health has been improving across much of the WHO European Region: average life expectancy at birth reached 75.4 by 2008 (WHO Regional Office for Europe 2007). However, this masks significant variations, as life expectancy ranges from just 66.7 in the Russian Federation to 82.2 in Switzerland. In general, health status is poorer in many of the countries in the central and eastern part of the region. In those countries that belonged to the EU before May 2004 (EU15) life expectancy in 2008 was 80.4. This compares with an average of 74.8 in the countries that joined the EU since May 2004 (EU12) and just 67.9 (2006) for countries in the Commonwealth of Independent States.

Lifestyle and environmental factors are key risk factors for mortality and morbidity in any population (Marmot and Wilkinson 2006). Noncommunicable

Table 6.1 Causes of disability-adjusted life-years by gender and European subregion

Cause	Percentage of disability adjusted life years (%)							
	Eur A		Eur B		Eur C		European Region	
	M	F	M	F	M	F	M	F
Communicable, maternal, perinatal and nutritional conditions								
Infectious and parasitic diseases	1.8	1.7	5.5	5.3	5.5	3.0	4.3	3.1
Respiratory infections	1.3	1.4	4.1	4.0	1.8	1.0	2.2	1.9
Perinatal conditions	1.0	0.9	4.4	4.0	1.0	1.1	1.9	1.8
Nutritional deficiencies	0.3	0.9	1.3	2.3	0.9	1.7	0.8	1.5
Maternal conditions	–	0.6	–	2.1	–	1.1	–	1.3
Total	**4.4**	**5.5**	**15.3**	**17.7**	**9.2**	**7.9**	**9.1**	**9.6**
Noncommunicable diseases								
Neuropsychiatric conditions	24.2	29.2	16.4	21.4	12.3	16.7	17.2	22.5
Cardiovascular diseases	18.3	15.7	22.2	21.1	26.9	31.1	23.0	22.8
Malignant neoplasms	17.2	15.8	9.0	8.4	8.0	9.8	11.3	11.6
Respiratory diseases	6.7	6.5	4.2	4.1	2.9	3.0	4.4	4.6
Sense organ diseases	4.3	5.3	3.5	5.1	2.6	5.0	3.4	5.1
Digestive diseases	4.9	4.4	5.3	4.7	4.9	5.3	5.0	4.8
Musculoskeletal diseases	3.2	5.4	3.1	5.1	1.9	5.0	2.6	5.2
Diabetes mellitus	2.0	2.3	1.3	1.7	0.6	1.3	1.2	1.8
Other noncommunicable diseases	4.3	4.9	4.6	5.0	2.8	4.0	3.6	4.7
Total	**85.1**	**89.5**	**69.6**	**76.6**	**62.9**	**81.2**	**71.7**	**83.1**
Injuries								
Unintentional	7.7	3.9	11.5	4.5	17.7	7.7	13.0	5.5
Intentional	2.8	1.1	3.6	1.2	10.2	3.3	6.2	1.9
Total	**10.5**	**5.0**	**15.1**	**5.7**	**27.9**	**10.9**	**19.1**	**7.4**

Source: World Health Organization 2004.
Notes: Eur A: European countries with very low child and very low adult mortality (Andorra, Austria, Belgium, Croatia, Cyprus, Czech Republic, Denmark, Finland, France, Germany, Greece, Iceland, Ireland, Israel, Italy, Luxembourg, Malta, Monaco, the Netherlands, Norway, Portugal, San Marino, Slovenia, Spain, Sweden, Switzerland, United Kingdom); Eur B: European countries with low child and low adult mortality (Albania, Armenia, Azerbaijan, Bosnia and Herzegovina, Bulgaria, Georgia, Kyrgyzstan, Montenegro, Poland, Romania, Slovakia, Tajikistan, the former Yugoslav Republic of Macedonia, Serbia, Turkey, Turkmenistan, Uzbekistan); Eur C: European countries with low child and high adult mortality (Belarus, Estonia, Hungary, Kazakhstan, Latvia, Lithuania, Republic of Moldova, Russian Federation, Ukraine); M: Male; F: Female.

disease accounts for most (77%) of the total disease burden in Europe, followed by external injuries and poisoning (14%) and communicable disease (9%) (Table 6.1) (World Health Organization 2004). Poor health in both men and women is dominated by cardiovascular diseases (23.0% in men and 22.8% in women), neuropsychiatric conditions (17.2% in men and 22.5% in women) and cancers (11.3% in men and 11.6% in women). Unintentional injuries are also substantial, accounting for 12.6% of the disease burden in men.

How can European policy-makers address these problems?

A key question for European policy-makers is to what extent should health systems help to facilitate investment in effective health promotion and prevention activities? There is good evidence that a substantial reduction in avoidable mortality might be achieved through preventive measures delivered within the health care system, for example vaccinations to prevent the spread of some communicable diseases or statins to reduce the risk of cardiovascular diseases (Nolte and McKee 2003; Treurniet, Boshuizen and Harteloh 2004; Korda and Butler 2006; see Chapter 5). However, it has long been recognized that any strategy to promote population health needs to take a broad perspective involving actions both within and outside the health system (World Health Organization 1986). In addition to biological and genetic characteristics, the socioeconomic environment in which individuals live can have a substantial impact on the risk of premature mortality and avoidable morbidity (Marmot and Wilkinson 2006).

A broad approach to promoting the health of the population could involve a combination of upstream and downstream interventions. The former may include measures that can help to promote health alongside other goals, such as income support, improvements in housing or increasing the amount of years in education. Although many of these actions will be delivered and funded by agencies outside the health system, it is critical that the health system liaises with them to emphasize the health impacts of their policies. In contrast, downstream interventions often are specifically concerned with health promotion and prevention, targeted at the population at large or at specific groups. This might include interventions such as diet and lifestyle advice programmes; tobacco and alcohol control policies; water and air quality monitoring; and legislative, regulatory and other safety measures against accidents and injury.

Constraints on space preclude a focus on one further aspect of any population health strategy, health protection. However, it is important to recognize that, in addition to routine vaccination campaigns, the health system must be able to react to emerging risks to population health such as the spread of new viral diseases. It must also provide support to prevent deterioration in the health of vulnerable populations in the aftermath of natural or man-made disasters.

Is there an economic argument for action?

The economic argument for preventive interventions makes use of at least three criteria: (i) evidence on the effectiveness of such interventions; (ii) information on the associated economic costs and benefits (see Chapter 5 on the economic costs of ill health); and (iii) if the public sector is expected to intervene (or to finance the intervention), can the existence of 'market failure' justify public sector action?

There is a growing body of evidence on the effectiveness of population health interventions, but much remains to be done to address the second and third criteria that relate to the economic argument. There is reason to believe that substantial economic benefits would accrue if a significant share of the existing burden of mortality and disease could be prevented. This expectation derives, for instance, from evidence of the wide-ranging economic benefits from better health in Europe in general (Suhrcke et al. 2006a) and more specifically from the economic benefits to be had from eliminating a significant share of the mortality that is caused (at least in principle) by modifiable risk factor behaviours (Table 6.2) (Suhrcke et al. 2007).

All too often, public health experts underestimate the importance of evidence on 'market failures' as a justification for government intervention. Put simply, market failures describe a scenario in which the unfettered activities of individuals in a free market have adverse implications for society as a whole. In theory, these implications could be mitigated by public sector intervention to correct some of these market inefficiencies. Perhaps the most obvious of these are the external costs that impact on the non-smoker as a result of passive smoking. Without government intervention (e.g. taxation) the price of cigarettes is unlikely to take account of these externalities. The benefits that the general population gains from herd immunity arising from a high uptake of vaccines is another area where financial incentives or regulations might be used to influence consumer behaviour.

In contrast to the well-established cases for vaccination or for smoking or alcohol abuse prevention, attention has only recent turned to market failures relating to many other lifestyle-related choices (Suhrcke et al. 2006b; Sassi and Hurst 2008). Often, this is seen as a matter of personal taste but there may be failures in the distribution of information that would inform choice. The positive/negative impacts of different lifestyles may not be fully conveyed to

Table 6.2 Potential economic benefits of actions against selected risk factors in Germany

Risk factor	Attributable deaths (2002)	Per capita benefit of 25% reduction (€)
Tobacco	61,548	950
High blood pressure	39,780	594
High cholesterol	29,124	428
High body mass index	25,556	374
Alcohol	16,845	243
Physical inactivity	13,749	198
Low fruit and vegetable intake	10,603	152

Source: Treurniet, Boshuizen and Harteloh 2004.

all groups in the population. Some individuals may take a myopic view of the very long-term risks of poor health arising from poor lifestyle choices. Others, such as children or people with learning difficulties, may not fully be able to weigh up the risks associated with different choices. Financial incentives or legislation might be appropriate in such cases in order to encourage some of these individuals towards greater consumption of health-promoting goods.

Even if market failures are shown to exist, there is a need to demonstrate that action will actually entail fewer costs than benefits so that society will be better off than in the absence of any intervention. Such information will also help policy-makers to maximize value for money, given the constraints of limited resources. The need to develop and strengthen the evidence on costs and benefits of public health interventions was highlighted in a review commissioned by the United Kingdom's Treasury to assess the potential impact of better population health. One key conclusion was that the evidence base on the costs and benefits of such interventions is limited, with robust evidence on cost-effectiveness available in only a small number of areas (Wanless 2004). While the evidence may be scarce compared with that for curative interventions, it should not be inferred that there is no such evidence. Some exemplary evidence of good value for money in prevention will be presented later in this chapter.

While considerable economic benefits may be derived from health-promoting and preventive measures, it does not follow that they are always economically more favourable than treating conditions as they arise. Economic analysis tends to discount both future costs and future benefits. All else being equal, a health-promoting intervention that potentially leads to substantial health gains in 20 years may not appear at all attractive. Future health gains are heavily discounted compared with health care interventions where much more modest health benefits are gained in the short term (Kenkel 2000). However, it can also be argued that there might be some more immediate non-health benefits, for example, health-promoting interventions can have favourable impacts on community cohesiveness (Hills, Elliot and Kowarzik 2007).

The role of economic evaluation

Systematic use of economic evaluation can help priority setting both within and outside health systems. Economic evaluation is widely used in the health care, environmental and transport sectors and can be defined as 'the comparative analysis of alternative courses of action in terms of both their costs and consequences' (Hale 2000; Drummond et al. 2005; Briggs, Schulpher and Claxton 2006). Economic evaluation acknowledges that scarcity is endemic to all societies and implies that investment in a specific project will mean a lost opportunity to use those resources elsewhere. Indeed, it can be argued that its aim is highly ethical – how to achieve the greatest benefits from a limited budget.

In the absence of long-term data on effectiveness, economic evaluation can use modelling techniques to estimate the long-term costs and consequences of different interventions and/or to identify the minimum level of effectiveness necessary for a strategy to be considered cost-effective. The decision is usually straightforward where a new intervention is both less costly and more effective than what is currently in place. An intervention that is both more effective and more costly requires policy-makers to make a value judgement. This will be influenced by the resources and infrastructure available – what may be deemed cost-effective in Ireland or France may not be cost-effective in Tajikistan or Georgia.

Economic evaluation provides substantial added value in both transparency and efficient use of available resources, but actual decision-making must consider other factors. Investment in the most cost-effective intervention might conflict with other policy goals, such as reducing inequalities in health between different sectors of the community. Other inputs into the deliberation process might include the wider economic consequences or local political concerns.

Economic evaluation methods

Although helpful in strengthening the case for investment, there are practical and methodological challenges to the application of existing methods of economic evaluation to population health interventions (Kelly et al. 2005; Drummond, Weatherly and Claxton 2007). The different approaches available all estimate costs in the same way but differ in how they measure outcomes. The simplest of these methods is cost minimization analysis. This evaluation assumes that effectiveness is the same for all alternatives and, therefore, concentrates on identifying the least costly. Cost-effectiveness analysis measures effects using a natural (e.g. disease-specific) measure, such as reductions in blood pressure or the symptoms of depression. While intuitively easy to understand, this approach makes it difficult to compare investment in public health with investment in other areas of health care, as no common outcome metric is used.

Guidelines from health technology assessment (HTA) bodies tend to recommend the use of cost utility analysis. Benefits are measured in utilities (the individual's preference for a specific level of health status or a specific health outcome) such as the quality-adjusted life-year (QALY) and the disability-adjusted life-year. Both adjust the value of years of life lived to take account of either the quality of life of those years or the level of disability experienced during that time period. This approach allows comparisons to be made on investment decisions within the health care system, but it does not capture what can be the substantial non-health impacts of population health interventions.

As cost utility analysis does not capture these non-health impacts, the National Institute for Health and Clinical Excellence (NICE) in England and Wales has developed specific public health guidance. This allows the use of cost consequences analysis in addition to cost utility analysis. This approach can present a range of natural health and non-health outcomes (e.g. heart attacks avoided as well as a reduction in crime rates). Non-health system costs, such as the impact on labour force productivity, can also be included in the analysis. Policy-makers must then judge which outcome (if any) may be of most importance.

Although this approach makes policy-makers more aware of the multiple impacts of interventions, it is not always easy to determine whether any investment will be worthwhile. An intervention might generate only modest health outcomes but have a much more positive impact on non-health outcomes. For example, the provision of free breakfast at school may lead to only a modest improvement in nutritional intake but generate additional positive benefits for the social and educational development of children (Shemilt et al. 2004; Murphy 2007).

Theoretically, cost–benefit analysis (CBA) should present a solution to these problems. This has the advantage of measuring both costs and benefits in monetary terms and is widely used in non-health sectors of the economy such as transport, the environment, agriculture and housing. The use of CBA enables comparisons between investments in different sectors of the economy. The analysis includes the value of both non-health and health gains and thus greatly aids decision-making – positive net benefits merit investment.

Use of CBA is intrinsically attractive, particularly for population health interventions in which many of the costs and benefits are incurred outside the health system. However, it can be problematic to conduct. For instance, it is difficult to elicit meaningful values on the public's willingness to see money spent on health improvements. Moreover, not only the general population but also the health care professionals may question the appropriateness of placing a monetary value on human life. Techniques used to obtain these values continue to be refined in order to overcome some of these limitations. They already play an important role in the economic evaluation of some population health interventions.

How might information on the cost-effectiveness of population health interventions be used in the policy-making process?

Many countries now have formal or semi-formal mechanisms that make use of economic evaluation as part of the HTA process. To date, the majority of such evaluations have concerned drugs (often costly and innovative), medical technologies and surgical techniques. In comparison, possibly because budgets for public health and health promotion appear so modest in Europe and indeed worldwide (from less than 1% of the health budget in Italy and Denmark to almost 6% in Canada; Organisation for Economic Co-operation and Development 2007), there appear to have been few incentives to undertake economic evaluations of public health and health-promoting interventions (Hale 2000; Godfrey 2001; Holland 2004; Kelly et al. 2005; McDaid and Needle 2006). (Note that it is far from straightforward to calculate an actual 'budget' for public health and health promotion because of the multisectoral nature of many population-based interventions. Here we refer to estimates compiled by the OECD.) In the United Kingdom, approximately 2.5% of research activities focus on the prevention of disease or the promotion of well-being. Only 20% of this research looked at primary prevention activities to modify behaviours compared with 36.8% of activity looking at vaccination (UK Clinical Research Collaboration 2006).

This situation is beginning to change. Perhaps most notably, NICE in England specifically broadened its remit in 2005 to consider public health interventions including those that are delivered and funded outside the health care sector. Recent evaluations have included assessments of mental and physical well-being programmes in the workplace as well as alcohol interventions delivered to children at school (UK National Institute for Health and Clinical Excellence 2006). Many of these initial evaluations have proved to be highly cost-effective.

Where capacity for such evaluation does not currently exist, it may be possible to adapt the results of specific evaluations from NICE and HTA bodies to other countries and settings. However, such generalizations of public health interventions are not always easy, particularly if the resources and institutional capacity within countries are very different. Nonetheless tools and guidance are being developed for this purpose, although to date none has focused on the highly contextual and specific nature of many health-promoting interventions (Boulenger et al. 2005).

Another approach may be to make use of data from the *CHOosing Interventions that are Cost-Effective* (WHO-CHOICE) project (World Health Organization 2005; see Chapter 5). This has built up a database of information on the cost-effectiveness of interventions over several years in order to tackle some of the leading elements of the global burden of disease. Compared with the more narrow evaluations conducted by NICE and other HTA bodies, WHO-CHOICE has the advantage of adopting a sectoral approach to economic evaluation: 'all alternative uses of resources are evaluated in a single exercise, with an explicit resource constraint' (Hutubessy, Chisholm and Edejer 2003). This allows a range of interventions (including those for prevention, treatment and rehabilitation) to be compared either in isolation or in combination to determine an optimal mix of resources within a health care system. These are compared against a situation where nothing is currently done and against the use of current practice. Results for each of the 17 WHO subregions are presented so as to show the probability of an intervention being cost-effective in situations of low, medium or high resources. They can be adapted to consider the issue of scaling up the use of existing resources, and by making use of local resource and population data they can be adapted to specific country contexts. The Centers for Disease Control and Prevention in the United States also collates information on a regular basis through the Community Guide and Task Force on Community Preventive Services programmes (Briss et al. 2000).

What do we know about the cost-effectiveness of interventions?

Contrary to some views (Wanless 2004), a number of recent reviews suggest that the evidence base is growing rapidly (Rush, Shiell and Hawe 2004; Winterthurer Institut für Gesundheitsökonomie 2004; McDaid and Needle 2006; Schwappach, Boluarte and Suhrcke 2007; Zechmeister, Kilian and McDaid 2008). One review of public health and health-promoting interventions

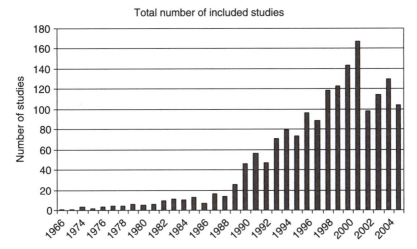

Figure 6.1   Growth in the use of economic evaluation in public health
Source: McDaid and Needle 2006.

attempted to map the literature since the 1960s systematically. It identified more than 1700 evaluations, the majority undertaken in the last 10 years (Fig. 6.1) (McDaid and Needle 2006).

Figure 6.2 gives an indication of the different areas of public health and health promotion in which economic evaluations have been conducted. Clearly, this is dominated by evaluations at the medical end of the public health spectrum. More than 60% of all the studies in this review have some focus on the prevention of communicable diseases (such as influenza) as well as the early detection of, and preventive measures against, cancer. Other areas of public health are more complex and economic evaluations are less frequent. Nonetheless, several hundred examples of broad health-promoting interventions (including the merits of exercise, smoking prevention, nutrition change and reduced drug/alcohol consumption) have been identified in past reviews (Rush, Shiell and Hawe 2004; McDaid and Needle 2006).

Another assessment of the reviews of economic studies of health promotion considered that investment in programmes targeted at promoting physical activity and healthy nutritional intake were highly cost-effective. It also recommended continued investment in measures to tackle stress, in anti-tobacco and alcohol campaigns, in HIV prevention measures and in broad vaccination programmes (Winterthurer Institut für Gesundheitsökonomie 2004). There have also been topic-specific reviews. For instance, one review of economic evaluations for the prevention of cardiovascular diseases was able to find a substantive body of evidence on clinical preventive measures (primarily lipid-lowering drugs) but little on health-promoting interventions (Schwappach, Boluarte and Suhrcke 2007). More recently a review of interventions to promote mental health found particularly encouraging economic evidence in favour of early childhood development programmes (Zechmeister, Kilian and McDaid 2008).

The discussion below reflects on what is known about the case for investment in interventions within some of these specific areas.

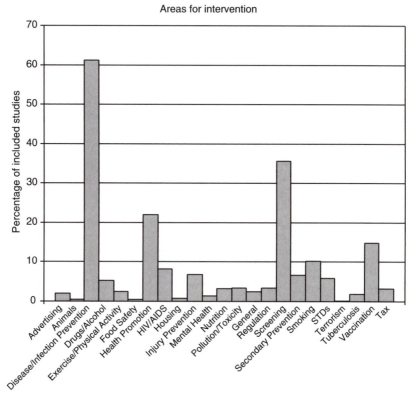

Figure 6.2 Areas addressed by economic evaluations of public health/health promoting interventions

Source: McDaid and Needle 2006.
Note: STDs: sexually transmitted diseases

Vaccination and screening studies

McDaid and Needle (2006) reported that more than 35% of all the studies they identified evaluated screening and early diagnostic tools, particularly for breast and colon cancer. These have been undertaken for many years, facilitated by the ease of measuring short-term outcomes in terms of true positive cases detected. For instance, one cost consequence analysis on the merits of screening schoolgirls for bacteriuria was published in 1975 (Edwards et al. 1975) and the first economic evaluation of breast cancer screening dates back to 1978 (Edinburgh Breast Screening Clinic 1978).

Immunization studies are also common. They are differentiated from many other public health interventions by the relative ease of measuring successful immunizations conducted. Also, the costs incurred can be identified and the lifetime benefits modelled. However, few evaluations of screening or immunization take account of the benefits of herd immunity or the value of reduced anxiety from having a lower risk of contracting a disease (Drummond, Chevat and Lothgren 2007).

Complex community-delivered health promotion programmes

The majority of complex community-delivered health promotion programmes seek to change individual behaviours. Several hundred interventions have been identified in reviews (Rush, Shiell and Hawe 2004; McDaid and Needle 2006). For example, Box 6.1 presents one study in England that suggests that exercise programmes can be a cost-effective way of promoting both the physical health and the mental well-being of older people (Munro et al. 2004).

Mental health promotion

Given its substantial contribution to the burden of ill health in Europe (Table 6.1), it is perhaps surprising that so little attention has been given to promoting mental well-being and the prevention of mental health problems. One recent review of economic evaluations of relevant interventions found the most compelling evidence related to interventions at early years that targeted children and their parents; some measures aimed at preventing depression and there was some limited evidence on suicide-prevention strategies (Zechmeister, Kilian and McDaid 2008). For instance, work in England to analyse group-based parenting interventions suggests that these interventions have the potential to be highly cost-effective, even if only very modest quality of life benefits can be

Box 6.1 Assessing the cost-effectiveness of a community-based exercise programme in those over 65 years of age in the United Kingdom

The objective of the study was to assess the cost-effectiveness of a community-based exercise programme as a population-wide public health intervention (Munro et al. 2004). Twelve general practices in Sheffield, England, were randomized to act either as one of four intervention practices or as one of eight control practices. Over a two-year period, the intervention practices offered all their sedentary male and female patients (aged 65 or older) the chance to attend free and locally organized exercise classes for 75 minutes twice per week. They focused on the improvement of joint mobility, muscle strength and endurance, balance coordination and cardiorespiratory fitness. Exercises were combined with fun activities such as tea dances, bowling or swimming in order to attract participants.

The benefit in the intervention group was 0.011 QALYs, resulting from a slower health decline over the two-year period. Benefits were seen in terms of mental well-being and in physical health. Costs were assessed from the perspective of the National Health Service and were estimated to be €128,302, €9.06 per participant (2004 prices). The incremental cost per QALY gained compared with usual care was €17,174. It was concluded that this cost per QALY compared well with investment in other funded curative and preventive interventions such as antihypertensive drug treatment.

Box 6.2 Evaluation of a parenting programme in Wales for parents of children at risk of developing conduct disorders

An economic evaluation was added to a randomized controlled trial of an initiative funded by the Welsh Ministry of Education and taking place in north and mid Wales. Parents of 116 children aged 36–59 months at risk of developing conduct disorders participated in the Webster–Stratton Incredible Years basic parenting programme or were placed on a six-month waiting list as controls. The incremental cost per unit of improvement on the intensity score of the Eyberg child behaviour inventory was €109. It would cost €8190 to bring the child with the highest intensity score to below the clinical cut-off point and €2006 to bring the average child in the intervention group within the non-clinical limits on the intensity score. Assuming a maximum limit for cost-effectiveness of €149 per point increase, there was an 83.9% chance of the intervention being cost-effective. The mean cost per parent attending the parenting group was €1924 in a group of 12 children, including initial costs and materials for training group leaders. The authors concluded that the parenting programme involves modest costs and demonstrates strong clinical effect, suggesting it would represent good value for money for public spending (Edwards et al. 2007).

gained (Dretzke et al. 2005). A Welsh study reported favourably on the cost-effectiveness of one specific group parenting programme (the Webster–Stratton Incredible Years basic parenting programme) (Box 6.2).

Several studies have also looked at interventions to prevent depression. Smit et al. (2006) in the Netherlands evaluated the cost-effectiveness of minimal-contact psychotherapy as a preventive measure for individuals at high risk of depression. At a cost-effectiveness threshold of €20,000 per case avoided, there was a 70% to 80% probability (depending on the costs included) that the intervention would be cost-effective. Additionally, there was a 40% to 60% probability that the intervention would be dominant compared with standard care (i.e. would have better outcomes at a lower cost). However, these calculations were based on results achieved over a short (one-year) period.

There is sparse evidence on the cost-effectiveness of suicide-prevention strategies. However, what is available suggests that this kind of preventive initiative may be highly cost-effective. Work in Scotland suggests that the national programme (with an annual investment of more than €7 million) would actually be cost-saving if just 1% of suicides could be avoided (McDaid et al. 2006). In England, it was also estimated that the National Suicide Prevention Strategy would be cost-saving rather than cost-effective if a 20% target for reduced suicides was attained. The savings were £700 million (€840 million) from avoidable deaths and £300 million (€360 million) from additional quality of life (Bevan et al. 2007).

Injury and accident prevention

There are a remarkable number of studies on injury and accident prevention. The extent to which such interventions need to be considered in a health system context is open to debate, but some can be highly cost-effective. These include road-safety interventions, such as the use of bicycle helmets or car seat-belts; home safety devices, such as smoke alarms (Box 6.3); and strengthening techniques and protective devices, such as hip protectors, to reduce the risk and/or consequence of accidents such as falls.

In New Zealand, an assessment by Guria (1999) in a setting where road traffic accidents were frequent found that enforcement and advertising campaigns against drink-driving, speeding and for seat-belt wearing all appeared to be highly cost-effective in reducing the number and severity of crashes. Investment in speed cameras has also been shown to be cost-effective in Canada (Box 6.4).

The context in which interventions are delivered can make a critical difference to cost-effectiveness. Looking again at road safety, one modelling study in the United States assessed the additional cost-effectiveness of installing air bags into new cars. The authors found them to be a cost-saving intervention once 50% of car occupants wear seat-belts. There was a marked difference in the incremental cost-effectiveness of installing driver-side and passenger-side air bags: US$ 24,000 and US$ 61,000 per QALY gained, respectively (Graham et al. 1997). Although air bags would be cost-effective in an American context they may not be so in low- and middle-income countries where other interventions

Box 6.3   Assessing the cost-effectiveness of a smoke alarm giveaway programme

Ten thousand smoke alarms were distributed free of charge in an area of Oklahoma City at high risk for residential fire injuries. The programme also included fire prevention education and battery replacement components. The costs of implementation were compared with fatal and non-fatal fire-related medical care costs and productivity losses averted over a five-year period. Overall, the programme was cost-saving. The total costs of implementation (US$ 531,000) were more than outweighed by more than $ 15 million of health and productivity costs avoided. Sensitivity analysis indicated that the programme would remain cost-effective even if effectiveness was reduced by more than half (Haddix et al. 2001).

A similar programme implemented in London was not found to be cost-effective. It was concluded that this was not because smoke alarms were ineffective, but rather that the alarms used long-life batteries which needed changing (rather than being battery free). Also, householders were relied on to fit the alarms themselves rather than having professional installation, and large numbers of non-English speakers in London may have been unable to read the information on how to fit alarms (Ginnelly et al. 2005).

Box 6.4   Do speed cameras produce net benefits?

A cost–benefit analysis of the implementation of a speed camera traffic safety programme, first introduced in 1996 in British Columbia, Canada, found that the programme cost US$ 21 million overall but the societal benefits gained were valued at US$ 109 million per annum. Results remained robust in sensitivity analysis and it was concluded that they would be likely applicable to other high-income countries with similar road infrastructures (Chen and Warburton 2006).

(such as greater use of seat-belts alone and encouraging children to ride in the back of cars may be more appropriate) (Graham et al. 1998).

Intervention settings

Workplace health promotion

Another way of looking at these health promotion interventions is to consider the setting in which they are delivered. McDaid and Needle (2006) reported that more than one-fifth (22%) of studies (where the setting could be identified) took place in the workplace (Table 6.3). This is one specialist area that has not only an extensive literature on effectiveness but also many studies of the resource consequences of poor employee health.

This raises more questions about the interface between health and other sectors of the economy. Clearly, investment in healthy workplaces can have beneficial impacts, not only for health systems but also for workforce productivity. Most information in the public domain comes from the United States, although some European evidence is available (Box 6.5) (Kreis and Bödeker 2004). Schemes

Table 6.3 Principal setting for intervention, where specified

Setting	Percentage of total studies
Community/local	34
Medical	26
Workplace	22
School	7
Transport	4
Military	3
Home	2
College/university	1
Prison/detention	1

Source: McDaid and Needle 2006.

Box 6.5   Evaluation of multicomponent workplace health promotion programme

Mills et al. (2007) used a quasi-experimental design delivered over a 12-month period to evaluate the effects of a multicomponent health promotion programme on changes in health risk status (including stress and depression) and work performance in 618 office-based employees in three units of Unilever PLC. The health promotion programme provided participants with a personalized health and well-being report, highlighted the personal health areas in need of improvement and gave practical suggestions on how to achieve the recommended changes. Intervention group participants were also given unlimited access to a password-protected personalized health, well-being and lifestyle web portal that included articles, assessments and interactive online behaviour-change programmes. Participants also received tailored e-mails every two weeks on relevant personal wellness topics, as well as packs of information and seminars on key health topics. Those in the intervention group were found to have significantly reduced health risks, reduced absenteeism and improved workplace performance. The cost of the intervention to the company was £70 per employee. These costs were more than outweighed by improvements in absenteeism and work performance.

evaluated include physical exercise programmes and the provision of lifestyle advice and workplace screening coupled with enhanced care management for people with depression and/or stress. With very few exceptions (and excluding screening as the evidence on this is mixed), where these studies have been evaluated they appear to be cost-effective (Pelletier 1991, 2001, 2005). Little information on the cost-effectiveness of measures to organize the workplace in such a way as to promote a healthy working environment could be identified (e.g. flexitime, access to child care, opportunities for promotion and initiative taking).

School-based interventions

Many school-based studies have been concerned with evaluating screening interventions (Lowin et al. 2000; Wang, Burstein and Cohen 2002; Chatterji et al. 2004; Konig and Barry 2004), although economic evaluations of interventions targeted at changing behavioural risk factors such as smoking (Elder et al. 1993) and unsafe sex (Berrios, Bedregal and Guzman 2004) can also be identified. There have also been a few economic evaluations of school-based interventions intended to impact on the chances of adult obesity. For example, one well-known experimental study conducted in the United States (Wang et al. 2003) examined the impact of an interdisciplinary curriculum intended to decrease television viewing and fatty food consumption and to increase intakes of fruit, vegetables and moderate exercise (Box 6.6).

Box 6.6   Economic evaluation of a school-based anti-obesity programme

A two-year randomized controlled trial involving 10 schools in Boston, MA, was undertaken to evaluate the impact on obesity of an intervention consisting of lessons on decreasing television viewing and consumption of fatty foods, increasing the intake of fruit and vegetables and increasing moderate/vigorous physical activity. The body mass index of participants was measured before and after the intervention. Models were then used to predict the transition from overweight at age 14 to obesity by age 40. A societal perspective was adopted in the economic analysis.

   The intervention had no impact on boys, but there was a 1.9% decrease in female students predicted to become overweight adults. Additional costs of the intervention were US$ 33,677 (US$ 14 per student) per year. In total, 4.1 discounted QALYs were saved by the programme, together with savings of US$ 15,887 in averted medical care costs and US$ 25,104 from averted lost productivity. These findings translated to a cost of US$ 4305 per QALY saved. The intervention remained cost-effective under all scenarios considered and cost-saving under many (Wang et al. 2003).

Regulatory and fiscal measures

Measures such as taxation, subsidies and regulation can also be used to promote health. In some cases (e.g. tobacco taxation) such measures may be justified by the existence of the above-mentioned market failures. Previous reviews indicate that these interventions can indeed play an important role in promoting and protecting health. In some respects, their simplicity may mean that they can have lower implementation costs than those observed for more complex interventions such as media campaigns (Sassi and Hurst 2008). However, such apparently financially costless measures often entail significant economic costs, but the benefits can be considerable. For instance, three-year data from the nationwide Fatal Accident Reporting System in the United States were examined to assess the impact of mandatory retesting of vision as a part of driver relicensing. The study concluded that sight tests were effective in reducing road-traffic fatalities and might avert more than US$ 31 million in costs, far exceeding the costs of administering the scheme (Shipp 1998).

   The role of potentially punitive legal action can also help to provide incentives for some employers to insulate themselves against such charges (e.g. through investment in health and safety measures in the workplace; Innes 2004). The effectiveness of legislation may be highly dependent on the degree to which it is enforced, and economic evaluation can be used to help policy-makers to determine whether such action is merited. This has been illustrated in the United States, where the law banning the sale of tobacco to children has been enforced actively. DiFranza and colleagues (2001) modelled the costs of quarterly inspections of all tobacco sales outlets, using different assumptions on the potential effectiveness of this measure. Although the scheme would cost

Box 6.7 Impact of tobacco tax reforms in Australia

> An evaluation assessed the impact of reforms to cigarette taxation in Australia introduced alongside a mass media national tobacco campaign that ran over a period of 42 months between 1997 and 2000 (Scollo et al. 2003). Prior to taxation reform, it had been possible for consumers to purchase cigarettes from supermarkets and specialist tobacconists at prices well below the recommended retail price. There was also a budget cigarette market as cigarettes that used less tobacco attracted less tax. Moreover, there had been opportunities for cross-border evasion of taxes between different Australian states. After reform, the tax was based on the number of cigarettes in a packet (rather than weight), there were additional sales taxes, and opportunities for cross-border tax evasion were eliminated.
>
> Using survey data, the evaluation reported that the new tax regime substantially reduced the affordability of budget cigarette brands. Consumers had not been able to find alternative lower cost options, with both average recommended retail price and average actual cigarette prices increasing by 25%. The fall in consumption in the last year of the campaign (when the tax reforms were in place) was considerably higher than would be expected on the basis of price rises alone. The authors hypothesized that the messages disseminated through the media campaign, coupled with increased taxation, may have helped to reduce demand further.

US$ 190 million per annum to implement, the study concluded that if this led to a 5% reduction in smoking by minors the intervention would be 10 times more cost-effective than investing in breast or colorectal cancer screening. Moreover, a 1% increase in cigarette tax would be sufficient to fund the scheme.

The use of taxation as a way of influencing behaviour has been studied extensively in respect of tobacco (Box 6.7) and harmful alcohol consumption. An econometric analysis based in the United States assessed the impact of increased restrictions on smoking in public places alongside changes in the price of cigarettes. This considered not only the impact on smoking but also the impact on the consumption of alcohol. The analysis suggested that there was a positive relationship between increases in the price of cigarettes and alcohol consumption (Picone, Sloan and Trogdon 2004).

Can cost-effectiveness evaluations be generalized to all countries?

The majority of economic analyses in the field of promotion and prevention (particularly of chronic health problems) have been dominated by studies conducted largely in the United States and other high-income countries. This raises questions about the extent to which this evidence base is appropriate for policy actions that could be implemented in the less-affluent countries of the European Region. Table 6.4 draws on data collected for WHO-CHOICE

Table 6.4 Selected population-based interventions

Condition	Intervention	Intervention description	Target population	Incremental cost-effectiveness ($/DALY)[a]
Alcohol abuse	Excise tax	50% increase in the current excise tax rate on alcoholic beverages	Adolescents and adults	Eur A 258 Eur B 489 Eur C 156
	Excise tax plus advertising ban	As above plus comprehensive advertising ban	Adolescents and adults	Eur A 570 Eur B 466 Eur C 209
	Excise tax, advertising ban and brief primary care advice	As above plus advice, education sessions and psychosocial counselling	Adolescents and adults	Eur A 2359 Eur B 616 Eur C 593
	Excise tax, advertising ban, brief primary care advice, random break testing	As above plus random driver breath testing	Adolescents and adults	Eur A 2690 Eur B 5070 Eur C 1168
Coronary artery disease	Legislation substituting 2% of trans-fat with polyunsaturated fat at US$ 0.50 to US$ 6 per adult	Legislation replacing 2% of dietary trans-fat from partial hydrogenation in manufactured foods with polyunsaturated fat, at a cost of US$ 6 per adult, and assuming a 7–40% reduction in coronary artery disease	Adults	48–838[b]
Diabetes, ischaemic heart disease and stroke	Legislation with public education to reduce salt content	Legislated reduction in salt content of manufactured foods and an accompanying public education campaign	All ages	1937[b]

	Media campaign to reduce saturated fat	Media campaign to reduce saturated fat content in manufactured foods and replace part of the saturated fat with polyunsaturated fat	All ages	2617[b]
Tobacco addiction	Excise tax 600% of supply price (double the regional rate)	Price increase in tobacco taxes to discourage tobacco use, prevent initiation (and subsequent addiction) among youths, increase the likelihood of cessation among current users, reduce relapse among former users and reduce consumption among continuing users	Adolescents and adults	Eur A: 32 Eur B: 21 Eur C: 5
	Excise tax at 600% supply price plus advertising ban	As above plus advertising bans on television, radio and billboards	Adolescents and adults	Eur A: 859 Eur B: 163 Eur C: 53
	Excise tax at 600% supply price, advertising ban, clean indoor air law enforcement, plus information dissemination	As above plus health information and health warning labels on tobacco products; banning smoking in public places	Adolescents and adults	Eur A: 1909 Eur B: 251 Eur C: 82
Traffic accidents	Increased speeding penalties, enforcement, media campaigns, speed bumps	Minimizing exposure to high-risk scenarios by installation of speed bumps at hazardous junctions, increased penalties for speeding, other effective road-safety regulations combined with media coverage and better law enforcement	Adults	21
	Enforcement of seat-belt laws, promotion of child restraints, random breath testing of drivers	Mandatory seat-belt and child-restraint laws, enforcement of drunk-driving laws, random breath testing of drivers	Adults	2449

Sources: World Health Organization 2003; Chisholm et al. 2004; Laxminarayan, Chow and Shahid-Salles 2006.
Notes: [a]2000 prices, using international dollars and age weighted unless indicated as differing; [b]2001 prices, using US dollars and unweighted for age; see Table 6.1 for WHO subgroups; DALY: Disability-adjusted life-years.

and the Disease Control Priorities projects. Focusing primarily on low- and middle-income countries, it provides examples of interventions that would be considered to be highly cost-effective even in the least affluent countries of the European Region (World Health Organization 2003; Chisholm et al. 2004; Laxminarayan, Chow and Shahid-Salles 2006). Again these include the use of fiscal policy to influence the consumption of alcohol and use of tobacco, legislation to restrict the use of salt and saturated fat in food and a whole range of traffic accident prevention measures that have also been considered in high-income countries.

Poorer health status in some of these countries means that the potential burden of ill health that might be averted can dwarf what can be achieved in high-income countries. For instance, recent analysis indicates that measures to limit salt and tobacco use could potentially avert substantial levels of avoidable mortality in some European countries, for example the Russian Federation (166), Poland (160) and Ukraine (153) with total implementation costs per person of US$ 0.66, US$ 1.04 and US$ 0.17, respectively (Asaria et al. 2007). Data from the WHO-CHOICE programme applied to Estonia also indicate that taxation would be the most cost-effective weapon in changing patterns of consumption of tobacco and alcohol (Lai et al. 2007).

Moving forward: strengthening the evidence base

While it is impossible to establish a universal economic case for all types of preventive intervention, it is clear that many interventions to promote population health do represent good value for money. Moreover, substantial non-health sector benefits often arise from these interventions. The rapid expansion of the evidence base in recent years and the growing interest of policy-makers attest further to the importance now being attached to this issue. How can different countries expand and make more use of economic evaluation in their deliberations on population health strategies? Potential ways forward are documented in detail elsewhere (McDaid, Drummond and Suhrcke 2008); three challenges are briefly considered here.

Strengthening the evidence base on the effectiveness of interventions

One challenge relates to what we know about the effectiveness of interventions. Many public health and health-promoting interventions are complex, involving a number of different mechanisms and usually delivered in a community setting. Often they do not lend themselves easily to randomized control trials. In many instances, evaluations conducted using other methods may be excluded from analyses and potentially useful sources of evidence may be overlooked.

While space does not permit a detailed discussion of the different ways of generating evidence, many different types of quantitative and qualitative evidence can be used to inform the policy-making process. Experimental studies help to reduce the chance of bias in evaluation, but the controlled conditions in which these studies are conducted may mean that results are not easily generalized. It should also be recognized that randomization may not be feasible in some population-based interventions that aim at fundamental changes to the environment in which individuals live, although a greater problem is an unwillingness of authorities to agree to randomization at community level. In this case, there is a reliance on observational data, although advanced statistical techniques can go some way to accounting for differences in intervention and control groups. Qualitative research can complement quantitative research by, for example, understanding the acceptability of interventions to different groups.

Augmenting the existing evidence base from economic evaluations

For some interventions, there is evidence of effectiveness but few economic evaluations have been conducted. Existing reviews indicate that the majority of work continues to focus on individual clinical interventions rather than more upstream health-promoting measures. One key reason for this is the limited opportunities for commercial advantage that accrue from many of these interventions.

Clearly, the private sector has an interest in demonstrating the (cost-) effectiveness of clinical products as it can subsequently appropriate much of the gains from its invention by selling patented products. Generally, this does not work in the case of non-clinical prevention (or, indeed, surgical techniques or new ways of delivering care, such as multidisciplinary teams). Any evidence on an effective or cost-effective health promotion programme would become a public good as soon as the evidence about its (cost) effectiveness was published. Everyone might use and benefit from this and could implement programmes without having to compensate researchers for the costs they incurred producing such knowledge. The social benefits of such evidence can thus be expected to be large but the private benefits to researchers will be small. The divergence between private and social costs/benefits leads to a suboptimal level of non-clinical preventive research, compared with a situation in which private and social costs/benefits are aligned.

This justifies a role for government intervention to correct this market failure, for example by promoting or undertaking research that everybody might benefit from but no one individually would do if left alone (Dranove 1998). One additional option might be to expand the remit of existing HTA bodies to assess the costs and effectiveness of population health interventions, akin to the expansion of the role of NICE in England or the Service Delivery and Organisation programme of research and development in the United Kingdom National Health Service.

Pragmatically, a more modest ambition would be retrospectively to add an economic dimension to those areas of public health where evidence on effectiveness is strong. Long used in the evaluation of health care interventions, decision analytical modelling can also play a critical role in helping to provide information on the potential long-term impacts of public health interventions.

Simple threshold analyses can be assessed. These look at the potential level of effectiveness that an intervention needs to demonstrate in order to make it cost-effective. Given the potential good value for money of many interventions, the level of improvement in effectiveness required may well be very modest.

However, it is not just a question of extending this evidence base on what works and at what cost. It is critically important to take account of context in understanding what influences individual behaviours and the uptake of interventions. Effective public health interventions from one setting may require careful adaptation before they can be implemented in different settings. Economic evaluations need to take account of this, as illustrated through the development of tools to allow country adaptation of data provided by WHO-CHOICE (Lai et al. 2007). Future methodological developments might consider how to enhance and increase the use of holistic approaches to economic evaluation that make use of qualitative methods to obtain contextual information on the implementation of interventions (Jan 1998; Jan et al. 2004). Approaches such as theory of change modelling merit further consideration. This involves the identification of why and how intervention planners believe that change in behaviour or practice will occur, and subsequently how this will link to changes in short-, mid- and long-term outcomes (Connell and Kubisch 1998).

Facilitating the implementation of evidence-informed population health strategies

The final key issue is implementation. What mechanisms are available to help to promote investment in cost-effective population health strategies, particularly when many of these will require buy in by stakeholders outside the health system, such as schools and workplaces? One helpful measure may be to ensure that economic evaluations of population health interventions take a broad perspective on costs and benefits. For example, an effective school-based health promotion programme might also foster better educational performance. In other cases, the non-health impacts might actually be detrimental.

Theoretically, well-conducted CBA studies could overcome the problem of multisector benefits and costs that cannot be addressed by cost-effectiveness analysis or cost utility analysis. In the absence of CBA, a range of health and non-health outcomes could be reported alongside costs in a cost consequences analysis so that decision-makers are at least given the opportunity to consider these factors. Where non-health benefits are modest but overall the intervention helps to improve social welfare, there may be a need for the sectors that will benefit most (e.g. health and social care) to transfer funds to those delivering the intervention. Health promotion in the workplace may require increased cooperation with the private sector, including the use of incentives such as tax breaks.

Other measures to improve effective implementation across sectors include improved communication between researchers and policy-makers, as well as awareness-raising measures on the health impacts of all policies. The formalized use of health impact assessment may be one way to improve awareness when looking at policy interventions across sectors. For instance, civil servants might be required to consider the health impacts of a new airport runway, traffic-calming measures or economic regeneration. Equally it might be prudent for policy-makers to assess the key non-health impacts when developing population health policies.

To date health impact assessment has been used in several high-income European countries, mainly at a local level. But the extent to which it has facilitated policy change remains unclear. One review of the effectiveness of this approach suggests that a lack of understanding of non-health sector issues by proponents may be a barrier to success. A key factor for success may be to ensure good links with decision-makers in order to institutionalize the health impact assessment process within their organizations, given the absence of a commonly agreed standard (Davenport, Mathers and Parry 2006).

Mechanisms to monitor implementation across sectors might facilitate change. Cross-sector, explicit measurable targets for population health improvement could provide additional incentives for action. Joint targets across government departments might be set and their progress monitored. Negative publicity from failing to achieve targets may also act as a powerful incentive for action.

Conclusions

Poor health can have profound personal, social and economic effects, many of which have impacts well beyond the health system. We have indicated that the economic case for investment in promotion/prevention activities is often justified by the presence of market failures. Moreover, there is a growing evidence base on effective and cost-effective interventions to promote health. Many of these compare very favourably with investment in clinical interventions. These include early years interventions to promote the physical and mental health of children, actions to promote health in the workplace, vaccination programmes, interventions to prevent road transport injuries, and smoking cessation/responsible alcohol consumption schemes. Some of these interventions can also have significant economic benefits beyond the health system, for instance linked to the improved educational performance of children or reduced absenteeism in the workplace.

One key limitation is the limited economic analysis reported for health promotion and prevention actions outside the United States. It is important to develop and adapt the evidence base to consider how interventions might be implemented in very different contexts (e.g. of culture, infrastructure and available human resources) across Europe. One way to expand the evidence base on cost-effectiveness might be to retrospectively quantify the costs of implementing interventions that have been demonstrated to be effective but which lack European evidence on cost-effectiveness.

It is also critical for health policy-makers to collaborate with other sectors. Many of the most cost-effective interventions may be both funded and delivered outside the health care system. Facilitating action across sectors may not only involve raising awareness of the health impacts of different interventions but also require flagging of any major non-health benefits that may be generated. Interventions that have modest non-health benefits but improve overall social welfare may require mechanisms that allow a transfer of funds from those sectors that benefit most (e.g. health and social care) to those that deliver the intervention.

References

Asaria, P., Chisholm, D., Mathers, C., Ezzati, M. and Beaglehole, R. (2007) Chronic disease prevention: health effects and financial costs of strategies to reduce salt intake and control tobacco use. *Lancet*, 370(9604): 2044–53.

Berrios, X., Bedregal, P. and Guzman, B. (2004) Costo-efectividad de la promocion de la salud en Chile. Experiencia del programa 'Mirame'! [Cost-effectiveness of health promotion in Chile. Experience with the 'Mirame!' programme.] *Revista Medica Chile*, 132(3): 361–70.

Bevan, G., Morton, A., Airoldi, M., Oliveira, M. and Smith, J. (2007) *Estimating Health and Productivity Gains in England from Selected Interventions*. London: The Health Foundation.

Boulenger, S., Nixon, J., Drummond, M., Ulmann, P., Rice, S. and Pouvourville, G. (2005) Can economic evaluations be made more transferable? *European Journal of Health Economics*, 6: 334–46.

Briggs, A.H., Schulpher, M.J. and Claxton, K. (2006) *Modelling Methods for Health Economic Evaluation*. Oxford: Oxford University Press.

Briss, P.A., Zaza, S. and Pappaioanou, M. for the Task Force on Community, Preventive Services (2000) *Developing an evidence-based guide to community preventive services—methods*. *American Journal of Preventive Medicine*, 18(Suppl. 1): 35–43.

Chatterji, P., Caffray, C.M., Crowe, M., Freeman, L. and Jensen, P. (2004) Cost assessment of a school-based mental health screening and treatment program in New York City. *Mental Health Services Research*, 6(3): 155–66.

Chen, G. and Warburton, R. (2006) Do speed cameras produce net benefits? Evidence from British Columbia, Canada. *Journal of Policy Analysis and Management*, 25(3): 661–78.

Chisholm, D., Rehm, J., van Ommeren, M. and Monteiro, M. (2004) Reducing the global burden of hazardous alcohol use: a comparative cost-effectiveness analysis. *Journal of Studies in Alcohol*, 65(6): 782–93.

Connell, J. and Kubisch, A. (1998) Applying a theory of change approach to the evaluation of comprehensive community initiatives: progress, prospects and problems, in K. Fulbright-Anderson, A. Kubisch and J. Connell (eds.) *New Approaches to Evaluating Community Initiatives*, Vol. 2: *Theory, Measurement, and Analysis*. Washington, DC: The Aspen Institute: 15–44.

Davenport, C., Mathers, J. and Parry, J. (2006) Use of health impact assessment in incorporating health considerations in decision making. *Journal of Epidemiology and Community Health*, 60(3): 196–201.

DiFranza, J., Peck, R.M., Radecki, T.E. and Savageau, J.A. (2001) What is the potential cost-effectiveness of enforcing a prohibition on the sale of tobacco to minors? *Preventive Medicine*, 32(2): 166–74.

Dranove, D. (1998) Is there underinvestment in R&D about prevention? *Journal of Health Economics*, 17(1): 117–27.

Dretzke, J., Davenport, C., Frew, E. et al. (2005) The effectiveness and cost-effectiveness of parent training/education programmes for the treatment of conduct disorder, including oppositional defiant disorder, in children. *Health Technology Assessment*, 9(50): iii, ix–x, 1–233.

Drummond, M., Chevat, C. and Lothgren, M. (2007) Do we fully understand the economic value of vaccines? *Vaccine*, 25(32): 5945–57.

Drummond, M., Weatherly, H.L.A. and Claxton, K. (2007) *Assessing the Challenges of Applying Standard Methods of Economic Evaluation to Public Health*. York: Public Health Research Consortium, University of York.

Drummond, M., Sculpher, M.J., Torrance, G.W., O'Brien, B.J. and Stoddart, G.L. (2005) *Methods for the Economic Evaluation of Health Care Programmes*, 3rd edn. Oxford: Oxford University Press.

Edinburgh Breast Screening Clinic (1978) Screening for breast cancer. *British Medical Journal*, ii: 175–8.

Edwards, B., White, R.H., Maxted, H., Deverill, I. and White, P.A. (1975) Screening methods for covert bacteriuria in schoolgirls. *British Medical Journal*, ii: 463–7.

Edwards, R.T., Céilleachair, A., Bywater, T., Hughes, D.A. and Hutchings, J. (2007) Parenting programme for parents of children at risk of developing conduct disorder: cost effectiveness analysis. *British Medical Journal*, 334: 646–82.

Elder, J.P., Wildey, M., de Moor, C. et al. (1993) The long-term prevention of tobacco use among junior high school students: Classroom and telephone interventions. *American Journal of Public Health*, 83(9): 1239–44.

Ginnelly, L., Sculpher, M., Bojke, C., Roberts, I., Wade, A. and Diguiseppi, C. (2005) Determining the cost effectiveness of a smoke alarm give-away program using data from a randomized controlled trial. *European Journal of Public Health*, 15(5): 448–53.

Godfrey, C. (2001) Economic evaluation of health promotion. *WHO Regional Publications European Series* 92: 149–70.

Graham, J.D., Thompson, K.M., Goldie, S.J., Segui-Gomez, M. and Weinstein, M.C. (1997) The cost-effectiveness of air bags by seating position. *Journal of the American Medical Association*, 27817): 1418–25.

Graham, J.D., Goldie, S.J., Segui-Gomez, M. et al. (1998) Reducing risks to children in vehicles with passenger airbags. *Pediatrics*, 102(1): e3.

Guria, J. (1999) An economic evaluation of incremental resources to road safety programmes in New Zealand. *Accident Analysis and Prevention*, 31(1–2): 91–9.

Haddix, A.C., Mallonee, S., Waxweiller, R. and Douglas, M.R. (2001) Cost effectiveness analysis of a smoke alarm giveaway program in Oklahoma City, Oklahoma. *Injury Prevention*, 7(4): 276–81.

Hale, J. (2000) What contribution can health economics make to health promotion? *Health Promotion International*, 15(4): 341–8.

Hills, D., Elliot, E. and Kowarzik, U. (2007) *The Evaluation of the Big Lottery Fund Healthy Living Centres Programme*. London: Big Lottery Fund.

Holland, W. (2004) Health technology assessment and public health: a commentary. *International Journal of Technology Assessment in Health Care*, 20: 77–80.

Hutubessy, R., Chisholm, D. and Edejer, T.T. (2003) Generalized cost-effectiveness analysis for national-level priority-setting in the health sector. *Cost Efficiency and Resource Allocation*, 1: 8.

Innes, R. (2004) Fines, appeals and liability in public enforcement with stochastic damage and asymmetric information. *Economica*, 71(283): 391.

Jan, S. (1998) A holistic approach to the economic evaluation of health programs using institutionalist methodology. *Social Science and Medicine*, 47(10): 1565–72.

Jan, S., Conaty, S., Hecker, R., Bartlett, M., Delaney, S. and Capon, T. (2004) A holistic economic evaluation of an Aboriginal community-controlled midwifery programme in Western Sydney. *Journal of Health Services Research and Policy*, 9(1): 14–21.

Kelly, M.P., McDaid, D., Ludbrooke, A. and Powell, J. (2005) *Economic Appraisal of Public Health Interventions*. London: National Institute for Health and Clinical Excellence.

Kenkel, D.S. (2000) Prevention, in A.J. Culyer and J.P. Newhouse (eds.) *Handbook of Health Economics*. Amsterdam: Elsevier Science: 1676–20.

Konig, H.H. and Barry, J.C. (2004) Cost-utility analysis of orthoptic screening in kindergarten: a Markov model based on data from Germany. *Pediatrics*, 113(2): e95–108.

Korda, R.J. and Butler, J.R. (2006) *Effect of Healthcare on Mortality: Trends in Avoidable Mortality in Australia and Comparisons with Western Europe. Public Health*, 120: 95–105.

Kreis, J and Bödeker, W. (2004) *Health-related and Economic Benefits of Workplace Health Promotion and Prevention. Summary of the Scientific Evidence*, IGA report 3e. Essen: BKK Bundesverband/Hauptverband der gewerblichen Berufsgenossenschaften.

Lai, T., Habicht, J., Reinap, M., Chisholm, D. and Baltussen, R. (2007) Costs, health effects and cost-effectiveness of alcohol and tobacco control strategies in Estonia. *Health Policy*, 84(1): 75–88.

Laxminarayan, R., Chow, J. and Shahid-Salles, A.A. (2006) Intervention cost effectiveness: overview of main messages, in D.T. Jamison, W.H. Mosley, A.R. Measham and J.L. Bobadilla (eds.) *Disease Control Priorities in Developing Countries*. New York: Oxford University Press: 35–86.

Lowin, A., Slater, J., Hall, J. and Alperstein, G. (2000) Cost effectiveness analysis of school based Mantoux screening for TB infection. *Australian and New Zealand Journal of Public Health*, 24(3): 247–53.

Marmot, M. and Wilkinson, R. (eds.) (2006) *Social Determinants of Health*, 2nd edn. Oxford: Oxford University Press.

McDaid, D. and Needle, J. (2006) *Economic Evaluation and Public Health: Mapping the Literature*. Cardiff: Welsh Assembly Government.

McDaid, D., Drummond, M. and Suhrcke, M. (2008) *How Can European Health Systems Support Investment in and Implementation of Population Health Strategies?* Copenhagen: WHO Regional Office for Europe.

McDaid, D., Halliday, E., Mackenzie, M. et al. (2006) *Issues in the Economic Evaluation of Suicide Prevention Strategies: Practical and Methodological Challenges*, discussion paper no. 2407. London: Personal Social Services Research Unit, London School of Economics and Political Science.

Mills, P.R., Kessler, R.C., Cooper, J. and Sullivan, S. (2007) Impact of a health promotion program on employee health risks and work productivity. *American Journal of Health Promotion*, 22(1): 45–53.

Munro, J.F., Nicholl, J.P., Brazier, J.E., Davey, R. and Cochrane, T. (2004) Cost effectiveness of a community based exercise programme in over 65 year olds: cluster randomised trial. *Journal of Epidemiology and Community Health*, 58(12): 1004–10.

Murphy, J.M. (2007) Breakfast and learning: an updated review. *Current Nutrition and Food Science*, 3(1): 3–36.

Nolte, E. and McKee, M. (2003) Measuring the health of nations: analysis of mortality amenable to health care. *British Medical Journal*, 327: 1129.

Organisation for Economic Co-operation and Development (2007) *OECD Health Data 2007*. Paris: Organisation for Economic Co-operation and Development.

Pelletier, K.R. (1991) A review and analysis of the health and cost-effective outcome studies of comprehensive health promotion and disease prevention programs. *American Journal of Health Promotion*, 5(4): 311–15.

Pelletier, K.R. (2001) A review and analysis of the clinical- and cost-effectiveness studies of comprehensive health promotion and disease management programs at the worksite: 1998–2000 update. *American Journal of Health Promotion*, 16(2): 107–16.

Pelletier, K.R. (2005) International collaboration in health promotion and disease management: implications of US health promotion efforts on Japan's health care system. *American Journal of Health Promotion*, 19(3): 216–29.

Picone, G.A., Sloan, F. and Trogdon, J.G. (2004) The effect of the tobacco settlement and smoking bans on alcohol consumption. *Health Economics*, 13(10): 1063–80.

Rush, B., Shiell, A. and Hawe, P. (2004) A census of economic evaluations in health promotion. *Health Education Research*, 19(6): 707–19.

Sassi, F. and Hurst, J. (2008) *The Prevention of Lifestyle-related Chronic Diseases: An Economic Framework*, working paper no. 32. Paris: Organisation for Economic Co-operation and Development.

Schwappach, D.L., Boluarte, T.A. and Suhrcke, M. (2007) The economics of primary prevention of cardiovascular disease – a systematic review of economic evaluations. *Cost Efficiency and Resource Allocation*, 5: 5.

Scollo, M., Younie, S., Wakefield, M., Freeman, J. and Icasiano, F. (2003) Impact of tobacco tax reforms on tobacco prices and tobacco use in Australia. *Tobacco Control*, 12(Suppl. 2): ii59–66.

Shemilt, I., Harvey, I. and Shepstone, L. et al. (2004) A National Evaluation of School Breakfast Clubs: Evidence from a Cluster Randomized Controlled Trial and an Observational Analysis. *Child Care and Health Development*, 30(5): 413–27.

Shipp, M.D. (1998) Potential human and economic cost-savings attributable to vision testing policies for driver license renewal, 1989–1991. *Optometry and Vision Science*, 75(2): 103–18.

Smit, F., Willemse, G., Koopmanschap, M., Onrust, S., Cuijpers, P. and Beekman, A. (2006) Cost-effectiveness of preventing depression in primary care patients: randomised trial. *British Journal of Psychiatry*, 188: 330–6.

Suhrcke, M., McKee, M., Stuckler, D., Sauto Arce, R., Tsolova, S. and Mortensen, J. (2006a) The contribution of health to the economy in the European Union. *Public Health*, 120(11): 994–1001.

Suhrcke, M., Nugent, R.A., Stuckler, D. and Rocco, L. (2006b) *Chronic Disease: An Economic Perspective*. London: Oxford Health Alliance.

Suhrcke, M., Urban, D., Moesgaard Iburg, et al. (2007) *The Economic Benefits of Health and Prevention in High Income Countries: The Example of Germany*, discussion paper sp 1 2007–302. Berlin: Wissenschaftszentrum.

Treurniet, H.F., Boshuizen, H.C. and Harteloh, P.P. (2004) Avoidable mortality in Europe (1980–1997): a comparison of trends. *Journal of Epidemiology and Community Health*, 58(4): 290–5.

UK Clinical Research Collaboration (2006) *UK Health Research Analysis*. London: Clinical Research Collaboration.

UK National Institute for Health and Clinical Excellence (2006) *The Public Health Guidance Development Process. An Overview for Stakeholders Including Public Health Practitioners, Policy Makers and the Public*. London: National Institute for Health and Clinical Excellence: 46.

Wang, L.Y., Burstein, G.R. and Cohen, D.A. (2002) An economic evaluation of a school-based sexually transmitted disease screening program. *Sexually Transmitted Diseases*, 29(12): 737–45.

Wang, L.Y., Yang, Q., Lowry, R. and Wechsler, H. (2003) Economic analysis of a school-based obesity prevention program. *Obesity Research*, 11(11): 1313–24.

Wanless, D. (2004) *Securing Good Health for the Whole Population: Final Report*. London: The Stationery Office.

WHO Regional Office for Europe (2007) *Health For All Database*. Copenhagen: WHO Regional Office for Europe.

Winterthurer Institut für Gesundheitsökonomie (2004) *Ökonomische Beurteilung von Gesundheitsförderung und Prävention*. Winterthur: Winterthurer Institut.

World Health Organization (1986) *Ottawa Charter for Health Promotion*. Geneva: World Health Organization.

World Health Organization (2003) CHO*osing* I*nterventions that are Cost E*ffective *(WHO-CHOICE)*. *WHO-CHOICE Interventions: Tobacco Use*. Geneva: World Health Organization, http://www.who.int/choice/interventions/rf_tobacco/en/index.html (accessed 8 September 2010).

World Health Organization (2004) *Global Burden of Disease Estimates*. Geneva: World Health Organization.

World Health Organization (2005) *CHOICE:* CHO*osing* I*nterventions that are Cost E*ffective. Geneva: World Health Organization, http://www.who.int/choice (accessed 8 September 2010).

Zechmeister, I. Kilian, R. and McDaid, D. (2008) Is it worth investing in mental health promotion and prevention of mental illness? A systematic review of the evidence from economic evaluations. *BMC Public Health*, 8: 20.

chapter seven

Evidence for strategies to reduce socioeconomic inequalities in health in Europe

Johan P. Mackenbach and Anton E. Kunst

Introduction

At the start of the twenty-first century, substantial inequalities in health persist within the populations of all European countries. Those with less education, in lower occupational groups or with lower incomes tend to have a higher prevalence of all kinds of health problem and to die younger. This produces remarkable variations in the number of years that people in different socioeconomic groups can expect to live in good health (health expectancy). In all European countries with available data, differences in health expectancy at birth typically vary by 10 years or more (Mackenbach 2006).

The Black Report was published in England in 1980 and documented health inequalities that were widening despite the creation of the National Health Service in 1948 and the rise of the welfare state in the decades after the Second World War. The Report recommended a number of specific policies to reduce them (Townsend and Davidson 1992). It also contributed to heightened awareness of health inequalities throughout Europe and in developed countries elsewhere. As a result, enormous amounts of descriptive data have been collected and analysed in many countries, confirming the existence of substantial inequalities in health in all countries that have good data.

The need to find entry points for policies and interventions to reduce health inequalities has shifted the emphasis of European research from description to explanation. Greater understanding of the causes of socioeconomic inequalities in health can inform policy-makers searching for strategies to reduce them. Countries are at widely different stages of policy development, but some (e.g. England) have taken political opportunities for large-scale implementation of policies to tackle health inequalities. Other countries (e.g. Sweden, the Netherlands and Norway) have developed comprehensive plans for tackling health inequalities; these are at various stages of implementation (Mackenbach and Bakker 2003).

Chapter outline

This chapter reviews the policy implications stemming from recent studies on health inequalities in European countries. The results of some descriptive and explanatory studies of socioeconomic inequalities in health and some reviews of the effectiveness of specific interventions and policies to tackle health inequalities are assessed, taking account of the variations in health, health determinants and socioeconomic conditions in Europe.

The first section presents a general framework based on the necessary ingredients of strategies to tackle health inequalities. Having ensured political commitment, such strategies need to formulate realistic objectives, identify and implement effective policies and monitor their progress. All these steps require evidence from descriptive, explanatory and evaluation studies.

The second section summarizes the results of overviews of health inequalities in different European countries and identifies opportunities and priorities for reducing them. This is useful for informing discussions about attainable objectives. The third section summarizes explanatory studies. Although mainly limited to health behaviours and welfare policies, these suggest that there are important intercountry differences and provide some important suggestions concerning entry points for policies to reduce health inequalities in Europe.

The fourth section summarizes evaluation studies and lists some of the main results of evaluations of policies and interventions in three fields: (i) labour market and welfare policies, (ii) interventions and policies to improve health-related behaviours, and (iii) health care interventions and policies. The fifth section presents a new strand of research, aimed at assessing the relevance of health inequalities for sectors other than health and health care. More specifically, this section presents estimates of the economic implications of health inequalities in the EU.

Finally, the chapter concludes by summarizing the main findings and their implications for strategies to reduce health inequalities. It ends with recommendations for further research and monitoring.

General framework for strategies to reduce health inequalities

Socioeconomic inequalities in health have been documented at least since the nineteenth century, but they can only be reduced substantially with a powerful, sustained and systematic effort. Several attempts have been made to develop systematic strategies to tackle health inequalities (Benzeval, Judge and Whitehead 1995; Acheson 1998; Programme Committee SEIH-II 2001; Mackenbach and Bakker 2003). Effective action requires the following elements: political commitment, attainable objectives, a package of effective policies and interventions, effective implementation, and evaluation and monitoring.

Political commitment

Reducing health inequalities requires action in many fields, and deciding which policies to pursue is essentially a political matter. Fortunately, such policies can be justified on the basis of a range of ideological perspectives, and not just the egalitarian perspectives that tend to dominate sociodemocratic political choices. A liberal perspective can also lead to an engagement with reducing health inequalities (particularly among children), for example on the basis of the need to achieve equal opportunity for social and economic success. Similarly, religiously inspired preferences for solidarity may also provide a basis for policies to reduce health inequalities (Whitehead 1990).

The recent history of efforts to tackle health inequalities in various European countries clearly shows the importance of political commitment. Without it, health inequalities may be largely ignored in policies to promote population health. For example, the Black Report received a cold reception from the incoming Conservative Government in the United Kingdom in 1989. Health inequalities only became a legitimate object of policy-making following the election of a Labour Government in the late 1990s (Benzeval 2002). Similar changes in political commitment have been observed elsewhere, for example in Spain where the Spanish equivalent of the Black Report was ignored by a conservative national government in the late 1990s (Benach, Borrell and Daponte 2002). In the Netherlands, a centre-right government largely ignored the recommendations of the Albeda committee between 2002 and 2007 (Stronks 2002).

Attainable objectives

Although socioeconomic inequalities in health have been found in all countries with available data, the existence of variations in the magnitude of health inequalities over time or between countries suggests that health inequalities are to some extent modifiable. Evidence from the United Kingdom suggests that inequalities in mortality were large in the early twentieth century, declined until 1950, and then started to rise again (Pamuk 1985), suggesting that if we identify the driving forces behind these changes we can reduce these inequalities once more. Previous studies by our group have shown that in the 1980s and 1990s there were clear differences between countries in the magnitude of health inequalities, in particular for specific diseases such as ischaemic heart disease (Mackenbach et al. 1997; Huisman et al. 2005), suggesting that if we identify the determinants of these variations we can reduce health inequalities where current inequalities are relatively large.

The WHO introduced quantitative target setting as a policy instrument by including a 25% reduction of health inequalities in its strategy for *Targets for Health for All by the Year 2000* (World Health Organization 1985). Variations in health inequalities can inform the formulation of quantitative targets, which, in turn, may help to steer policy and provide a benchmark for evaluation. For this reason, several European countries have introduced quantitative targets in their health policies, including those to reduce health inequalities (Droomers et al. 2007; Bauld, Day and Judge 2008).

Package of effective policies and interventions

Strategies to reduce health inequalities should be evidence based. This implies that entry points are chosen carefully (e.g. the determinant addressed by the policy or intervention plays a key role in generating health inequalities) and that interventions can be expected to work (e.g. there is theoretical and/or empirical support for their effectiveness).

Studies seeking to explain health inequalities in various European countries have identified a wide range of entry points, for example reducing inequalities in income and other resources, providing extra health care to disadvantaged population groups, and reducing exposure to specific health determinants such as smoking and occupational risk factors in lower socioeconomic groups (Mackenbach and Bakker 2002). There is no agreement about which level provides the best entry point, but it is likely that strategies that simultaneously address a range of entry points will be most effective.

Few studies have investigated the effectiveness of policies and interventions to reduce health inequalities (MacIntyre et al. 2001) as the need for such evidence has been recognized only recently. This requires intercountry exchanges of research findings and systematic assessments of the available evidence. The size of the task and the practical barriers to collect this evidence mean that no single country has the resources for rapid construction of a satisfactory evidence base.

Effective implementation

There is often a large gap between policy-makers' intentions and the actual delivery of policies and interventions to the populations concerned. This is a particular problem for strategies to reduce health inequalities, where it is essential to reach large sections of the population with policies and interventions delivered according to specific standards. This has important implications for resources, delivery modes and quality assurance procedures.

Very few countries have experience of delivering policies and interventions that explicitly aim to reduce health inequalities. England is the most important exception, having developed a systematic approach to implementation. A regular stream of official reports that set out the rationale for interventions, the progress being made and audits of practical developments have been critical to this process of implementation (Department of Health 2003, 2005, 2007).

Evaluation and monitoring

Currently, only a very limited number of policies and interventions have been shown to be effective in reducing health inequalities. New policies and interventions are needed and, perhaps more importantly, those that have been implemented should be evaluated carefully.

Even when strategies to reduce health inequalities employ packages of policies and interventions that are known to be effective, it is still necessary to assess whether the strategy helps to reduce health inequalities at the population level. Continuous monitoring of health inequalities and interventions is essential and also helps to sustain the political will to reduce health inequalities over an extended period (Kunst, Bos and Mackenbach 2001).

Variations in health inequalities between European countries

Although no individual can escape death, there are important differences in the average age of dying between men and women, between inhabitants of town or country, between native people and immigrants and between population groups classified according to many other characteristics. Some of the largest inequalities in premature mortality are found when individuals are classified according to their socioeconomic position. This section provides an overview of the results of recent European overviews of inequalities in mortality. Where appropriate we also summarize evidence on inequalities in general health or health-related quality of life.

Ubiquity of health inequalities

International overviews have consistently shown that socioeconomic inequalities in health are substantial throughout the EU, in terms of both premature mortality and self-assessed health (Mackenbach et al. 2008). For example, recent analyses of the European Social Survey of 2002–2004 demonstrated that educational and occupational inequalities in general health are about equally large in all parts of Europe (Eikemo et al. 2008a,b).

Since the mid 1980s, there has been no clear tendency for health inequalities to narrow over time. On the contrary, some health inequalities, particularly relative inequalities in mortality, have been increasing in many European countries (Mackenbach and Bakker 2003). The widening relative gap in death rates generally results from differences between socioeconomic groups. While mortality declined in all groups, the decline has been proportionally faster in the higher socioeconomic groups, generally as a result of faster mortality declines for cardiovascular diseases (Mackenbach and Bakker 2003). In the 1980s and 1990s, many developed countries saw substantial reductions in deaths associated with cardiovascular diseases. These resulted from improvements in health-related behaviours (e.g. less smoking, modest improvements in diet, more physical exercise) and the introduction of effective health care interventions (e.g. detection and treatment of hypertension, surgical interventions, thrombolytic therapy). These improvements have been taken up to some extent by all socioeconomic groups but higher socioeconomic groups have tended to benefit more.

Although there are good opportunities for reducing health inequalities, their ubiquity shows that we should not be too optimistic about the feasibility of achieving substantial reductions within a short period. Even highly developed welfare states like those in the Nordic countries have substantial inequalities in health, on both relative and absolute scales (Mackenbach et al. 2008). Universal welfare policies may effectively reduce inequalities in income, access to adequate housing, access to health care and so on, but they do not guarantee the elimination of health inequalities. They may be considered to be necessary but insufficient measures to reduce health inequalities. This clearly points to the need to develop innovative approaches that are geared to the nature of health inequalities in modern industrialized societies.

Variations in the magnitude of health inequalities: scope for intervention

The fact that some countries exhibit much wider health inequalities than others suggests that inequalities are not inevitable. In recent studies, we found that the smallest inequalities in mortality (on both relative and absolute scales) are seen in some southern European populations (Turin, Italy; Barcelona, Madrid and the Basque country, Spain) (Mackenbach et al. 2008). This illustrates how health inequalities are not immutable and that substantial improvements in the European region as a whole are theoretically possible.

Intercountry variations in the magnitude of health inequalities are much more striking when specific diseases, such as ischaemic heart disease, various cancers and injuries, are considered. Both on a relative and an absolute scale the variations are immense. For ischaemic heart disease, inequalities in mortality are almost negligible in some southern European populations, comparatively speaking, and the same applies to lung cancer in Sweden, and cerebrovascular disease and injuries in England (Avendano et al. 2004; Avendano, Aro and Mackenbach 2005; van der Heyden et al. 2009). If the narrowest inequalities in mortality from a disease observed anywhere in Europe could be achieved everywhere then inequalities in mortality could be almost eliminated. Of course, this presupposes that we know how some populations have succeeded where others have failed. While this is not yet possible, these variations provide some tantalizing suggestions.

More effort is needed to understand the patterns and dynamics of health inequalities. Better understanding of differences between countries and temporal variations in health inequalities would help to identify opportunities to tackle them and to see what degree of health inequalities might be avoidable.

Large health inequalities in some populations: priorities for intervention

Recent studies have drawn attention to the wide relative and absolute inequalities in mortality in many eastern European populations (Stirbu et al. 2007, 2010; Mackenbach et al. 2008). Following the political changes around 1990, mortality rates have changed dramatically in many countries in eastern Europe – sometimes improving (e.g. in the Czech Republic) but often worsening, at least temporarily (e.g. in Hungary and Estonia), particularly among men (Leinsalu, Vågerö and Kunst 2003; Shkolnikov et al. 2006; Leinsalu et al. 2009). This probably reflects a combination of interlinked factors: more economic insecurity and poverty; the breakdown of protective social, public health and health care institutions; and a rise in excessive drinking and other risk factors for premature mortality. In countries with available data, it is clear that these changes in mortality vary between socioeconomic groups: mortality rates have generally improved less (or deteriorated more) in the lower socioeconomic groups. Apparently, those with higher levels of education have been able to protect themselves better against increased health risks, and/or have been able to benefit more from new opportunities for health gains. All this suggests that tackling health inequalities is a particularly urgent priority for public health policy in eastern Europe. Multilateral agencies such as the WHO or EU could support national and local policies in these countries by recognizing this priority in their own policies for public health and other areas (e.g. structural funds).

Specific diseases contribute to health inequalities between national populations; for example, ischaemic heart disease largely drives mortality inequalities in north and west Europe but cancer is relatively more important in the south. In eastern Europe, injuries are relatively more important as a cause of inequalities in mortality (Mackenbach et al. 2008; Menvielle et al. 2008). These findings show that different countries need different policies to address the specific determinants of health inequalities. Hence, interventions to reduce inequalities in ischaemic heart disease are required in northern Europe but should not be a priority (for health equity) in the south.

Determinants of health inequalities in European countries

Great progress in unravelling the determinants of health inequalities has been made since the mid 1990s. Further research is certainly necessary but our understanding of the causes of health inequalities has reached a stage where rational approaches to reduce health inequalities are becoming feasible.

Social stratification is associated with inequalities in access to various resources, both material and immaterial. It is generally recognized that the link between socioeconomic position and health rests mainly on a *causal effect* through inequalities in access to various resources. This is likely to be largely indirect: the result of a number of more specific health determinants that are differentially distributed across socioeconomic groups. Also, *selection effects* reinforce the link between socioeconomic position and health. Health-related selection may act through greater opportunities for upward social mobility for healthy people or greater risks of downward mobility for those with poor health (Davey Smith, Blane and Bartley 1994).

The role of specific health determinants

Many risk factors for diseases are more prevalent in lower socioeconomic groups. These inequalities in exposure to specific health determinants should be seen as the main explanation of health inequalities. Three sets of determinants are addressed here: (i) material, (ii) psychosocial and (iii) behavioural.

There is no doubt of the effects of *material factors* (i.e. low incomes and health risks in the physical environment). All European countries have large inequalities in income. According to Eurostat, the 20% of the population with the highest income in the EU (EU25) received 4.5 times more than the 20% of the population with the lowest income in 2001. Within the EU as a whole, 15% of the population was at risk of poverty (defined as having an income less than 60% of the national average). Income and poverty rates differ between countries, partly as a result of differences in taxation and social security schemes, but it is quite likely that financial inequalities play an important role in the explanation of health inequalities in all developed countries. Financial disadvantage may affect health through various mechanisms: psychosocial stress and subsequent risk-taking behaviours (e.g. smoking, excessive alcohol consumption) or reduced access to health-promoting facilities and products (e.g. fruits and vegetables, sports, preventive health care services). Risks related to occupations (e.g. exposure to chemicals, accidents, physically strenuous work) and housing (overcrowding, damp, accidents) are other examples of material factors that have been shown to make important contributions to some health inequalities (Marmot and Wilkinson 2006; Siegrist and Marmot 2006).

Psychosocial factors also contribute to health inequalities. On average, people in low socioeconomic groups experience more psychosocial stress, in the form of negative life events (e.g. loss of loved ones, financial difficulties), day-to-day problems, effort–reward imbalances (high levels of effort without appropriate reward) and a combination of high demands and low control. These forms of psychosocial stress can lead to ill health through biological (e.g. affecting the endocrine or immune systems) or behavioural (e.g. inducing risk-taking behaviours) pathways. Psychosocial factors related to work organization (e.g. job strain) have been shown to play an important role in the explanation of socioeconomic inequalities in cardiovascular health (Marmot and Wilkinson 2006; Siegrist and Marmot 2006).

The third group of contributory factors are *behavioural* (e.g. smoking, inadequate diet, excessive alcohol consumption and lack of physical exercise). In many developed countries, one or more of these lifestyle factors are more prevalent in the lower socioeconomic groups. This is discussed further below. Disease-specific patterns of health inequalities (e.g. marked international variations in mortality from ischaemic heart disease) also suggest that a substantial contribution is made by health-related behaviours (Avendano et al. 2004; Avendano, Aro and Mackenbach 2005).

Finally, it is important to note that these three groups of explanatory factors are interlinked. For example, the greater frequency of material disadvantage in lower socioeconomic groups may partly explain the higher frequency of psychosocial stress or lack of leisure time and physical exercise.

Health-related behaviours and socioeconomic inequalities: international patterns

Recent international overviews have paid extensive attention to socioeconomic inequalities in the prevalence of health-related behaviours. These studies show wide variations in the prevalence of specific health determinants, smoking being the best documented case. These intercountry variations in specific health determinants have implications for the understanding of health inequalities and the strategies needed to tackle them effectively.

In most European countries, smoking is strongly patterned by educational level, occupational class, income level and wealth (Schaap, van Agt and Kunst 2008). There are important differences between countries in the social patterning of smoking, particularly among women. Some of these variations may be explained by differences in gender emancipation (Schaap et al. 2009) and in the intensity of national tobacco-control policies (Schaap et al. 2008). Our findings suggest that these differences in social patterning play an important role in explaining international patterns of health inequalities, particularly for mortality (Mackenbach et al. 2008; van der Heyden et al. 2009). This confirms the findings of many studies at the individual level and suggests that smoking is an important entry point for policies to tackle health inequalities in many European countries, particularly those in the north, west and east. In southern Europe, policies to prevent the uptake of smoking in lower socioeconomic groups may help to prevent larger health inequalities appearing in the future.

Smoking is clearly bad for health but alcohol is a more complex risk factor – both abstinence and excessive alcohol consumption have adverse consequences for health. Abstinence is usually more common in lower socioeconomic groups (in men and women) but the pattern of excessive alcohol consumption is more variable. Many studies report a higher prevalence in lower socioeconomic groups, particularly among men, but the results for women are far from consistent (Droomers et al. 1999). These inconsistencies may well reflect real intercountry differences in the social patterning of excessive alcohol consumption. In the Nordic and several eastern European countries, for example, binge drinking (drinking more than, say, 8 units on a single occasion) is a more serious source of health problems than regular overconsumption of alcohol. In these countries, binge drinking tends to be more common in lower socioeconomic groups and is likely to contribute to health inequalities, through higher rates of ischaemic heart disease, stroke and injury mortality (Mäkelä, Valkonen and Martelin 1997). In southern countries, excessive regular consumption is likely to be more important. Whatever the pattern, the consequences for health inequalities appear similar in each region. Recent international overviews of mortality from alcohol-related causes of death showed higher mortality risks among lower educational groups (men and women) in all European populations (van Oyen et al. 2007; Menvielle et al. 2008).

Many other health-related behaviours may provide possible entry points for policy. For example, obesity is strongly socially patterned, particularly by education, among women and in southern Europe (Roskam and Kunst 2008; Roskam et al. 2010). Interestingly, this is one of the very few aspects of health where patterns of social inequalities are clearer for women. Among women, overweight and obesity are more prevalent in lower socioeconomic groups in all countries with available data, whereas the patterns are more variable among men (Roskam and Kunst 2008). Except for diabetes, we have not been able to study obesity's role in generating health inequalities (Espelt et al. 2008a) but it is likely that it will contribute to increasing health inequalities and is, therefore, an important entry-point for policy in many countries, particularly in southern Europe. This is also true for leisure-time physical activity, which we found to be strongly socially patterned in many European countries (Demarest et al. 2007). Lack of leisure-time physical activity also tends to be more common in lower socioeconomic groups (Roskam and Kunst 2008).

Comparable data on dietary behaviour by socioeconomic status are more difficult to obtain. Diet is notoriously difficult to measure and it is costly to collect nationally representative data on diet by socioeconomic position from a range of countries. The few comparative studies that have been conducted show that men and women in lower socioeconomic groups tend to eat fresh vegetables less frequently, particularly in the north of Europe. Differences in fresh vegetable consumption are smallest in the south, perhaps because of the larger availability and affordability of fruits and vegetables in Mediterranean countries (Prättälä et al. 2009). A similar north–south gradient has been found for fruit consumption (Cavelaars, Kunst and Mackenbach 1997). Literature reviews have shown that it is likely that many other aspects of diet (such as consumption of meat, dairy products and various fats and oils) are socially patterned in many European countries but with intercountry differences (López-Azpiazu et al. 2003).

Effectiveness of interventions and policies

Researchers have different opinions about how much evidence is required to justify strategies designed to reduce health inequalities. Some argue that the urgent need to tackle inequalities demands that interventions are initiated on the basis of plausibility (Petticrew et al. 2004); political windows of opportunity are usually short (four years at most) and may close before careful evaluations can be conducted (Whitehead et al. 2004). Others argue that this strategy has serious risks. There are many historical examples of 'plausible' interventions and policies that did not work, or even had adverse effects (MacIntyre et al. 2001). It could be argued that any investment to reduce health inequalities should be justified on the basis of its cost-effectiveness compared with other possible investments in health and well-being. This requires credible evidence (Oliver 2001) and indicates the need for systematic collection of the evidence on the (cost-)effectiveness of interventions and policies to reduce health inequalities (MacIntyre et al. 2001). This section provides brief reviews of the recent evidence for interventions in three areas: (i) the labour market and welfare policies, (ii) interventions and policies to improve health-related behaviours, and (iii) health care interventions and policies.

Labour market and welfare policies

Health inequalities are responsive to labour market regulations and working conditions. Swedish labour market policies enforce strong employment protection and active promotion of labour market participation for citizens with chronic illness. A comparison with England suggested that these policies were effective in protecting vulnerable groups from labour market exclusion during the recession of the 1990s (Burström 2000). In France, occupational health services are mandatory and include an annual health check for every employee. This provides a good setting for introducing preventive activities for those who may have few other medical contacts, particularly those in manual occupations. Randomized controlled trials within this setting have shown that interventions aimed at the detection and treatment of hypertension and smoking cessation were successful (Lang et al. 2000). Past improvements in working conditions have made important contributions to reducing health inequalities but much remains to be done. In the Netherlands, a recent intervention involving task rotation among garbage collectors (truck driving and mini-container loading) reduced sickness absenteeism by reducing physical load and (possibly) increasing job control (Kuijer, Visser and Kemper 1999).

Most of the available evidence suggests that universal welfare transfers and services (including universal health care services) contribute to improving the health of populations, particularly vulnerable subpopulations (Navarro et al. 2006). However, there is less clear evidence about their impact on inequalities in health between socioeconomic groups (Dahl et al. 2006). In our recent international work, we performed a number of studies to compare the magnitude of socioeconomic inequalities in health between groups of countries with different types and levels of welfare provision (e.g. Scandinavian or social-democratic; Anglo-Saxon or liberal; continental or Bismarckian welfare regimes) (Eikemo et al. 2008c; Mackenbach et al. 2008; Bambra and Eikemo 2009), or with different political traditions that could be expected to impact on labour market and welfare policies (e.g. countries which have been governed mainly by Social- or Christian-Democratic parties or recently became democracies) (Espelt et al. 2008b; Borrell et al. 2009). A few findings were in line with expectations, for example inequalities in self-assessed health appeared to be larger in some of the countries in southern Europe that later became democracies (Espelt et al. 2008b; Borrell et al. 2009). However, there were also a number of important counter-intuitive findings. For example, health inequalities do not appear to be systematically smaller in the north of Europe (Eikemo et al. 2008a,b; Mackenbach et al. 2008; Bambra and Eikemo 2009).

There may be several explanations (Dahl et al. 2006). There is the possibility that higher socioeconomic groups have benefited more from these welfare policies, just as most new improvements in population health tend to start earlier in higher socioeconomic groups. If this is the case, then there is a need to combine universal policies that affect the whole population with more targeted policies aimed at vulnerable populations.

We believe that this important question urgently requires further study. Special attention should be paid to policies aimed at encouraging participation in the labour market, universal services and transfers, the reduction of income inequalities, interventions in working conditions, and environmental and consumer protection policies. It has been suggested that these socioeconomic and political determinants have great relevance in explaining the level of population health (Navarro et al. 2006); consequently, there is a strong case for analysing their impact on reducing health inequalities.

Interventions and policies to improve health-related behaviours

Health-related behaviours like smoking, food consumption and physical exercise contribute to socioeconomic inequalities in health. In many countries, smoking is increasingly concentrated in lower socioeconomic groups and a variety of policies and interventions can be effective in reducing smoking in these groups (Kunst, Giskes and Mackenbach 2004). In an international comparative project, we found some evidence that the implementation of comprehensive tobacco control policies is associated with lower smoking rates in lower socioeconomic groups. Higher prices and advertising bans are important ingredients of these policies (Schaap, van Agt and Kunst 2008). Price measures (raising excise taxes) are very effective and any regressive impact on the poorest smokers with established addictions can be counteracted by active promotion of nicotine replacement therapy and other cessation support. It is particularly difficult to change the smoking behaviour of women in low-income groups. A promising Scottish initiative combined various approaches (community development, drama and poetry, fitness, cessation services and social support) (Gaunt-Richardson et al. 1999).

An evaluation of the British National Health Service stop smoking services suggests that equity-oriented smoking policies and services can make a modest contribution to reducing socioeconomic inequalities in health (Bauld, Judge and Platt 2007). These services were introduced after a major strategy for tobacco control was set out in the 1985 White Paper *Smoking Kills*. Treatment services were made available to all smokers and typically consisted of six to eight weeks of group or individual counselling plus nicotine replacement therapy. Huge efforts were made to encourage disadvantaged smokers, implementing positive discrimination so that the provision of services was skewed towards smokers living in deprived areas. Although partly successful, the effects were limited by the use of a standard package of care to all service recipients. This resulted in lower cessation rates among disadvantaged smokers. Nevertheless, these experiences show that if services can be tailored to the specific needs and circumstances of smokers in poor socioeconomic conditions, there is a very real prospect of a substantial reduction in inequalities in smoking (Bauld, Judge and Platt 2007).

For most other health-related behaviours there is a paucity of evidence on the effectiveness of interventions targeted specifically at lower socioeconomic groups. One of the few incidental studies with encouraging results comes from Finland, where nutrition policies have followed the general principle of universality within Nordic welfare ideology. Schoolchildren, students and employees received free or subsidized meals at school or in the workplace. These follow special dietary guidelines to ensure the use of low-fat food products and have probably contributed to the favourable trend of narrowing socioeconomic inequalities in the use of butter and high-fat milk in Finland (Prättälä, Berg and Puska 1992).

Health care interventions and policies

Universal access to high-quality health care can help to reduce health inequalities, regardless of income or other forms of social disadvantage. Unequal access to health care services may cause or aggravate socioeconomic inequalities in health. At the European level, there is evidence that lack of access to good quality health care is part of the causal chain that leads from low socioeconomic position to premature mortality because there are important socioeconomic differences in mortality from conditions amenable to medical intervention (Mackenbach and Bakker 2003; Stirbu et al. 2010). These differences are found everywhere but are particularly apparent in some countries in eastern Europe, suggesting that improving access to good quality health care should be a high priority there. Chapter 5 provides a more detailed review of avoidable mortality patterns in Europe.

International overviews based on survey data show that higher socioeconomic groups make more frequent use of many forms of health care. In most or perhaps all European countries, those in higher socioeconomic groups use specialist care for their health problems more often (Mielck et al. 2007). Also, those in lower socioeconomic groups more often report that they have forgone health care because of cost or because these services were not accessible (Mielck et al. 2009). In many countries, those in lower socioeconomic groups also make less use of preventive care, such as flu vaccination and breast cancer screening (Stirbu et al. 2007).

A review of studies evaluating different financing schemes confirmed that direct payments (including informal co-payments) for health care increase the risk of inequalities in health care utilization (Gelormino et al. 2007). Also, a review of studies evaluating the effect of different ways of organizing female cancer screening programmes showed that population-based programmes, active recruitment strategies, the involvement of primary care physicians and strategies based on well-established theoretical models are effective in reducing socioeconomic inequalities in attendance rates (Spadea et al. 2010). Finally, analysis of inequalities in the utilization of preventive services among the elderly suggests that well-implemented national programmes with high coverage rates leave little room for inequalities in uptake (Stirbu et al. 2007).

Health care can contribute to reducing health inequalities not only by offering dedicated services to lower socioeconomic groups but also by taking the lead in working with other agencies. In England during the first decade of the twenty-first century, health service reforms gave local health authorities the lead responsibility for working with other agencies to improve health and reduce inequalities. The key integrating device is the production of a three-year rolling plan for health. This feeds into a wider community strategy that commits all the local public sector services to a programme to improve the economic, social and environmental well-being of each area (Department of Health 2003). The forthcoming abolition of these health authorities by the new Conservative government raises questions about the future of such initiatives (Bowling and McKee 2010).

In this way, improvements in the health care system can play an important role in reducing health inequalities. Policies that promote financial, geographical and cultural access to good quality health care services for people with low socioeconomic status should be a priority for health care policy in all European countries – but a particular priority in eastern Europe.

Economic implications of health inequalities in Europe

Strategies to reduce health inequalities require the active engagement of not only the public health and health care systems but also those in other sectors such as education, social security, working life and city planning (Whitehead 2007). A fruitful dialogue may be facilitated by highlighting the economic benefits of reducing health inequalities.

There is growing attention to the potential economic benefits of improvements in population health in general. This is far from new – the origins of the public health movement lie in the awareness that the prosperity of nations is partly dependent on the health of their populations (Rosen 1993). This awareness received a new stimulus with the 2001 publication of the WHO Commission on Macroeconomics and Health report (Commission on Macroeconomics and Health Working Group Five 2001). This was followed (in 2005) by an overview of evidence concerning health's impact on the economy in high-income countries, particularly in the EU (Suhrcke et al. 2005). The latter report concluded that there are good economic arguments for investing in health. Greater investments in human capital are necessary if Europe is to become more competitive globally. The economic consequences of ill health and their implications are addressed in detail in Chapter 4.

It is not possible to estimate the economic benefits of investing in equality in health as this requires insight into the costs and effects of policies to reduce health inequalities – which is not yet available (MacIntyre et al. 2001). However, a first step would be to quantify the current economic losses that health inequalities generate. Mackenbach, Meerding and Kunst (2007) quantified the potential economic impact of improving the health of groups with a lower socioeconomic status to that of the more advantaged sections of the population in the EU25. This included estimates of the impact on personal earnings and GDP, health care costs, costs of social security benefits and total welfare.

The analysis of the European Community Household Panel (ECHP) showed large differences in the level of personal earnings according to general health. The earnings of those with 'very good' or 'good' health were about four times higher than those of people with 'poor' and 'very poor' health. The main cause of lower earnings among those with poor health was their lower participation in the labour force. The effects of health on labour force participation, the number of hours worked and hourly wages were generally larger (in relative terms) among persons with lower educational levels. These effect estimates were used in a levelling-up counterfactual scenario in which the prevalence of 'very good' or 'good' health in lower educational groups was assumed to increase up to the level of higher educational groups. On the basis of this scenario, an estimated 2.8% of average personal income was lost through health inequalities in the EU. This translated into an approximately 1.4% loss in GDP, or €141 billion for the EU as a whole (Mackenbach, Meerding and Kunst 2007).

The analysis of ECHP data also confirmed that poor health was consistently associated with more general practitioner visits, specialist visits and hospitalization rates. People with 'very poor' health had more than six times the visits to the general practitioner and more than nine times more specialist visits than those with 'very good' health, after adjustment for confounders. In the levelling-up scenario, the number of general practitioner and specialist visits decreased by 16%; and the number of nights in hospital decreased by 22%. The costs of the impact of health inequalities on health care was estimated at €26 billion for physician services and €59 billion for hospital services. If the empirical results for physician visits and hospitalizations applied to total health care, the impact of health inequalities would represent €177 billion, around 20% of total health care costs in the EU25.

The analysis of the ECHP panel data confirmed that poorer health is strongly associated with receipt of unemployment benefits and, especially, with the receipt of disability benefits. People with 'very poor' health receive, on average, about 20 times more disability benefits than those with 'very good' health, after adjustment for confounders. On the basis of the levelling-up counterfactual scenario, it was estimated that education-related health inequalities account for 25% of the costs of disability benefits (representing €55 billion annually) and 3% of the costs of unemployment benefits (about €5 billion annually) in the EU as a whole. The €60 billion total corresponds to 15% of the total costs of social security systems.

In a final step, health was considered as an independent component of population welfare (*consumption good*) instead of as a determinant of economic outcomes (*capital good*). First, the years of life lost through inequalities in mortality were counted and valued. The number of life-years lost through inequalities in mortality were estimated to be 11.4 million, using a levelling-up counterfactual scenario. If each of these life-years was valued at €77,000 and a standard discount rate of 1.5% per annum over an average of 16 years was applied, the total value of this lost life would amount to €778 billion. Inequalities-related losses to self-assessed health were estimated to be equivalent to about 4.3 million years of life lost – 40% of the mortality effect of 11.4 million years. This would, therefore, add another €280 billion to the welfare impact of health inequalities.

These estimates suggest a substantial economic impact from socioeconomic inequalities in health. While the estimates of inequalities-related losses to personal income and GDP seem to be modest in relative terms (1.4% of GDP), they are large in absolute terms (€141 billion). When health is valued as a consumption good it becomes clear that the economic impact of socioeconomic inequalities in health is really huge – approximately €1000 billion. The separate calculations of the impacts on the costs of social security, health care systems and health care support these conclusions. Inequalities-related losses to health account for 15% of the costs of social security systems and 20% of the costs of health care systems in the EU as a whole. It is important to emphasize that all these estimates represent yearly values and as long as health inequalities persist, these losses will continue to accumulate.

These results imply that there are likely to be important economic benefits from investing in strategies to reduce health inequalities. Although relatively little is known about the effectiveness of these strategies, it is possible to make some educated guesses about their potential economic impact in the EU. For example, further analyses suggested that a substantial impact would be generated by implementing a number of equity-oriented anti-tobacco policies to reduce the prevalence of smoking by 33% in the lower socioeconomic groups and 25% in the higher (Kunst, Giskes and Mackenbach 2004; Giskes et al. 2007). This would considerably reduce health inequalities as well as some 7% of the economic costs of mortality and general health, including the costs of health care and social security benefits. The inequalities-related losses to health as a consumption good (through mortality) would be reduced by about €75 billion per year for the EU25 as a whole; inequalities-related losses to health as a capital good would be reduced by almost €9 billion (Mackenbach, Meerding and Kunst 2007).

This is still largely uncharted scientific territory. However, the numbers highlighted by these analyses indicate that there is likely to be a good economic case for reducing health inequalities – in addition to the more self-evident case for population health.

General conclusions

Summary and main policy implications

Substantial socioeconomic inequalities in health throughout Europe represent one of the main challenges for public health policy in all individual countries and throughout the region. Improving the health of people with lower levels of education, occupational class or income will reduce these health inequalities and produce substantial gains in overall population health. However, although the impact of socioeconomic inequalities in health on the economy of WHO European Region Member States cannot yet be determined with precision, the implications are very likely to be substantial. This warrants significant investment in policies and interventions to reduce socioeconomic inequalities in health, by those within and outside the public health and health care sectors.

Intercountry variations in the magnitude of health inequalities (particularly for specific diseases) strongly suggest that a reduction of health inequalities is feasible. At the same time, the ubiquity of health inequalities across Europe and their persistence over time warns against too much optimism and indicates that innovative policies and great determination will be required. There has been good progress in unravelling the determinants of health inequalities, and a number of specific determinants (particularly material, psychosocial and lifestyle factors) have been found to contribute. Further research is necessary, but current understanding of the causes of health inequalities makes it feasible to undertake rational approaches to reduce health inequalities.

Powerful, sustained and systematic strategies are required in order to reduce health inequalities. Their development requires political will, attainable objectives, effective policies and interventions, effective implementation, and evaluation and monitoring. Some European countries have been making important steps in developing (and sometimes implementing) such strategies since the mid 1990s, but much more needs to be done. Policies and interventions to reduce health inequalities should be tailored to the specific pattern of health inequalities that prevail in each country. There are marked intercountry differences in the diseases and determinants that make the largest contribution to inequalities in overall health. Special attention should be given to countries with relatively large health inequalities, particularly in eastern Europe.

Wider policies that address people's socioeconomic positions (including labour market, income and welfare policies) are necessary ingredients of strategies to reduce health inequalities. However, the persistence of health inequalities in countries with universal welfare systems warns that these alone are not sufficient. Policies that address more specific determinants and risk factors are also needed.

Health-related behaviours (particularly smoking and excessive alcohol consumption) are important contributors to health inequalities in many countries. They represent important entry points for reduction strategies. The available evidence suggests that comprehensive approaches and new and innovative methods are needed to tackle health-related behaviours in lower socioeconomic groups.

Lack of access to good quality health care is likely to contribute to the poorer health of people in disadvantaged socioeconomic positions, particularly in eastern Europe. Avoiding inequalities in access to health care is a key element of strategies to reduce health inequalities. This requires no (or few) direct payments by consumers as well as organizational measures to improve access to good quality health care, including prevention programmes.

It may not be realistic to eliminate health inequalities in the foreseeable future but it is certainly possible to reduce them to more acceptable levels. This requires a genuine determination to follow the logic of emerging evidence and apply it to the health outcomes of greatest concern in any particular setting. Health inequalities can be reduced if the will is there.

Recommendations for further research and monitoring

The description and continued monitoring of health inequalities should be improved in many countries. All European countries should be able to monitor socioeconomic inequalities in mortality, general health, diseases and determinants on a routine basis, following generally accepted monitoring guidelines. The EU and WHO should promote this by including the socioeconomic dimension in their health monitoring systems. A European-level databank should be created to allow comparisons of health inequalities between countries and over time.

Explanatory research still faces many challenges. One puzzling finding that needs further research is the lack of a clear association between the magnitude of health inequalities and the labour market and welfare policies of different European countries. This requires the development of monitoring systems that collect detailed information on policies that potentially impact on health inequalities. There is a lack of good quality longitudinal data that are comparable across different countries; these would permit investigation of the links between health inequalities, welfare state arrangements and other contextual characteristics.

There is a general paucity of evaluations of the effectiveness of policies and interventions among lower socioeconomic groups. Further research is needed to increase evidence on the effectiveness of interventions to reduce health inequalities and to evaluate ongoing and newly developed policies and interventions. Where possible, evaluations should assess not only the effectiveness but also the costs of interventions tailored or targeted at lower socioeconomic groups. Funding is essential for studies that take advantage of variations in policies or practices between European countries in order to assess outcomes.

This is a complex task. The practical barriers for conducting evaluation studies mean that no single country has the capacity to build a comprehensive evidence base for tackling health inequalities. It is, therefore, essential to create opportunities for mutual intercountry learning by constructing a systematic evidence base. A clearing house for proactive identification, thorough evaluation and quick dissemination of evidence from around Europe, would enable policy-makers at the European, national and local levels to develop rational strategies for tackling health inequalities.

Acknowledgements

This paper is largely based on recent investigations that have been funded by the Health and Consumer Protection Directorate General of the EU, including the projects EUROTHINE Tackling Socioeconomic Inequalities in Health in Europe (contract no. 2003125) and the Economic Implications of Socioeconomic Inequalities in Health in the European Union (contract no. SANCO/2005/C4/Inequality/01).

References

Acheson, D. (1998) *Independent Inquiry into the Inequalities in Health Report*. London: HMSO.

Avendano, M., Aro, A.R. and Mackenbach, J.P. (2005) Socio-economic disparities in physical health in 10 European countries, in A. Börsch-Supan, A. Brugiavini, H. Jürges, J.P. Mackenbach, J. Siegrist and G. Weber (eds.) *Health, Ageing and Retirement in Europe. First Results from SHARE*. Mannheim: Mannheim Research Institute for the Economics of Aging: 89–94.

Avendano, M., Kunst, A.E., Huisman, M. et al. (2004) Educational level and stroke mortality: a comparison of 10 European populations during the 1990s. *Stroke*, 35: 432–7.

Bambra, C. and Eikemo, T.A. (2009) Welfare state regimes, unemployment and health: a comparative study of the relationship between unemployment and self-reported health in 23 European countries. *Journal of Epidemiology and Community Health*, 63: 92–8.

Bauld, L., Day, P. and Judge, K. (2008) Off target: a critical review of setting goals for reducing health inequalities in the United Kingdom. *International Journal of Health Services*, 38: 439–54.

Bauld, L., Judge, K. and Platt, S. (2007) Assessing the impact of smoking cessation services on reducing health inequalities in England: observational study. *Tobacco Control*, 16: 400–4.

Benach, J., Borrell, C. and Daponte, A. (2002) Spain, in J.P. Mackenbach and M.J. Bakker (eds.) *Reducing Inequalities in Health: A European Perspective*. London: Routledge: 262–73.

Benzeval, M. (2002) England, in J.P. Mackenbach and M.J. Bakker (eds.) *Reducing Inequalities in Health: A European Perspective*. London: Routledge: 201–13.

Benzeval, M., Judge, K. and Whitehead, M. (eds.) (1995) *Tackling Inequalities in Health: An Agenda for Action*. London: The King's Fund.

Borrell, C., Espelt, A., Rodríguez-Sanz, M. et al. (2009) Analyzing differences in the magnitude of socioeconomic inequalities in self-perceived health by countries of different political tradition in Europe. *International Journal of Health Services*, 39: 321–41.

Bowling, A. and McKee, M. (2010) Unequal access to health care in England. *British Medical Journal*, 341: c3726.

Burström, B. (2000) Inequality in the social consequences of illness: how well do people with long-term illness fare in the British and Swedish labor markets? *International Journal of Health Services*, 30: 435–51.

Cavelaars, A.E.J.M., Kunst, A.E. and Mackenbach, J.P. (1997) Socio-economic differences in risk-factors for morbidity and mortality in the European Community. An international comparison. *Journal of Health Psychology*, 2: 353–72.

Commission on Macroeconomics and Health Working Group Five (2001) *Improving health outcomes of the poor*. Geneva: World Health Organization Commission on Macroeconomics and Health.

Dahl, E., Fritzell, J., Lahelma, E. et al. (2006) Welfare state regimes and health inequalities, in J. Siegrist and M. Marmot (eds.) *Health Inequalities in Europe*. Oxford: Oxford University Press: 193–222.

Davey Smith, G., Blane, D. and Bartley, M. (1994) Explanations for socioeconomic differentials in mortality. Evidence from Britain and elsewhere. *European Journal of Public Health*, 4: 131–44.

Demarest, S., Roskam, A.-J., Cox, B. et al. (2007) Socioeconomic inequalities in leisure time physical activity, in J.P. Mackenbach, A.E. Kunst, I. Stirbu, A. Roskam and M. Schaap (eds.) *Tackling Health Inequalities in Europe: An Integrated Approach (Eurothine)*. Rotterdam, Erasmus MC: 445–54.

Department of Health (2003) *Tackling Health Inequalities: A Programme for Action*. London: The Stationery Office.

Department of Health (2005) *Tackling Health Inequalities: Status Report on the Programme for Action*. London: The Stationery Office.

Department of Health (2007) *Review of the Health Inequalities Infant Mortality PSA Target*. London: COI for the Department of Health.

Droomers, M., Schrijvers, C.T., Stronks, K., van de Mheen, D. and Mackenbach, J.P. (1999) Educational differences in excessive alcohol consumption: the role of psychosocial and material stressors. *Preventive Medicine*, 29(1): 1–10.

Droomers, M., Judge, K., Mackenbach, J.P. et al. (2007) Quantitative targets to reduce social health inequalities and tools to monitor progress in Europe, in J.P. Mackenbach, A.E. Kunst, I. Stirbu, A. Roskam and M. Schaap (eds.) *Tackling Health Inequalities in Europe: An Integrated Approach (Eurothine)*. Rotterdam, Erasmus MC: 546–66.

Eikemo, T.A. Huisman, M., Bambra, C. and Kunst, A.E. (2008a) Health inequalities according to educational level in different welfare regimes: a comparison of 23 European countries. *Sociology of Health and Illness*, 30: 565–82.

Eikemo, T.A., Kunst, A.E., Judge, K. and Mackenbach, J.P. (2008b) Class-related health inequalities are not larger in the East: a comparison of 4 European regions using the new socio-economic classification. *Journal of Epidemiology and Community Health*, 62: 1072–8.

Eikemo, T.A., Bambra, C., Joyce, K. and Dahl, E. (2008c) Welfare state regimes and income-related health inequalities: a comparison of 23 European countries. *European Journal of Public Health*, 18: 593–9.

Espelt, A., Borrell, C., Rodriquez-Sanz, M. et al. (2008a) Socioeconomic inequalities in diabetes mellitus across Europe at the beginning of the 21st century. *Diabetologia*, 51: 1971–9.

Espelt, A., Borrell, C., Rodríguez-Sanz, M. et al. (2008b) Inequalities in health by social class dimensions in European countries of different political traditions. *International Journal of Epidemiology*, 37: 1095–105.

Gaunt-Richardson, P., Amos, A., Howie, G., McKie, L. and Moore, M. (1999) *Women, Low Income and Smoking: Breaking Down the Barriers*. Edinburgh: ASH Scotland/Health Education Board for Scotland.

Gelormino, E., Bambra, C., Spadea, T., Kunst, A., Bellini, S. and Costa, G. (2007) The effects of health care reforms on health inequalities: a review and analysis of the European evidence base, in J.P. Mackenbach, A.E. Kunst, I. Stirbu, A. Roskam and M. Schaap (eds.) *Tackling Health Inequalities in Europe: An Integrated Approach (Eurothine)*. Rotterdam, Erasmus MC: 524–44.

Giskes, K., Kunst, A., Ariza, C. et al. (2007) Applying an equity lens to tobacco-control policies and their uptake in six western-European countries. *Journal of Public Health Policy*, 28: 261–80.

Huisman, M., Kunst, A.E. and Bopp, M. et al. (2005) Educational inequalities in cause-specific mortality in middle-aged and older men and women in eight western European populations. *Lancet*, 365: 493–500.

Kuijer, P.P., Visser, B. and Kemper, H.C. (1999) Job rotation as a factor in reducing physical workload at a refuse collecting department. *Ergonomics*, 42: 1167–78.

Kunst, A.E., Bos, V. and Mackenbach, J.P. (2001) Guidelines for monitoring health inequalities in the European Union. Rotterdam: Department of Public Health.

Kunst, A.E., Giskes, K. and Mackenbach, J.P. (2004) Socioeconomic inequalities in smoking in the European Union: applying an equity lens to tobacco control policies. Brussels: European Network for Smoking Prevention.

Lang, T., Nicaud, V., Slama, K. et al. (2000) Smoking cessation at the workplace. Results of a randomised controlled intervention study. Worksite physicians from the AIREL group. *Journal of Epidemiology and Community Health*, 54: 349–54.

Leinsalu, M., Vågerö, D., Kunst, A.E. (2003) Estonia 1989–2000: enormous increase in mortality differences by education. *International Journal of Epidemiology*, 32: 1081–7.

Leinsalu, M., Stirbu, I., Vågerö, D. et al. (2009) Educational inequalities in mortality in four Eastern European countries: divergence in trends during the post-communist transition from 1990 to 2000. *International Journal of Epidemiology*, 38: 512–25.

López-Azpiazu, I., Sánchez-Villegas, A., Johansson, L., Petkeviciene, J., Prättälä, R. and Martínez-González, M.A. (2003) FAIR-97–3096 Project 2003. *Journal of Human Nutrition and Dietetics*, 16: 349–64.

MacIntyre, S., Chalmers, I., Horton, R. and Smith, R. (2001) Using evidence to inform health policy: case study. *British Medical Journal*, 322: 222–5.

Mackenbach, J.P. (2006) *Health Inequalities: Europe in Profile*. London: UK Presidency of the European Union.

Mackenbach, J.P. and Bakker, M.J. (eds.) (2002) *Reducing Inequalities in Health: A European Perspective*. London: Routledge.

Mackenbach, J.P. and Bakker, M. (2003) Tackling socioeconomic inequalities in health: an analysis of recent European experiences. *Lancet*, 362: 1409–14.

Mackenbach, J.P., Meerding, W.J. and Kunst, A. (2007) *Economic Implications of Socioeconomic Inequalities in Health in the European Union.* Luxembourg: Directorate-General for Health and Consumer Protection of the European Commission.

Mackenbach, J.P., Kunst, A.E., Cavelaars, A.E., Groenhof, F. and Geurts, J.J. (1997) Socioeconomic inequalities in morbidity and mortality in western Europe. *Lancet,* 349: 1655–9.

Mackenbach, J.P., Stirbu, I., Roskam, A.J. et al. (2008) Socioeconomic inequalities in mortality and morbidity: a cross-European perspective. *New England Journal of Medicine,* 358: 2468–81.

Mäkelä, P., Valkonen, T. and Martelin, T. (1997) Contribution of deaths related to alcohol use of socioeconomic variation in mortality: register based follow up study. *British Medical Journal,* 315(7102): 211–16.

Marmot, M. and Wilkinson, R.G. (2006) *Social determinants of health,* 2nd edn. Oxford: Oxford University Press.

Menvielle, G., Kunst, A.E., Stirbu, I. et al. (2008) Educational differences in cancer mortality among women and men: a gender pattern that differs across Europe. *British Journal of Cancer,* 98: 1012–19.

Mielck, A., Kiess, R., Stirbu, I. and Kunst, A.E. (2007) Educational level and the utilisation of specialist care: results from nine European countries, in J.P. Mackenbach, A.E. Kunst, I. Stirbu, A. Roskam and M. Schaap (eds.) *Tackling Health Inequalities in Europe: An Integrated Approach (Eurothine).* Rotterdam, Erasmus MC: 456–70.

Mielck, A., Kiess, R., von dem Knesebeck, O., Stirbu, I. and Kunst, A.E. (2009) Association between foregone care and household income among the elderly in five Western European countries: analyses based on survey data from the SHARE-study. *BMC Health Services Research,* 9: 52.

Navarro, V., Muntaner, C., Borrell, C. et al. (2006) Politics and health outcomes. *Lancet,* 368: 1033–7.

Oliver, A. (2001) Health inequalities policy: do we need evidence on effectiveness? [letter to the editor]. Rapid response to: Davey Smith *et al.* How policy informs the evidence. *British Medical Journal,* 322: 184–5.

Pamuk, E. (1985) Social class inequality in mortality from 1921 to 1972 in England and Wales. *Population Studies,* 39: 17–31.

Petticrew, M., Whitehead, M., Graham, H., Macintyre, S. and Egan, M. (2004) Evidence for public health policy on inequalities I: the reality according to policymakers. *Journal of Epidemiology and Community Health,* 58: 811–16.

Prättälä, R., Berg, M.-A. and Puska, P. (1992) Diminishing or increasing contrasts? Social class variation in Finnish food consumption patterns 1979–1990. *European Journal of Clinical Nutrition,* 42(Suppl): 16–20.

Prättälä, R., Hakala, S., Roskam, A.-J.R. et al. (2009) Association between educational level and vegetable use in nine European countries. *Public Health Nutrition,* 12: 2174–82.

Programme Committee SEIH-II (2001) *Reducing Socioeconomic Inequalities in Health. Final Report and Policy Recommendations of the Programme Committee SEIH-II.* The Hague: ZorgOnderzoek Nederland.

Rosen, G. (1993) A history of public health, expanded edition. Baltimore, MD: Johns Hopkins University Press.

Roskam, A.J. and Kunst, A.E. (2008) The predictive value of different socioeconomic indicators for overweight in nine European countries. *Public Health of Nutrition,* 11: 1256–66.

Roskam, A.J., Kunst, A.E., van Oyen, H. et al. (2010) Comparative appraisal of educational inequalities in overweight and obesity among adults in 19 European countries. *International Journal of Epidemiology,* 39: 392–404.

Schaap, M.M., van Agt, H.M. and Kunst, A.E. (2008) Identification of socioeconomic groups at increased risk of smoking in European countries: looking beyond educational level. *Nicotine and Tobacco Research*, 10: 359–69.

Schaap, M.M., Kunst, A.E., Leinsalu, M., et al. (2008). Effect of nationwide tobacco control policies on smoking cessation in high and low educated groups in 18 European countries. *Tobacco Control*, 17: 248–55.

Schaap, M.M., Kunst, A.E., Leinsalu, M. et al. (2009) Female ever-smoking, education, emancipation and economic development in 19 European countries. *Social Science and Medicine*, 68(7): 1271–8.

Shkolnikov, V.M., Andreev, E.M., Jasilionis, D., Leinsalu, M., Antonova, O.A. and McKee, M. (2006) The changing relation between education and life expectancy in central and eastern Europe in the 1990s. *Journal of Epidemiology and Community Health*, 60: 875–81.

Siegrist, J. and Marmot, M. (eds.) (2006) *Health Inequalities in Europe*. Oxford: Oxford University Press.

Spadea, T., Bellini, S., Kunst, A., Stirbu, I. and Costa, G. (2010) The impact of interventions to improve attendance in female cancer screening among lower socioeconomic groups: a review. *Preventive Medicine*, 50: 159–64.

Stirbu, I., Kunst, A.E., Mielck, A. and Mackenbach, J.P. (2007) Educational inequalities in utilization of preventive services among elderly in Europe, in J.P. Mackenbach, A.E. Kunst, I. Stirbu, A. Roskam and M. Schaap (eds.) *Tackling Health Inequalities in Europe: An Integrated Approach (Eurothine)*. Rotterdam, Erasmus MC: 483–99.

Stirbu, I., Kunst, A.E., Bopp, M. et al. (2010) Educational inequalities in avoidable mortality in Europe. *Journal of Epidemiology and Community Health*, 64: 913–20.

Stronks, K. (2002) The Netherlands, in J.P. Mackenbach and M.J. Bakker (eds.) *Reducing Inequalities in Health: A European Perspective*. London: Routledge: 249–61.

Suhrcke, M., McKee, M., Sauto Arce, R., Tsolova, S. and Mortensen, J. (2005) *The Contribution of Health to the Economy in the European Union*. Brussels: European Commission.

Townsend, P. and Davidson, N. (eds.) (1992) The Black Report 1982, in P. Townsend, N. Davidson and M. Whithead (eds.) *Inequalities in Health: The Black Report and the Health Divide*, 2nd edn. London: Penguin Books: 29–213.

van der Heyden, J.H., Schaap, M.M., Kunst, A.E. et al. (2009) Socioeconomic inequalities in lung cancer mortality in 16 European populations. *Lung Cancer*, 63: 322–30.

van Oyen, H., Demarest, S., Borrell, C. et al. (2007) Inequalities in alcohol-related mortality by educational level in 16 European countries, in J.P. Mackenbach, A.E. Kunst, I. Stirbu, A. Roskam and M. Schaap (eds.) *Tackling Health Inequalities in Europe: An Integrated Approach (Eurothine)*. Rotterdam, Erasmus MC: 104–22.

Whitehead, M. (1990) *The Concepts and Principles of Equity and Health*. Copenhagen: WHO Regional Office for Europe.

Whitehead, M. (2007) A typology of actions to tackle social inequalities in health. *Journal of Epidemiology and Community Health*, 61: 473–8.

Whitehead, M., Petticrew, M., Graham, H., Macintyre, S., Bambra, C. and Egan, M. (2004) Evidence for public health policy on inequalities II: assembling the evidence jigsaw. *Journal of Epidemiology and Community Health*, 58: 817–21.

World Health Organization (1985) *Targets for Health for All by the Year 2000*. Geneva: World Health Organization.

chapter eight

Being responsive to citizens' expectations: the role of health services in responsiveness and satisfaction

Reinhard Busse, Nicole Valentine,
Suszy Lessof, Amit Prasad and
Ewout van Ginneken

Introduction

The World Health Report 2000 (WHR2000); (World Health Organization 2000) on the performance of health systems posited responsiveness to citizens' expectations as a fundamental goal. It pushed forward a debate that framed responsiveness as a valued and desired outcome of health system interventions regardless of the extent to which those interventions lead to health improvement. Health services reforms in many countries thus place ever-increasing emphasis on meeting citizens' expectations, improving responsiveness to patients and increasing both population and patient satisfaction.

In recent years, many countries have introduced reforms to enhance transparency, patient rights and entitlements and to provide choice of provider and access to services – all core elements of responsiveness. Attempts to boost efficiency (by introducing market forces), improve access and increase the quality of the services are also intended to improve each system's responsiveness to the justified expectations of the population, albeit that some of the reforms respond primarily to the articulate and advantaged.

The European Observatory's book on social health insurance (SHI) systems in western Europe (Saltman, Busse and Figueras 2004) marshals evidence on this issue. Figueras et al. (2004) showed that, on average, these systems are associated with higher levels of responsiveness. However, they hypothesized that this correlation is not directly attributable to the funding mechanism but rather results from other factors that are more pronounced in countries using SHI. For example, the benefit basket of services covered (i.e. the entitlements of the insured) have been defined more clearly. In addition, SHI countries spend, on average, a higher percentage of their GDP on health care than tax-funded systems. Such extra costs are justifiable only if they recognize the value of responding to citizens' expectations.

This chapter initially explores the basic concepts behind *responsiveness*, *satisfaction* and related terms. and the major organizations involved in this area of work, primarily WHO, but also the EU and the Picker Institute, which has developed a questionnaire for use in inpatient care (Coulter and Cleary 2001; Jenkinson, Coulter and Bruster 2002), and the European Task Force on Patient Evaluations of General Practice (EUROPEP), with its instrument to assess responsiveness in primary care (Grol et al. 2000). The chapter then describes research on comparative methodology. For example, the basic terms 'responsiveness to the legitimate expectations of the population in their interaction with the health system' and 'satisfaction of the overall population with the health system' are different but overlapping. Recently, other dimensions have been added to the debate (e.g. 'generosity of the system'), particularly through initiatives such as the Health Consumer Powerhouse.

The chapter continues by shedding some light on the objectives and achievements of some recent reforms aimed at increasing responsiveness in European health systems; it concludes with some reflections about the significance of making responsiveness a health system goal and its instrumental value in achieving other goals. For example, higher responsiveness should result in higher utilization of services and better adherence to long-term treatment plans, and therefore better health outcomes (assuming that services are effective and appropriate).

Responsiveness and satisfaction: conceptual and measurement issues

Both responsiveness and satisfaction are terms that aim to capture the degree to which health systems, or their components, are successful in responding to the expectations of the general population or a subgroup of patients within a population. A wide range of methods has been used to measure responsiveness and/or satisfaction over the last decades, most visibly in work by Blendon et al. (1990), population satisfaction questions in Eurobarometer surveys since 1996 (European Commission 1996, 1998, 1999, 2000, 2002), the Picker Institute's development of inpatient satisfaction surveys (Coulter and Cleary 2001; Jenkinson, Coulter and Bruster 2002), the EUROPEP instrument to assess general practice (Grol et al. 2000) and the measures used in WHR2000 (World Health Organization 2000).

Responsiveness and satisfaction are different but overlapping concepts. WHO defines responsiveness as meeting 'the legitimate expectations of the population for their interaction with the health system'. This implies that there can be illegitimate or unjustified expectations too, but the instrument only captures those that are regarded as legitimate. The 'satisfaction of the overall population with the health system' may be influenced by other expectations (which experts or policy-makers may consider illegitimate) and factors outside the direct control of the health care system (such as government in general). Therefore, satisfaction is likely to be more dependent on expectations than responsiveness surveys: the lower the expectations, the higher the satisfaction with the actual system and vice versa. WHO initially used vignettes in its responsiveness methodology in order to correct for different expectations but this approach was dropped because of the complex data requirements. It is extremely difficult to adjust for variations in expectations between countries and this has not been achieved with any approach to date.

Responsiveness captures detailed aspects of the system that users encounter. Satisfaction can include the satisfaction of the whole population – regular (e.g. those with chronic illness) and irregular users as well as those who do not utilize the system (but still pay for it). Unlike similar measures in the quality-of-life and satisfaction domains, responsiveness has an additional criterion that requires self-reports to be based on one (or several) actual experience(s) with health services in the respondents' recent past (e.g. previous year). Usually these experiences are based on some type of interaction with the health system – with a specific person, a communication campaign or another type of event or action that did not entail direct personal interactions.

The WHO instrument focuses on what happened during actual contact rather than eliciting a respondent's satisfaction with, or expectations of, the health system in general. Consequently, it has much in common with patient satisfaction instruments such as those developed by the Picker Institute. These usually contain a question regarding a general assessment of the care received but are based on patients' assessments of specific, predefined dimensions of care. They may rather more accurately be termed patient responsiveness surveys.

All the responsiveness and satisfaction surveys mentioned so far are based on surveys among health system users and/or the general population rather than (for example) expert opinion or facility audits. This differentiates them from approaches based on an expert assessment of published data and health system characteristics. The most high profile of these approaches is the annual *Euro Health Consumer Index* produced by the Health Consumer Powerhouse (Health Consumer Powerhouse 2006, 2007, 2008, 2009) (discussed below).

Responsiveness to legitimate expectations: methodology and results

The WHO measure aims to capture the responsiveness of the whole health system to the whole population (so far it has been applied mostly to those with ambulatory and/or inpatient encounters) by examining what actually happens when the system comes into contact with an individual. This is conceptually different from either a population's general satisfaction with its health system or patients' satisfaction with the care they receive (Üstün et al. 2001).

Conceptualizing and measuring responsiveness

In preparation for WHR2000, an extensive literature review, drawing on disciplines including sociology, anthropology, ethics, health economics and management, sought to elicit what people value most in their interactions with the health system (De Silva 2000). This was used to select a common set of seven dimensions (or domains) that characterize the concept of responsiveness. Three were grouped under 'respect for persons' (dignity, confidentiality and autonomy) and four under 'client orientations'.

The data presented in the WHR 2000 (World Health Organization 2000) were based on expert opinions but WHO consequently undertook two large population surveys in a number of countries. The Multicountry Survey Study in 2000/2001 (MCS study; Üstün et al. 2001) and the World Health Survey in 2002 (WHS; Üstün et al. 2003) used mainly interviews but also partly postal surveys (in the MCS study). Both surveys include two major categories (inpatient and ambulatory care) within responsiveness, each with a total of eight domains; 'communication' was added as an eighth dimension (most closely related to the 'respect for persons' group). The detailed descriptions of the dimensions, the weighing of each dimension in the WHR 2000 as well as the questions used in the two surveys are given in Table 8.1.

Interviewees in the MCS study were asked to rate their experiences over the past 12 months. While the questions regarding six of the eight domains were relevant for both inpatient and ambulatory care, only inpatients were asked about social support and only outpatients about the quality of basic amenities. All domains included a summary rating question (scaled 1–5, from very good to very bad). In addition, several domains included questions on how often a particular experience had occurred during encounters with the health system (scaled 1–4, from always to never).

Table 8.2 shows the available results for 13 of the EU15 countries (belonging to the EU before May 2004) in the MCS survey: five SHI countries (Luxembourg, Germany, Belgium, France, the Netherlands), seven tax-financed systems (Ireland, United Kingdom, Sweden, Finland, Spain, Italy, Portugal) and a mixed system (Greece). The WHO's weights were derived from the frequencies with which respondents ranked the different elements first. Prompt attention was perceived as the most important and choice of provider the least. When these are applied to the different components of responsiveness, the United Kingdom scored best for inpatient care (followed by Luxembourg and Ireland); Ireland scored highest for ambulatory care (followed by Germany and the United Kingdom). Unfortunately, no longitudinal data are available yet so interpretation of the results for the impact of system characteristics and reforms on responsiveness should be cautious.

Except for confidentiality, the SHI countries scored (on average) 2% to 8% higher than tax-funded countries. The greatest and most relevant advantages are seen in the area of choice. Clearly, this is not a consequence of the SHI funding mechanism itself but rather of deliberate decisions to allow patient choice of provider in these countries (introduced later and often more restricted in other countries).

Table 8.1 Dimensions of responsiveness set by WHO and questions used to measure it in two population surveys

Dimension	WHR2000 grouping (weighting, %)	MCS study 2000/2001: questions used	WHS 2002: questions used
Dignity: respectful treatment and communication	Respect for persons (16.7)	How often did doctors, nurses or other health care providers treat you with respect? How often did the office staff, such as receptionists or clerks there, treat you with respect? How often were your physical examinations and treatments done in a way that your privacy was respected? How would you rate your experience of being treated with dignity?	How would you rate: your experience of being greeted and talked to respectfully? the way your privacy was respected during physical examinations and treatments?
Confidentiality: confidentiality of personal information	Respect for persons (16.7)	How often were talks with your doctor, nurse or other health care provider done privately so other people who you did not want to hear could not overhear what was said? How often did your doctor, nurse or other health care provider keep your personal information confidential? This means that anyone whom you did not want informed could not find out about your medical conditions.	How would you rate: the way the health services ensured you could talk privately to health care providers? the way your personal information was kept confidential?
Autonomy: involvement in decisions	Respect for persons (16.7)	How often did doctors, nurses or other health care providers involve you in deciding about the care, treatment or tests? How often did doctors, nurses or other health care providers ask your permission before starting the treatment or tests? Rate your experience of getting involved in making decisions about your care or treatment.	How would you rate: your experience of being involved in making decisions about your health care or treatment? your experience of getting information about other types of treatment or tests?
Communication: clarity of communication	Not included	How often did doctors, nurses or other health care providers listen carefully to you? How often did doctors, nurses or other health care providers explain things in a way you could understand? How often did doctors, nurses or other health care providers give you time to ask questions about your health problem or treatment? Rate your experience of how well health care providers communicated with you in the last 12 months.	How would you rate: the experience of how clearly health care providers explained things to you? your experience of getting enough time to ask questions about your health problem or treatment?

(continued)

Table 8.1 Dimensions of responsiveness set by WHO and questions used to measure it in two population surveys *(continued)*

Dimension	WHR2000 grouping (weighting, %)	MCS study 2000/2001: questions used	WHS 2002: questions used
Prompt attention: convenient travel and short waiting times	Client-orientation (20)	How often did you get care as soon as you wanted? How would you rate your experience of getting prompt attention at the health services?	How would you rate: the travelling time? the amount of time you waited before being attended to?
Quality of basic amenities: surroundings	Client-orientation (15)	How would you rate the basic quality of the waiting room, for example space, seating and fresh air? How would you rate the cleanliness of the place? How would you rate the quality of the surroundings, for example space, seating, fresh air and cleanliness of the health services?	How would you rate: the cleanliness of the rooms inside the facility, including toilets? the amount of space you had?
Access to family and community support: contact with outside world and maintenance of regular activities	Client-orientation (10)	How big a problem, if any, was it to get the hospital to allow your family and friends to take care of your personal needs, such as bringing you your favourite food, soap, etc? How big a problem, if any, was it to have the hospital allow you to practise religious or traditional observances if you wanted to? How would you rate your experience of how the hospital allowed you to interact with family, friends and to continue your social and/or religious customs?	How would you rate: the ease of having family and friends visit you? your [your child's] experience of staying in contact with the outside world when you [your child] were in hospital?
Choice: choice of health care provider	Client-orientation (5)	How big a problem, if any, was it to get a health care provider you were happy with? How big a problem, if any, was it to get to use other health services other than the one you usually went to? How would you rate your experience of being able to use a health care provider or service of your choice?	How would you rate: the freedom you had to choose the health care providers that attended to you?

Source: World Health Organization 2000; Valentine et al. 2003.
Notes: WHR2000: *World Health Report 2000* (World Health Organization 2000); MCS: Multicountry Survey Study, 2000/2001 (Üstün et al. 2001); WHS: World Health Survey, 2002 (Üstün et al. 2003).

Table 8.2 WHO's components of responsiveness used for EU15 countries in the Multicountry Survey Study 2000/2001

| | Respect for persons | | | | | | | | Client orientation | | | | | | Country-weighted mean | | Relative order | |
| | Dignity | | Confidentiality | | Autonomy | | Communication | | Prompt attention | | Quality of basic amenities | Access to family and community support | Choice | | | | | |
	In	Amb	In	Amb	In	Amb	In	Amb	In	Amb	Amb	In	In	Amb	In	Amb	In	Amb
Ireland	91	98	92	94	75	87	91	94	82	95	88	90	88	98	87	94	2	1
United Kingdom	94	95	90	96	81	81	85	85	82	81	77	95	93	98	88	87	1	3
Sweden	97	95	88	86	81	83	89	88	74	82	74	95	87	94	86	86	4	4
Luxembourg	92	91	83	82	83	83	90	81	83	82	74	94	88	98	87	85	2	9
Germany	85	90	83	87	74	84	74	85	85	94	83	89	85	98	82	89	8	2
Belgium	88	92	79	81	75	79	87	87	73	84	75	91	97	100	83	86	5	4
France	91	95	83	85	71	71	88	89	72	81	77	90	96	100	83	86	5	4
Netherlands	87	94	75	77	72	80	82	85	85	89	72	96	88	97	83	86	5	4
Finland	85	95	83	86	76	84	86	88	81	86	72	87	60	83	79	86	9	4
Spain	85	83	83	83	61	64	84	79	78	83	71	80	82	85	79	79	9	10
Italy	74	73	68	69	53	58	74	73	78	75	61	79	90	98	74	73	11	11
Portugal	66	71	70	71	66	67	71	76	71	76	65	74	78	85	71	73	12	11
Greece	61	63	79	81	44	48	49	53	61	71	59	78	71	72	62	64	13	13

Sources: Modified from Figueras et al. 2004; based on data in Valentine et al. 2003.
Notes: Countries are sorted by average level of overall responsiveness for inpatients and outpatients; no data are available for other countries; In: Inpatient care; Amb: Ambulatory care.

The large differences within the country groups confirm that the funding mechanism is not the determinant of higher levels of responsiveness. Countries that choose SHI contributions rather than taxation put more emphasis on certain dimensions of responsiveness, particularly on choice and autonomy, followed by dignity, access to family and community support and quality of basic amenities. On average, they also scored higher on communication and prompt attention. However, France, for example, scored lower for prompt attention in inpatient care than most tax-financed countries, while the United Kingdom scored higher than almost all of the SHI countries for both autonomy and choice.

Given the more restricted character of choice in the United Kingdom compared with SHI countries, this raises the question of intercountry comparability. Can the same level of care receive comparatively high responsiveness scores when lower expectations are met but lower responsiveness scores if expectations are high and therefore not met? This question is addressed below.

Responsiveness and population expectations

The WHS 2002 (Üstün et al. 2003) collected data on responsiveness, as well as other aspects related to health systems performance. Data were collected from 69 countries globally, including 29 Member States of the WHO European Region.

As described above, respondents were asked to rate their last encounter with the (ambulatory or inpatient) health care system on a five-point scale across eight domains. In addition, the survey contained vignettes depicting a variety of situations that might arise in interactions with the health care system. Respondents were asked to rate these hypothetical experiences on a five-point scale ranging from very bad to very good, so as to be able to assess comparability of responses. Five vignettes were used for choice and ten vignettes for every other domain. Available data on both responsiveness and expectations are given in Table 8.3. The data show wide variations in responsiveness scores – from 55.8 to 91.5 in outpatient care and from 51.6 to 90.3 for inpatient care. However, there were far fewer variations in expectations (56.3–64.3 in ambulatory care; 56.6–64.3 in inpatient care).

Table 8.4 depicts the five countries with the highest average expectations for each of the eight domains, grouped by 'respect for persons' (including 'communication') and 'client orientation').

On average, Norwegians reported the highest expectations for respect-for-persons domains. While Sweden and Denmark also featured commonly among the five countries with the highest expectations in these domains, there is a different pattern of expectations for client-orientation domains. Spain had the highest expectations for prompt attention and basic amenities but people from central and eastern European and former Soviet countries also reported relatively high expectations for these domains.

It is noteworthy that Austria showed both the lowest (overall) expectation scores and the highest responsiveness score. The country with the lowest responsiveness score (Ukraine) had comparatively high expectation scores.

Table 8.3 WHO's components of responsiveness for 29 available European countries in the World Health Survey 2002

Country	Overall responsiveness (average ambulatory and inpatient score)	Ambulatory responsiveness score	Inpatient responsiveness score	Ambulatory expectations score	Inpatient expectations score
Austria	90.6	91.5	89.7	56.3	56.6
Luxembourg	90.4	90.4	90.3	62.3	61.4
Belgium	90.2	91.4	88.9	62.3	61.7
Denmark	85.9	89.2	82.5	62.5	62.3
Greece	85.2	85.3	85.0	59.7	59.2
France	85.6	89.1	82.1	62.2	61.6
Netherlands	84.3	89.1	79.4	60.1	59.5
Czech Republic	84.3	84.9	83.6	60.8	60.2
Ireland	84.2	82.2	86.1	61.0	60.6
Germany	83.9	86.9	80.8	60.1	60.1
United Kingdom	82.5	83.8	81.1	61.4	61.4
Israel	81.8	83.1	80.4	60.3	59.4
Finland	81.7	88.3	75.0	62.0	61.8
Georgia	80.0	81.5	78.4	60.9	60.1
Spain	79.2	81.0	78.3	64.3	63.7
Bosnia and Herzegovina	78.1	77.2	79.0	62.0	61.6
Slovenia	77.8	80.4	75.1	63.2	63.0

(continued)

Table 8.3 WHO's components of responsiveness for 29 available European countries in the World Health Survey 2002 *(continued)*

Country	Overall responsiveness (average ambulatory and inpatient score)	Ambulatory responsiveness score	Inpatient responsiveness score	Ambulatory expectations score	Inpatient expectations score
Sweden	77.6	77.1	78.1	63.6	63.3
Hungary	77.0	79.2	74.8	59.0	58.6
Norway	76.9	80.3	73.4	64.3	64.3
Slovakia	75.8	75.4	76.1	59.2	59.0
Portugal	73.2	68.2	78.1	60.5	61.0
Estonia	72.5	74.5	70.5	62.6	62.1
Italy	70.7	73.6	67.7	62.4	61.7
Latvia	70.4	72.5	68.2	64.2	63.7
Kazakhstan	69.5	68.7	70.2	61.5	60.9
Croatia	64.9	70.7	59.0	63.5	63.2
Russian Federation	57.7	55.8	59.5	62.4	61.9
Ukraine	55.6	59.5	51.6	62.9	62.1

Source: Üstün et al. 2003.
Note: Countries sorted by level of overall responsiveness.

Table 8.4 Five countries with the highest expectations for each responsiveness domain under respect for persons and client orientation

Domain	Countries
Dignity	Norway, Sweden, Belgium, Denmark, Luxembourg
Confidentiality	Norway, Sweden, United Kingdom, Italy, Denmark
Autonomy	Norway, Sweden, Ireland, Spain, United Kingdom
Communication	Norway, Spain, Slovenia, Latvia, Denmark
Prompt attention	Spain, Ukraine, Latvia, Croatia, Russian Federation
Basic amenities	Spain, Luxembourg, France, Belgium, Italy
Social support	Portugal, Norway, Slovenia, Sweden, Croatia
Choice	Bosnia and Herzegovina, Norway, Georgia, Latvia, Croatia

Source: Üstün et al. 2003 (World Health Survey 2002).

This suggests that people with different expectations rate similar experiences differently. For example, those with low expectations may rate their last experience as good while those with higher expectations may rate an experience with similar characteristics and quality as only moderate.

Figure 8.1 shows the average responsiveness score when the 29 countries of WHO European Region were divided into three approximately equal groups (10, 10 and 9 countries) according to their differing levels of expectations –

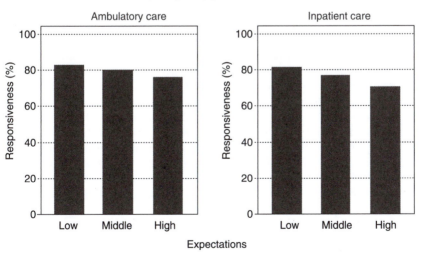

Figure 8.1 Relationship between overall responsiveness and population expectations for 29 countries of the WHO European Region

Source: Üstün et al. 2003 (World Health Survey 2002).

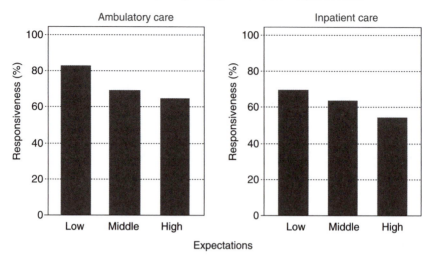

Figure 8.2 Relationship between responsiveness for choice of health care provider and population expectations for 29 countries of the WHO European Region

Source: Üstün et al. 2003 (World Health Survey 2002).

from low to high. For both, ambulatory and inpatient care, the responsiveness score (which is not adjusted for expectations) decreases as the population expectations increase. Also, the *t*-test for equality of means reveals that the average responsiveness scores for countries with high expectations are significantly different from those for countries with low expectations.

Only prompt attention, communication and choice show a statistically significant association within individual domains. Figure 8.2 shows an example of choice of health care provider. Populations with low expectations about choice described substantially higher responsiveness in terms of choice in ambulatory care than populations with higher expectations. For inpatient care, responsiveness also decreased with increasing expectations.

In a survey conducted by the Picker Institute around the same time, respondents in eight countries were interviewed about the communication with their physician, their involvement in treatment decisions (autonomy) and choice of providers (Coulter and Jenkinson 2005). The study showed that expectations between countries differed quite markedly; for example Spaniards expected considerable less autonomy than Germans. Table 8.5 shows that Swedes expected very little choice of specialists (only 31%), while almost all Germans expected such choice (97%). Spaniards ranged between these but were the most satisfied regarding their actual opportunities to make choices (even though they were not satisfied that they were getting sufficient information to do so), with both Swedes and Germans only moderately satisfied in this regard. Polish respondents' expectations were as high as those of the Germans but were met to a much less extent.

Table 8.5 Expectations for and rating of choice of different types of provider in eight European countries, 2002: countries sorted from left to right by responsiveness rating

	Spain	Switzerland	Germany	Italy	Sweden	Slovenia	United Kingdom	Poland
Expectation (% answering yes)								
Primary care doctor	89	93	98	86	86	98	87	98
Specialist	86	84	97	83	31	87	79	95
Hospital	78	85	94	85	54	86	80	94
Information to support choice of provider (% answering yes)								
Primary care doctor	30	52	52	53	31	45	40	43
Specialist	23	41	42	53	23	25	28	32
Hospital	32	52	42	54	36	30	35	35
Rating (average; 1 very bad; 5 very good)	3.93	3.86	3.35	3.28	3.19	3.05	3.05	2.67

Source: Coulter and Jenkinson 2005.
Notes: Questions asked: *Expectation*: 'In general, if you need to [consult a primary care doctor/ consult a specialist doctor/go to hospital] do you think you should have a free choice?'; *Information to support choice of provider*: 'Do you feel you have sufficient information about [primary care doctors/specialist doctors/hospitals] to choose the best one for you?'; *Rating*: 'Overall, how would you rate the opportunities for patients in this country to make choices about their health care?' (average of answer categories: 1, very bad; 2, bad; 3, moderate; 4, good; 5, very good).

Three main conclusions for European countries can be drawn from the analyses above.

- Some intercountry variations in responsiveness may be explained by differences in population expectations.[1] This indicates that expectations-based adjustment to the scores may be necessary before meaningful intercountry comparisons can be made.
- For a smaller set of domains, there was a significant correlation between responsiveness and expectations. These included choice, prompt attention and communication.
- Some country populations have relatively higher expectations of certain domains of responsiveness than others, signalling that there might also be differences regarding the valuation of which dimensions are most – and thus least – important.

Health care expenditure and responsiveness

The situation with SHI countries noted above raises the question of whether the amount spent on health care explains differences in responsiveness. Keeping all other factors constant, well-resourced health systems should be able to afford better quality care and receive better responsiveness ratings. A simple correlation for the result for each responsiveness domain (keeping development contexts constant by looking at correlations within World Bank country-income groups) was used to analyse whether higher health expenditures are associated with higher responsiveness (Valentine et al. 2009). In general, the results show a positive association across many of the domains for most country-income groupings. Especially for high-income countries, there are clear correlations between total health care expenditure and levels of responsiveness. If public expenditure alone is taken into account, there are correlations with even more domains. This suggests a more direct impact on levels of responsiveness – in other words, that private expenditure does not (or only marginally) contributes to higher levels of responsiveness. However, increasing levels of health expenditures are no guarantee that responsiveness will improve. Conversely, lower responsiveness is associated with lower coverage and greater inequity in access.

Population satisfaction: methodology and results

In principle, the concept of population satisfaction with the whole health system is straightforward. In fact, it is difficult to measure satisfaction as the answers to all questionnaires depend on the specific wording of the question asked as well as the response categories provided. In the circumstances discussed in this chapter, these answers depend particularly on factors not yet well understood: (i) the context in which a survey takes place (e.g. coloured by recent media coverage of scandals, fraud or underprovision of services), (ii) no differentiation between the system as a whole and certain subsectors about which the respondent may be more knowledgeable, and (iii) the inability to differentiate between the health care system and government in general.

These caveats need to be kept in mind when drawing international comparisons. Comparisons of absolute levels of satisfaction should be treated with great caution. Satisfaction data incorporate underlying expectations so that low satisfaction may mean high expectations that are unmet. Satisfaction would be higher in other countries with similar health care but lower expectations.

Table 8.6 incorporates data from different population surveys over the last decades. All but one share a common focus on the broader health system, but the actual questions – and, therefore, the range of answers which can be considered positive or negative – differ between surveys (see notes to Table 8.6). In the final column (L), results of a survey focusing on the local area of the respondents are presented; they can be contrasted with the results regarding the national systems acquired at the same time (column K).

The actual percentages of those answering that they are satisfied are – in addition to varying expectations and their assessment of the situation at any given point in time – dependent on (i) the exact phrasing of the question and (ii) the number of answer categories. Denmark provides a good example of the former: In 1998, 91% of respondents were satisfied 'with the way health care runs' (*Eurobarometer 49*; European Commission 1998), while only 48% were satisfied 'with health services' (*Eurobarometer 50.1*; European Commission (1999); apparently Danes see a distinct difference between these terms. Regarding the latter, the relatively high 2008 Gallup results (Brown and Khoury 2009) should be treated with caution as only two response categories were possible (positive and negative), while all other surveys presented at least three possibilities. Given such semantic and methodological complexities, most attention should be devoted to the relative position of countries within the particular surveys.

In this respect, the positive development in Austria is most striking. Austrians were only fairly satisfied in the 1970s (rank 4 of 6) and as late as 1996 (7/15) but were much more satisfied in 1998 (3/15), 1999/2000 (1/15), 2002 (2/15) and 2008 (3/15). Similar positive trends can be seen in Belgium (5/15 in 1996, 3/15 in 1999/2000 and 2002, 2/15 in 2008) and Spain[2] (albeit at a lower level), while Finland has high scores continuously (in spite of the drastic cuts in public health finances in the first half of the 1990s). In contrast, (relative) satisfaction figures have decreased in the United Kingdom (moving from first position in the 1970s to 11/15 in 1996, 9/15 in 1999/2000, 11/15 in 2002 and 10/15 in 2008), Ireland and, to a lesser degree, Germany (from 3/6 in the 1970s, 7/15 in 1996, 10/15 in 1999/2000 and 8/15 in 2002 to 12/15 in 2008). Greece, Italy and Portugal (the last at least until recently) score continuously low, with Italy never higher than 12/15 and Greece never higher than 14/15.

The 2008 Gallup poll (Brown and Khoury 2009) is interesting as it is the only one where respondents were asked to differentiate between the 'national health care or medical system' and 'health care in their city or area'. While the answers are similar for many countries, there are striking differences in both directions: While 87% of the Germans were very satisfied with the local availability of quality health care (the fifth highest result in the EU15), the positive rating of the system was more than 30 percentage points lower. In contrast, 85% of Finns were satisfied with their system, but only 66% with health care in their area (only 11th place in the EU15), possibly reflecting access problems in a sparsely populated country – or that the performance of responsible authorities at different levels are rated differently (i.e. the municipalities responsible for providing services get much worse marks than the national government for steering and regulating the system).

Patient surveys of providers: methodology and results

As mentioned above, patient surveys of particular providers constitute a third pillar of data. Usually, they belong more to responsiveness than to satisfaction as they are based on (i) predetermined domains and (ii) patients' actual health service encounters. They are shown here as they partly contradict the responsiveness data described in the previous section. Surveys are available for

Table 8.6 Satisfaction (%) with country's health care system or availability of quality health care in city/area in EU15 countries, various surveys 1973/1976–2008; countries sorted according to results of 2008 survey

	Country's health care system										Health care in city or area	
	1973/76 (A)	1988/91 (B)	1996 (C)	1998 (D)	1998 (E)	1999/2000 (F)	2002 (G)	2004 (H)	2007 (I)	2008 (J)	2008 (K)	2008 (L)
Luxembourg			71	67	50	72	58				90	90
Belgium			70	63	57	77	65				88	91
Finland	71		86	81	78	74	73				85	66
Austria	79		63	73	71	83	67				84	93
France		41	65	65	59	78	64	65		23	83	83
Sweden		32	67	58	46	59	48				79	77
Denmark			90	91	48	76	52				77	86
Netherlands	84	47	73	70	70	73	46		42		77	89
Spain		21ᵃ	36	43	31	38	46	42		37	77	74
United Kingdom	85	27	48	57	49	56	31	32	26	17	73	85
Portugal			20	16	6	24	14				58	64
Germany	81	41	66	58	43	50	47	28	20	20	54	87
Italy	38	12	16	20	15	26	31	21	20	13	53	57
Greece			18	16	11	19	19				45	52
Ireland			50	58	23	48	20				40	64

Sources: A: Pescosolido, Boyer and Tsui 1985; B: Blendon et al. 1990, 1991; C: European Commission 1996 (Eurobarometer 44.3, conducted February–April 1996); D: European Commission 1998 (Eurobarometer 49, conducted April–May 1998); E: European Commission 1999 (Eurobarometer 50.1, conducted November–December 1999); F: European Commission 2000 (Eurobarometer 52.1, conducted November–December 1999); G: European Commission 2002 (Eurobarometer 57.2, conducted April–June 2002); H: Taylor 2004 (Harris Poll conducted in June 2004; I: Taylor 2008 (Harris Poll conducted in January 2008; J: Schoen et al. 2007 (Commonwealth Fund International Health Policy Survey 2007; K,L: Brown and Khoury 2009 (Gallup World Poll 2008).

Notes: A: level of satisfaction very good or good; B,G,l: 'On the whole the system works pretty well, and only minor changes are necessary to make it work better' (as opposed to 'There are some good things in our health care system, but fundamental changes are needed to make it work better' and 'Our health care system has so much wrong with it that we need to completely rebuild it'); C,D: 'In general, would you say you are very satisfied, fairly satisfied, neither satisfied nor dissatisfied, fairly dissatisfied or very dissatisfied with the way health care runs in (our country)?', very or fairly satisfied; E: 'And, on a scale from 1 to 10, how satisfied are you with health services in (our country)?', answers 7, 8, 9 or 10; F: 'Please tell me whether you are very satisfied, fairly satisfied, not very satisfied or not at all satisfied with each of the following? ... (our country)'s health-care system in general', very or fairly satisfied; H: 'Feel positively about health care system (in my country)'; J: 'How do you think (country) is doing in regard to health care?: very well, well or neither well nor badly' (as opposed to 'badly' and 'very badly'); K: 'Have confidence in (own) national health care or medical system' (as opposed to 'no confidence'); L: 'Satisfied with the availability of quality health care in (own) city or area' (as opposed to 'dissatisfied').

inpatient and for general practitioner care, the latter being the most important component of ambulatory care.

Inpatient care

Satisfaction surveys among inpatients have become regular features in many countries of the European region but are seldom comparable, either within or, especially, between countries. The Picker Institute questionnaire is an exception. This survey asks inpatients to describe a range of aspects of their care upon discharge. It distinguishes seven dimensions of patient-centred care that overlap with the areas of responsiveness but draws different boundaries between them.

Information, communication and education. This includes clinical status, progress and prognosis, processes of care, facilitation of autonomy, self-care and health promotion.

Coordination and integration of care. This includes clinical care, ancillary and support services, and front-line care.

Physical comfort. This encompasses pain management, help with activities of daily living, surroundings and hospital environment.

Emotional support and alleviation of fear and anxiety. This includes clinical status, treatment and prognosis, impact of illness on self and family and the financial impact of illness.

Respect for patients' values, preferences and expressed needs. This includes impact of illness and treatment on quality of life, the patient's involvement in decision-making and their dignity, needs and autonomy.

Involvement of family and friends. This includes social and emotional support, involvement in decision-making, support for caregiving, and impact on family dynamics and functioning.

Transition and continuity. This last includes information about medication and danger signals to look out for after leaving hospital; coordination and discharge planning; and clinical, social, physical and financial support.

Results collected between 1998 and 2000 showed that patients in the United Kingdom reported more problems than those in Germany, for example (Table 8.7), even though their responsiveness was higher according to the data presented in Table 8.2. It has to be borne in mind, however, that the Picker instrument was used in fewer than 10 hospitals in each European country, which clearly differs from the population-oriented sampling strategy used in WHO responsiveness surveys.

Care by general practitioners

The results of an evaluation of general practice care differ from those of WHO MCS survey. EUROPEP surveyed more than 17,000 patients in 10 European countries on 23 items. Table 8.8 depicts selected results, namely for the four items with the highest overall scores and for the four items with the lowest

Table 8.7 Percentage of patients reporting problems with hospital, 1998–2000: countries sorted by overall evaluation from left to right

	Switzerland	Germany	Sweden	United Kingdom
Overall level of care NOT GOOD	4	7	7	9
Problems with:				
information and education	17	20	23	29
coordination of care	13	17	n/a	22
physical comfort	3	7	4	8
emotional support	15	22	26	27
respect for patients' preferences	16	18	21	31
involvement of family and friends	12	17	15	28
continuity and transition	30	41	40	45
Would not recommend this hospital to friends/family	4	5	3	8

Source: Modified from Figueras et al. 2004; based on data in Coulter and Cleary 2001.
Notes: No data are available for other countries; n/a: Not available.

overall scores (Grol et al. 2000). In comparison with the data on outpatient care responsiveness, the comparatively bad results are particularly contradictory for the United Kingdom. Sweden achieved worse results than Germany, Belgium and the Netherlands (even though it scored roughly the same as those countries in the responsiveness surveys reported in Table 8.2). Again, this may reflect the sampling strategy, the EUROPEP was only used by patients in a limited number of practices (around 36 per country), or it may reflect the more specific questions asked.

In summary, different questionnaires with different items reach different results. In some instances, this has a large impact on rankings. All methodologies are, therefore, rightly subject to further extensive critical debate.

Comparative methodology and results

The WHO concept of responsiveness was developed following an extensive literature review covering disciplines such as sociology, anthropology, ethics, health economics and management and was designed to elicit what people value most in their interactions with the health system. This review formed the basis of the set of eight domains mentioned above (De Silva 2000). Many of these domains are present in existing patient questionnaires (e.g. the Picker surveys or the EUROPEP evaluation), but none of these adequately captures all of the dimensions that emerged from the literature review. Therefore, WHO developed an instrument (questionnaire) specific to responsiveness in order to cover all of the dimensions valued by individuals when they interact with health systems.

Table 8.9 demonstrates that the questions on the population's satisfaction with the health system in general (or the need to reform it) are in a separate

Table 8.8 Evaluations of general practice care in 10 European countries, circa 1998 (%): countries sorted from left to right by overall evaluation

	Switzerland	Slovenia	Germany	Belgium	Iceland	Netherlands	Sweden	Norway	Denmark	United Kingdom
Overall evaluation	91	89	88	87	83	80	78	76	74	72
1. Keeping records and data confidential	96	97	94	97	97	95	88	91	96	91
2. Listening to you	96	95	92	93	93	89	85	85	79	83
3. Making you feel you had time during consultations	96	92	90	92	93	88	85	78	75	80
4. Providing quick services for urgent problems	96	89	95	93	86	85	84	83	81	71
. . . 15 other items										
20. Offering you services for preventing disease	84	85	85	77	74	76	75	67	68	74
21. Getting through to the practice on the telephone	96	92	95	93	75	71	67	56	53	62
22. Being able to speak to the GP on the telephone	91	93	87	90	72	72	65	54	59	51
23. Waiting time in the waiting room	79	60	70	66	70	61	65	57	59	50

Source: Modified from Figueras et al. 2004; based on data in Grol et al. 2000.
Notes: No data are available for other countries; GP: General practitioner.

Table 8.9 Important 'prototypical' questionnaires/studies/surveys/rankings with questions on the responsiveness domain; sorted by date of first use

	Blendon and Eurobarometer[a]	Picker inpatient survey[b]	EUROPEP GP practice evaluation[c]	WHR 2000[d]	MCS study, WHS[e]	Euro Health Consumer Index[f]	Gallup Poll[g]
Data sources used	A	B	B	C, D	E	C, D	A
Outcomes							
Health-adjusted life years				X			
Potential years of life lost						X	
Specific health-related outcomes						X[h]	
Responsiveness/satisfaction							
Respect for dignity		X	X	X	X		
Respect for confidentiality		X	X	X	X		
Respect for autonomy		X	X	X	X	X	
Communication		X	X		X		
Access to prompt attention/waiting			X	X	X	X	
Basic amenities			X	X	X		
Access to social support networks		X		X	X		
Choice of institution/care provider				X	X	X	
Patients rights and information						X	
Range of benefit basket ('generosity' of system)						X	
Access to pharmaceuticals						X	
Satisfaction with country's health system	X						X
Satisfaction with local availability of health care							X
Fairness in financing				X			

Source: Based on [a]Blendon et al. 1990; European Commission 1996, 1998, 1999, 2000, 2002; [b]Jenkinson, Coulter and Bruster 2002; [c]Grol et al. 2000; [d]World Health Organization 2000; [e]Üstün et al. 2001, 2003; [f]Health Consumer Powerhouse 2006, 2007, 2008, 2009; [g]Brown and Khoury 2009.
Notes: A: Randomly selected population; B: Patients treated by certain providers; C: Routine data; D: Experts; E: Randomly selected population with health care encounter; [h]See Table 8.10 for details.

category in the Blendon, Eurobarometer and Gallup surveys and do not overlap directly with any of WHO responsiveness domains, which, in turn, were an expansion over the previously developed patient surveys. The more recent *Euro Health Consumer Index* only partially overlaps with WHO responsiveness domains; its overlap with the 'respect for persons' domains is particularly weak as only aspects of autonomy are covered. Table 8.9 also includes information on the data sources; that is, whether the results are based on a survey (general population or patients), routine data or expert judgement.

Besides autonomy, the *Euro Health Consumer Index* retains the main contents of WHO's dimensions of prompt attention and choice (even they are named differently), but it expands the 'client-orientations' by adding the dimensions of patient rights and information (with questions on the existence of patient rights legislation, right to a second opinion, access to own medical record, readily available register of doctors, or a provider catalogue with quality listing); e-health (e.g. on penetration of electronic medical records); range and reach of services provided (until 2007, generosity of public health care), with indicators relating to the number of publicly paid cataract operations and kidney transplants or the inclusion of dental care in the benefit basket; and pharmaceuticals (including the degree of cost sharing or the speed with which new cancer drugs are deployed in the system). The *Euro Health Consumer Index* also includes several dimensions related to outcomes, the results of which also influence its overall ranking; for example, in the 2009 index, Sweden is only placed 7th because of its number one ranking in the outcomes – without these, it would have scored considerably lower. Table 8.10 provides a full listing of the indicators used in the so-called sub-disciplines as well as their weighing in the 2006–2009 versions.

Different dimensions may very well produce different results that reflect the selection of weights, domains and indicators (i.e. surveys capture different phenomena), differences in the methodology of data collection (e.g. sampling) and interpretation, or actual differences resulting from changes in the various health systems over time.

Table 8.11 provides data on the ranks of the EU15 countries in the EUROPEP instrument to evaluate general practitioner practices; the WHO responsiveness surveys on outpatient and inpatient care, respectively; the *Eurobarometer 57.2* question on satisfaction; the Gallup Poll questions on satisfaction with national and local health care; and the 2007–2009 versions of the *Euro Health Consumer Index*.

The results of these assessments are sometimes inconsistent or contradictory and are difficult to interpret. Overall, no individual survey enables any clear conclusions to be drawn about the differences in the degree of responsiveness between health systems and even less about the health system strategies that may explain them. Taken together, they provide a slightly clearer picture (particularly for countries that score consistently high or low) but still do not provide conclusive advice about the characteristics of the health systems that 'explain' the differences.

For example, regarding our initial conclusion that responsiveness seems to be higher in SHI countries, the data show that, on average, these countries (i.e. Austria, Belgium, France, Germany, Luxembourg and the Netherlands) fare

Table 8.10 Weighing and indicators used in the sub-disciplines of the Euro Health Consumer indices 2006–2009

Sub-discipline	Weighing of sub-discipline and indicators used			
	2006	*2007*	*2008*	*2009*
Outcomes	26.7%	26.7%	25%	25%
	Avoidable deaths (potential years of life lost)			
	Acute myocardial infarction (AMI) mortality			
	Infant deaths			
	MRSA infections			
	Breast cancer mortality	Cancer 5-year survival		Ratio of cancer deaths to incidence 2006
	Colorectal cancer mortality		Relative decline of suicide rate	
			% of diabetes patients with high HbA1c levels	
Waiting time for treatment	26.7%	26.7%	20%	20%
	Family doctor same day access			
	Direct access to specialist			
	Cancer therapy waiting time			
	Bypass/PTCA waiting time	Major non-acute operations waiting time		
	Knee/hip joint operations waiting time	MRI examination waiting time		CT scan waiting time
Patient rights and information	20%	20%	15%	17.5%
	Patients' rights-based health care law			
	Patient organizations involved in decisions			
	No-fault malpractice insurance			
	Right to second opinion			
	Access to own medical record			
	Web or 24–7 telephone health care information			
	Patient ombudsman	Register of legitimate doctors		
	Provider catalogue with quality ranking (in 2008 under 'e-Health')			
	Repetitive prescriptions available		Cross-border care information	Cross-border care financed from home
	e-mail address of family doctor			

(continued)

Table 8.10 Weighing and indicators used in the sub-disciplines of the Euro Health Consumer indices 2006–2009 *(continued)*

Sub-discipline	Weighing of sub-discipline and indicators used			
e-Health			10%	7.5%
	Electronic patient record penetration (in 2007 under 'patient rights and information')			
		e-transfer of medical data (between providers)		
		e-prescriptions		
				Laboratory test results communicated direct to patients via e-health
				Patients access to on-line booking of appointments
				On-line access to check how much doctors/clinics charge insurers
Provision levels ('generosity')/ from 2008: range and reach of services provided	13.3%	13.3%	15%	15%
	Cataract operations, age adjusted			
	Infant poliomyelitis vaccination	Infant four-disease vaccination		
	Dental care affordability			
		Kidney transplants		
			Mammography reach	
			Informal payments to doctors	
				Equity of health care systems
Pharmaceuticals	13.3%	13.3%	15%	15%
	Treatment subsidy (%)			
	Layman-adapted pharmacopoeia			
	New cancer drugs deployment speed			
	Access to new drugs (time to subsidy)			

Source: Based on Health Consumer Powerhouse 2006, 2007, 2008, 2009.
Notes: MRSA: Methicillin-resistant *Staphylococcus aureus*; HbA1c: Glycated haemoglobin; PTCA: Percutaneous transluminal coronary angioplasty; MRI: Magnetic resonance imaging; CT: Computed tomography.

Table 8.11 Rankings of the EU15 countries in selected surveys/rankings, 1998–2009

	GP evaluation[a]	Responsiveness outpatient[b]	Responsiveness inpatient[b]	Satisfaction with health system[c]	Satisfaction with health system[d]	Satisfaction with local health care[d]	Euro Health Consumer Index[e]		
	1998	2000/01	2000/01	2002	2008	2008	2007	2008	2009
Austria	n/a	n/a	n/a	2	4	1	1	3	3
Belgium	2	4	5	3	2	2	8	9	8
Denmark	5	n/a	n/a	6	7	6	7	2	2
Finland	n/a	4	9	1	3	11	6	9	9
France	n/a	4	5	4	5	8	3	8	5
Germany	1	2	8	8	12	5	4	6	4
Greece	n/a	13	13	14	14	15	15	14	15
Ireland	n/a	1	2	13	15	12	11	11	10
Italy	n/a	11	11	12	13	14	13	12	12
Luxembourg	n/a	9	2	5	1	3	9	4	6
Netherlands	3	4	5	9	7	4	2	1	1
Portugal	n/a	11	11	15	11	12	13	15	13
Spain	n/a	10	9	10	7	10	10	13	14
Sweden	4	4	4	7	6	9	5	5	7
United Kingdom	6	3	1	11	10	7	12	10	11

Sources: Based on [a]Grol et al. 2000; [b]Valentine et al. 2003; [c]European Commission 2002; [d]Brown and Khoury 2009; [e]Health Consumer Powerhouse 2006, 2007, 2008, 2009.

Notes: n/a: Not available; GP: General practitioner.

better in all surveys – even if some of them rank lower in particular surveys, while mainly tax-financed countries such as Ireland and the United Kingdom in the 2001/2002 responsiveness ratings or Denmark in the latest Health Consumer Powerhouse indices do well. This does not appear to be a result of the funding mechanism per se (i.e. whether a population contributes to the health system through SHI contributions or taxes) because the difference becomes larger when consumer-orientation dimensions (i.e. generosity of the system), rather than actual patient experience with the encounter, are weighted. Assuming that the results are collected in a (relatively) valid manner, it can be interpreted that SHI countries put more emphasis on consumer orientation (such as choice of provider and purchaser; clearly defined entitlements; patient rights, including the right to claim entitlements). In turn, this leads to better results if these dimensions are taken into account.

It is important to accept that these surveys exist and will appear increasingly on the public's agenda. Policy-makers have to deal with the pressures exerted by such league tables. They cannot simply dismiss the data as unreliable even when they are used to call for ineffective, inequitable or inefficient changes in the health care system.

Health care reforms that aim to increase responsiveness

In many (if not all) European countries, policy-makers have begun to react to the greater emphasis on – and the populations' greater demand for – responsiveness in the health care system. Important strategies include:

- defining patients' rights and entitlements and making them transparent (e.g. definition of benefit baskets and patient rights charters);
- enlarging the benefit basket with services that primarily address dignity (particularly palliative care) rather than health gain;
- addressing the issue of waiting lists;
- introducing or enlarging choice of provider and purchaser.

Strategies to increase the first four WHO dimensions of responsiveness (dignity, autonomy, confidentiality and communication) also include changes in organizational and policy development. Staff education and training have been refocused to promote greater respect for human dignity, to ensure that members of staff communicate effectively and to foster the appropriate application of confidentiality policies. Information sharing has been made more effective and mechanisms put in place to allow patients a more autonomous role and to participate more in clinical decision-making, as legitimate co-producers of care. Such improvements can be expected to result in better compliance with treatment and care (particularly among patients with chronic conditions) and can be secured without necessarily requiring significant additional investment.

An indirect approach to influencing provider behaviour involves broader regulatory initiatives such as the enactment of patient rights legislation or patient charters (Nys and Goffin 2010); specific service guarantees, for example on waiting times; or an ombudsman function. Patients rights are subject to numerous international and regional declarations and conventions. The increasing complexity of the health care sector, the technological developments in medicine and the introduction of market elements in the health care system have increased the need to guarantee patient rights by law. Some commentators have questioned an emphasis on legal approaches to patient rights but an explicit consideration of the patient's perspective fits well with a general democratic evolution in many countries.

The concept of patient rights is moving from a focus on individual rights – that is, restricting state intervention in the individual's right to life and privacy – to a focus on the collective right to health care. In addition to ensuring access to health services, the right to health care has also been interpreted as including consumer participation via procedural mechanisms to implement their preferences, for example the International Labour Organization Convention No.130, also known as the European Social Code. The WHO took up the subject of citizen participation and collective rights as early as 1994. Its publication, *A Declaration on the Promotion of Patients' Rights in Europe*, states that 'patients have a collective right to some form of representation at each level of the health care system in matters pertaining to the planning and evaluation of services, including the range, quality and functioning of the care provided' (WHO Regional Office for Europe 1994; den Exter 2005).

Another measure to ensure transparency and clarity about patient rights is an explicit definition of a benefit basket. This development is usually seen in the context of the health system's goal to improve health, as a benefit basket will be designed primarily to ensure that effective and cost-effective technologies are covered while those that are ineffective or less cost-effective are omitted. In order to ensure responsiveness it is also important to remember the right to die in dignity and that most people want to do this at home. This requires additional palliative-care services, which should be part of the benefit basket. However, palliative care and hospices have to be treated separately from the usual health technology assessment evaluation mechanisms, as these (with their emphasis on health gain and cost-effectiveness) may disadvantage such services.

It is perhaps even more challenging to create a climate that encourages health service personnel to treat patients well. Health workers typically value professionalism but where pay fails to meet legitimate expectations they may become unmotivated and fail to deliver the highest quality care. Those that are paid particularly badly may raise money illicitly, responding only to informal payments and creating barriers to access. Maintaining responsiveness, therefore, implies providing adequate resources – a potentially challenging proposition. It may be expensive to increase pay but it creates an opportunity to refocus management and specify expectations. However, health system managers must be aware of the evidence that policies that seek to micromanage clinical behaviour can lead to a loss of professional identity and undermine autonomy and motivation, resulting in health workers doing exactly what they are meant to, but no more.

Other dimensions of responsiveness (i.e. those that primarily improve the client orientation of services) are also likely to require a considerable commitment of resources. This is particularly true if capacity is to be increased in order to reduce waiting times or facilities are to be improved; it is also the case if new client information systems or new complaints procedures are required. In combination or separately, policy-makers may also advance responsiveness by including explicit requirements to meet clients' expectations in contractual arrangements (where these apply) or by building them into service delivery strategies.

It has been argued that, in principle, waiting times can be reduced through supply-side policies if the volume of surgery is considered inadequate and by demand-side policies if it is not (Hurst and Siciliani 2003). Supply-side policies include raising public capacity by increasing the number of specialists and beds, or by using capacity available in the private sector. They also include increasing productivity by funding extra activity, fostering day-surgery and linking the remuneration system of doctors and hospitals to the activity performed. On the supply side, the pronounced reductions in long waits for coronary revascularization surgery in Denmark have been achieved by significant increases in activity, backed up by increases in capacity. Hospitals that breach the one-month waiting-time target must bear the expense of the patient's choice of a different public or private provider (even outside the country).

The striking reductions in long waiting times in England and Spain have resulted from a combination of maximum waiting-time targets, additional activity and changed incentives. In addition, there appears to have been a marked fall in mean waiting times for patients requiring various procedures in Spain after financial incentives were linked to the achievement of waiting-time targets in 1998. Many OECD countries have implemented visible improvements in the efficiency of surgical units, particularly by increasing the share of day surgery. However, increased activity to reduce waiting times is often swiftly followed by increased demand, which returns waiting times to near their original levels. Any strategy to tackle waiting times is, therefore, a combination of increased capacity and approaches aimed at both providers (financial incentives to provide more services and/or disincentives for failing to meet targets) and patients (increased choice).

Client orientation can be viewed from two perspectives. First, the collective and individual influences on care decisions occurs either when citizens influence the package of care and benefit coverage or the power of individual patients to get the care they desire or deem necessary is increased. The second perspective looks at the mechanisms available to citizens to influence health care decisions. Following Hirschman's (1970) notions on organizational behaviour, these can be grouped into voice and exit. Voice is essentially a political or administrative category, whereas exit is market based. Voice mechanisms include information, consultation and assessment of public views, advocacy groups, formal representation and patient rights. Exit revolves around consumer choice, which is often portrayed as a core issue that touches on fundamental rights and is instrumental in increasing responsiveness.

Choice can apply to providers and/or purchasers. Consumers in most countries have the right to choose their primary care providers (Table 8.12). In SHI systems, consumers can also choose ambulatory specialists and hospitals (although gatekeepers are used in some countries such as the Netherlands). Choices are more restricted in countries with a national health service system, although this is changing rapidly in many countries. For example, patients in

Table 8.12 Choice of provider for primary and secondary care and of purchaser

Member State	Provider		Purchaser
	Primary care	*Secondary care*	
Austria	Only contracted doctors	Free among public hospitals if no additional costs arise	No
Belgium	Free	Free among approved hospitals	Yes
Cyprus	Free choice of government doctors, not obliged to register with one GP	Free, on referral to hospital where doctor is employed	No
Czech Republic	Free	Free choice of contracted hospitals	Yes
Denmark	Group 1: Only GPs that joined collective agreement; Group 2: Free	Free for public hospitals. If waiting time exceeds 1 month also private and abroad	No
Estonia	Free	Partly free choice with direct access (e.g. gynaecologists, psychiatrists); partly on referral with free choice	No
Finland	Determined by district of residence	Determined by district of residence	No
France	Free	Free among public and private (approved) hospitals	No
Germany	Free among contracted sickness fund doctors (97% of all)	Free choice among contracted public and private hospitals (99% of all beds)	Yes
Greece	In urban regions: insured choose doctor from a list. In rural areas: no free choice, insured goes to local insurance institute doctor	Only public hospital and registered clinic designated by the insurance institute or in hospital of social insurance institute	No
Hungary	Free choice of contracted doctors	No free choice (only in case of emergency)	No
Ireland	Persons with full eligibility choose from list of local GPs	Limited	No, only for those insured under VHI
Italy	Free in region for approved GPs	Free for public hospitals and contracted private hospitals	No
Latvia	Free	On referral, patients can choose between contracted hospitals	No
Lithuania	Free	Free on referral	No

(continued)

Table 8.12 Choice of provider for primary and secondary care and of purchaser *(con't)*

Member State	Provider		Purchaser
	Primary care	*Secondary care*	
Luxembourg	Free	Free	No
Malta	Free	Free, however, because of size only limited number of hospitals available (e.g. only two general hospitals)	No
Netherlands	Free	Free, but co-payment for uncontracted care may be needed in case of a benefits-in-kind policy	Yes
Poland	Free among contracted GPs	Free choice of contracted hospitals	No
Portugal	Free among contracted GPs	Free among public hospitals, and, if there is a waiting list, institutions approved by the ministry of health	No
Slovakia	Free among contracted GPs	Free, on referral	Yes
Slovenia	Free	Free choice of public hospital and contracted private hospitals	No
Spain	Free in area	No choice, according to region (except in case of emergency)	No
Sweden	Free	Free choice of regional public hospitals and approved private establishments	No
United Kingdom	Free	Patients can choose from a minimum of four local providers	No

Sources: Based on data in Busse, van Ginneken and Wörz 2011.
Notes: GP: General practitioner; VHI: Voluntary health insurance.

Sweden and Norway are allowed to choose any hospital outside their county of residence; in Denmark, this is permissible only if waiting times are not met. Patients within the English system have also seen their hospital choices increase. Increased consumer choice of providers clearly increases responsiveness, but there is debate over its negative impact on other social objectives, notably equity, cost-containment and allocative efficiency. There is evidence that choice tends to benefit the more affluent (and usually better-informed) classes and thus may lead to increasing health inequalities. The policy response should not necessarily be to reduce choice in line with the equity in poverty argument but rather to focus efforts to ensure wider access to information and support choice among the underprivileged.

In countries where choice has been extended or there is essentially a free choice of provider, there are concerns about the resulting fragmentation of care and duplication of investigations. For example, consumers may choose different primary and ambulatory care providers for the same episode. While this responds to the expectations of users, it is clinically undesirable as it gives rise to poorer health outcomes and undermines efficiency by overutilizing services. Also, patients value some 'treatments', therapeutic interventions and medicaments that are neither efficacious nor cost-effective. These pose a direct conflict between responsiveness and efficiency. Policy-makers need to manage these trade-offs, although there is growing evidence that they overestimate the importance that patients attach to unlimited choice.

Several countries have also introduced a free choice of insurer (notably Switzerland, Germany, the Netherlands). The evidence on whether this free choice enhances consumers' capacity to choose and increases efficiency is rather disappointing. It suggests that the choice of insurer might not function well for all (particularly for bad risks) and that the information is not always adequate to support informed choices. Moreover, consumer reluctance to switch insurers has not heightened competition. There has been little increase in the quality of health services, either because the funds lack the instruments to do so, as in Germany, or because they do not use the available instruments, such as selective contracting in the Netherlands. In contrast, Busse (2001) concluded that (generally speaking) the introduction of individual free choice of insurer in Germany was successful, since it raised the funds' accountability and stimulated their development from payers to more active purchasers. However, there is no conclusive evidence that this has increased the responsiveness of the system.

In a review of trade-offs, equity is certainly another key consideration that has potentially very significant conflicts with responsiveness. Measures to increase responsiveness (e.g. those that focus on choice) may favour those sectors of the population that are better able to compare and choose between options. This tendency to benefit the younger, healthier, more affluent and better educated (who can negotiate the services they want) has been termed the inverse law of participation – widening the equity gap.

Again policy-makers need to be explicit about how they balance competing issues and to be proactive in pursuing equity, widening access to information about services and using positive discrimination strategies to increase access and choice for the socioeconomically disadvantaged. Policy-makers may also make use of other equity considerations. There is explicit evidence on disparities in responsiveness, particularly towards ethnic minority populations. One of the best-documented examples is the widespread discrimination against Roma populations across Europe. Direct and indirect strategies on equity in responsiveness will tend to improve access and so reduce health inequalities. These may be exacerbated if strategies overlook the ability of different population groups to benefit from responsiveness initiatives like choice.

All trade-offs need to be considered within the wider context and the part that responsiveness can play in producing societal well-being. As always, context is hugely important. This is an area in which culture plays a very significant part in shaping perceptions, making it particularly difficult to extrapolate from one country or population group to another. Policy-makers will need to adjust the priority they attach to responsiveness and the measures they take to achieve it in order to reflect societal norms and expectations as well as the availability of resources. However, it is not inevitable that resource constraints (and a commitment to equity) lead to levelling down to the lowest common (responsiveness) denominator.

Conclusions

Ten years after the publication of WHR2000, it is undisputed that responsiveness (i.e. the reaction of the health system and health service providers to 'the legitimate expectations of the population for their interaction with the health system') is a value in and of itself and a dimension of health systems that is genuinely valued by patients and citizens. It can involve significant extra expenditure, which begs the question of how much more societies are prepared to pay for responsiveness, and how much will they pay for equity of responsiveness. However, many strategies that increase responsiveness are also cost-effective in health gain terms. For example, responsiveness leads to better compliance with treatment, which is particularly significant for chronic disease treatments. The role of health system stewards, therefore, must be to promote (as always) good governance, transparency and accountability; to refine the use of existing resources to enhance responsiveness; and to manage the trade-offs between goals when they arise.

Policy-makers need to be aware, that – while the importance of the concept of 'responsiveness' is more or less undisputed – considerable methodological issues remain regarding its measurement and interpretation. Policy-makers, therefore, might begin work to enhance responsiveness simply by addressing some of the concerns above and taking steps to improve the quality and comparability of assessments. Certainly, ensuring transparency in the composition of indices and the attribution of weights, flagging up underlying values and promoting rigour in interpretation of results are all areas where health stewardship could (and should) take a lead and which will support efforts to improve the way health services treat citizens. Policy-makers will also need to play their role in offering and interpreting information on responsiveness, empowering populations to contribute to decision-making (including that on trade-offs), and in assessing the opportunity cost of investing in responsiveness rather than other health system goals.

Endnotes

1. Although not tested in this analysis, variations in responsiveness across population groups such as poor/not poor, educated/uneducated within a country may also occur (at least) partly due to differences in expectations.
2. Data cover the entire period of the transition from a system based largely on social security contributions via a tax-funded national health service type of system to a tax-funded regionalized system.

References

Blendon, R., Leitman, R., Morrison, I. and Donelan, K. (1990) Satisfaction with health systems in ten nations. *Health Affairs*, 9(2): 185–92.

Blendon, R.J., Donelan, K., Jovell, A., Pellise, L. and Costas Lombardia, E. (1991) Spain's citizens assess their health care system. *Health Affairs*, 10(3): 216–28.

Brown, I.T. and Khoury, C. (2009) In OECD countries, universal healthcare gets high marks. *Gallup*, 20 August, http://www.gallup.com/poll/122393/oecd-countries-universal-healthcare-gets-high-marks.aspx (accessed 22 September 2011).

Busse, R. (2001). Risk structure compensation in Germany's statutory health insurance. *European Journal of Public Health*, 11(2): 174–7.

Busse, R., van Ginneken, E. and Wörz, M. (2011) Access to health care services within and between countries of the European Union, in M. Wismar, W. Palm, J. Figueras, K. Ernst and E. van Ginneken (eds.) *Cross-Border Health Care in the European Union: Mapping and Analysing Practices and Policies*. Copenhagen: WHO Regional Office for Europe on behalf of the European Observatory on Health Systems and Policies: 47–90.

Coulter, A. and Cleary, P.D. (2001) Patients' experiences with hospital care in five countries. *Health Affairs*, 20(3): 43–53.

Coulter, A. and Jenkinson, C. (2005) European patients' views on the responsiveness of health systems and healthcare providers. *European Journal of Public Health*, 15: 355–60.

De Silva, A. (2000) *A Framework for Measuring Responsiveness*, GPE discussion paper no. 32. Geneva: World Health Organization, http://www.who.int/responsiveness/papers/paper32.pdf (accessed 13 February 2010).

den Exter, A.P. (2005) Purchasers as the public's agent, in J. Figueras, E. Jakubowski and R. Robinson (eds.) *Purchasing to Improve Health Systems Performance*. Maidenhead: Open University Press: 122–39.

European Commission (1996) *Eurobarometer 44.3*. Brussels: European Commission.

European Commission (1998) *Eurobarometer 49*. Brussels: European Commission.

European Commission (1999) *Eurobarometer 50.1*. Brussels: European Commission.

European Commission (2000) *Eurobarometer 52.1*. Brussels: European Commission.

European Commission (2002) *Eurobarometer 57.2*. Brussels: European Commission.

Figueras, J., Saltman, R.B., Busse, R. and Dubois, H.F.W. (2004) Patterns and performance in social insurance systems, in R.B. Saltman, R. Busse and J. Figueras (eds.) *Social Health Insurance Systems in Western Europe*. Buckingham: Open University Press: 81–140.

Grol, R., Wensing, M., Mainz, J. et al. (2000) Patients in Europe evaluate general practice care: an international comparison. *British Journal of General Practice*, 50: 882–7.

Health Consumer Powerhouse (2006) *Euro Health Consumer Index 2006*. Stockholm: Health Consumer Powerhouse, http://www.healthpowerhouse.com/media/RaportEHCI2006en.pdf (accessed 22 September 2011).

Health Consumer Powerhouse (2007) *Euro Health Consumer Index 2007*. Stockholm: Health Consumer Powerhouse, http://www.healthpowerhouse.com/media/Rapport_EHCI_2007.pdf (accessed 22 September 2011).

Health Consumer Powerhouse (2008) *Euro Health Consumer Index 2008*. Stockholm: Health Consumer Powerhouse, http://www.healthpowerhouse.com/files/2008-EHCI/EHCI-2008-report.pdf (accessed 22 September 2011).

Health Consumer Powerhouse (2009) *Euro Health Consumer Index 2009*. Stockholm: Health Consumer Powerhouse, http://www.healthpowerhouse.com/files/Report%20EHCI%202009%20091005%20final%20with%20cover.pdf (accessed 22 September 2011)

Hirschman, A. (1970) *Exit, Voice and Loyalty*. Cambridge, MA: Harvard University Press.

Hurst, J. and Siciliani, L. (2003) *Tackling Excessive Waiting Times for Elective Surgery: A Comparison of Policies in Twelve OECD Countries*, health working papers no. 6. Paris: Organisation for Economic Co-operation and Development.

Jenkinson, C., Coulter, A. and Bruster, S. (2002) The Picker Patient Experience Questionnaire: development and validation using data from in-patient surveys in five countries. *International Journal for Quality in Health Care*, 14: 353–8.

Nys, H. and Goffin, T. (2011) Mapping national practices and strategies relating to patients' rights, in M. Wismar, W. Palm, J. Figueras, K. Ernst and E. van Ginneken (eds.) *Cross-Border Health Care in the European Union: Mapping and Analysing Practices and Policies*. Copenhagen: WHO Regional Office for Europe on behalf of the European Observatory on Health Systems and Policies: 159–216.

Pescosolido, B.A., Boyer, C.A. and Tsui, W.Y. (1985) Medical care in the welfare state: a cross-national study of public evaluations. *Journal of Health and Social Behavior*, 26: 276–97.

Saltman, R.B., Busse, R. and Figueras, J. (eds.) (2004) *Social Health Insurance Systems in Western Europe*. Buckingham: Open University Press.

Schoen, C., Osborn, R., Doty, M.M., Bishop, M., Peugh, J. and Murukutla, N. (2007) Toward higher-performance health systems: adults' health care experiences in seven countries, 2007. *Health Affairs*, 26(6): w717–34.

Taylor, H. (2004) In the 5 largest European countries, French health care system most popular at home and most admired abroad. *Health Care News*, 4(12), http://www.harrisinteractive.com/news/newsletters/healthnews/HI_HealthCareNews2004Vol4_Iss12.pdf (accessed 22 September 2011).

Taylor, H. (2008) Majorities in United States and three of five largest European countries believe health care is doing badly in their countries. *Health Care News* 8(3), http://www.harrisinteractive.com/news/newsletters/healthnews/HI_HealthCareNews2008Vol8_Iss3.pdf (accessed 22 September 2011).

Üstün, T.B., Chatterji, S., Mechbal, A., Murray, C.J.L. and WHS Collaborating Groups (2003) The world health surveys, in C.J.L. Murray and D.B. Evans (eds.) *Health Systems Performance Assessment: Debates, Methods and Empiricism*. Geneva: World Health Organization: 797–808.

Üstün, T.B., Chatterji, S., Villanueva, M. et al. (2001) *WHO Multi-country Survey Study on Health and Responsiveness 2000–2001*, GPE discussion paper no. 37. Geneva: World Health Organization, http://www.who.int/responsiveness/papers/gpediscpaper37.pdf (accessed 13 February 2010).

Valentine, N.B., Prasad, A., Rice, N., Robone, S. and Chatterji, S. (2009) Health systems responsiveness: a measure of the acceptability of health-care processes and systems from the user's perspective, in P.C. Smith, E. Mossialos, I. Papanicolas and S. Leatherman (eds.) *Performance Measurement for Health System Improvement: Experiences, Challenges and Prospects*. Cambridge: Cambridge University Press: 138–86.

Valentine, N.B., de Silva, A., Kawabata, K., Darby, C., Murray, C.J.L. and Evans, D.B. (2003) Health system responsiveness: concepts, domains and operationalization, in C.J.L. Murray and D.B. Evans (eds.) *Health Systems Performance Assessment: Debates, Methods and Empiricism*. Geneva: World Health Organization: 573–96.

WHO Regional Office for Europe (1994) *A Declaration on the Promotion of Patients' Rights in Europe*. Geneva: World Health Organization.

World Health Organization (2000) *The World Health Report 2000. Health Systems: Improving Performance*. Geneva: World Health Organization.

nine

Assessing health reform trends in Europe

Richard B. Saltman, Sara Allin,
Elias Mossialos, Mathias Wismar and
Joseph Kutzin

Introduction

A growing number of health systems across Europe are in the midst of a long-term process of structural and organizational reform. Both tax-funded systems and social health insurance systems, in western European countries and the countries of central and eastern Europe (CCEE), are re-thinking and often re-configuring important organizational and institutional structures for delivering both individual clinical and population-based public health services. They are also exploring initiatives to encourage actors in other sectors to influence health determinants. While the broad policy objectives being pursued by most countries have remained relatively constant, the strategies and mechanisms by which policy-makers are trying to reach them have undergone considerable change.

This wide-ranging debate about reform has been underway since the late 1980s in western Europe and since the early 1990s in central Europe (Saltman and Figueras 1997, 1998). What began as a relatively small number of limited initiatives has now broadened into a complex, many-pronged endeavour that includes discussion of a wide range of measures at multiple levels within and beyond the formal health system structure.

This expanded health reform process was set in motion by, as well as facilitated and made possible through, a series of ongoing policy developments in six parallel areas. Although each area has evolved separately along its own pathway, all six together have served to lay the groundwork for debate about broad health sector reform. These six parallel areas of policy development are:

- *evidence-based medicine*, providing a systematic framework to evaluate the effectiveness and appropriateness of clinical procedures and interventions and organizational developments;

- *market-based mechanisms*, particularly among providers, emphasizing competition, cost reductions and patient responsiveness and satisfaction;
- *total quality management*, previously developed in manufacturing industries, leading in health care to re-engineering of the service production process, emphasizing high quality of care, good outcomes and enhanced patient safety;
- *integrated care and provider substitution*, requiring sophisticated coordination between acute, primary, nursing home and home care in response to an ageing population and rising rates of chronic disease; in the process, helping to shift power in health systems from inpatient specialists towards outpatient, primary care and primary health care arenas;
- *health promotion and disease prevention*, seeking to move personnel and resources upstream towards the behavioural, organizational and societal sources of ill health;
- *information technology*, facilitating the digitalization of clinical, financial and managerial information to support major new organizational efficiencies and organizational strategies.

Together, these clinical, epidemiological, financial and organizational developments, interwoven in a complexly evolving pattern, have re-shaped the health policy discourse in Europe over the past twenty years. Public decision-makers now expect to generate and manage a multidimensional set of activities at various levels of their health systems and, simultaneously, to draw upon and utilize a dramatically expanded range of policy tools and mechanisms to influence processes and outcomes within as well as beyond the health sector. One key question that emerges from this new situation is how well the expanded range of policy tools and mechanisms has improved the overall delivery of health services; specifically, whether it has generated systematic improvements in the efficiency, efficacy, quality and acceptability of care. This topic will be taken up in the section on stewardship and governance below.

A growing number of countries in Europe now have considerable experience with this broad, multipronged process of health reform. Confronted by a difficult set of epidemiological, demographic, economic and social challenges, national policy advisers have sought to apply the available evidence from both academic research and country experience about how best to position their health care and public health systems for the next decades. Policy-makers in all countries can benefit from nearly 20 years of effort both in analysing the nature of particular problems and in testing the usefulness of different reform strategies and mechanisms. Drawing on this practical experience-based foundation, the current debate across Europe has evolved into a more targeted and focused process, in which the core characteristics and components of reform are widely known, and the resulting policy discussions tend to revolve around how, when and where to apply specific approaches.

This chapter provides a broad overview of the expanded health policy landscape, reviewing the main reform strategies that have been explored in countries of the European region. The examination of these strategies is grouped following the four main functions of the health systems framework introduced in Chapter 2: health service delivery, resource generation, financing and stewardship. The chapter then contrasts the current state of health system reform in Europe with the status of reforms at the time of the 1996

Ljubljana Ministerial Meeting on Health Care Reform (Saltman and Figueras 1998). The chapter concludes with two brief observations regarding the overall development of the health reform process in Europe.

A major caveat is necessary before continuing. This chapter cannot provide a comprehensive overview of health system reforms in Europe. Despite the best efforts of organizations such as the European Observatory on Health Systems and Policies, WHO, World Bank, Bertelsmann Foundation and OECD, as well as many individual researchers and research teams, there is still a scarcity of rigorous evaluations that can ascertain how effective many of the reforms described have actually been.

Health service delivery: delivering services cost-effectively

Service delivery activities have been the focus of a great many reform measures and strategies. They bear, in particular, the brunt of both demographic change and the ageing of the population, and of the consequent rapid increase in chronic disease (Nolte and McKee 2008). They also have been the locus of multiple efforts to shift services when possible from intensive and/or inpatient care to less-intensive outpatient, primary care and primary health care settings. Indeed, all six of the major health policy developments noted above directly affect the content and process of service delivery. Policy-makers, confronted by continued upwards pressure on expenditures linked to ageing populations and changing technologies, have sought new strategies and mechanisms to streamline the production of individual patient services in hospitals and to more fully integrate the growing number of chronic care and elderly services across tertiary/secondary/primary care boundaries and at the health–social interface.

The wide range of service delivery reforms currently underway across Europe fall into five general categories:

- *integrating and coordinating services* across hospital/primary care, hospital/home care and curative/social care boundaries, and substituting nurse practitioners and other specially trained staff in order to assure an appropriate continuum of care, particularly for elderly and/or chronic care;
- *restructuring publicly operated providers* (hospitals and primary health centres) from passively (or politically) administered to actively managed organizations, also seeking to give publicly employed professionals a personal stake in the organization's clinical and financial effectiveness, often through patient choice of provider institution and physician;
- *enhancing quality of care*, including process and outcome in clinical services, patient safety and responsiveness/satisfaction of patients;
- *assessing health technologies* systematically for their effectiveness and cost-effectiveness;
- *strengthening public health, prevention, and health promotion* activities, improving equity and incorporating separate vertical programmes and other similar activities where possible into existing primary care activities.

This section will briefly review key initiatives in each of these five categories.

Integrating and coordinating services

A key objective in many countries across Europe has been to integrate clinical services for patients across hospital and primary care boundaries (Starfield 1998; Dowling and Glendinning 2003). This strategy seeks to re-equilibrate the balance of financial and decision-making power within the overall health system by empowering primary care, often by giving some or all of the hospital sector budget to organizations in which primary care plays a prominent role (municipal health and social boards in Finland, subcounty district health boards in Sweden, Primary Care Trusts in the United Kingdom). This has sometimes been referred to as 'putting primary care in the driver's seat' (Saltman, Rico and Boerma 2006). Another popular strategy has been to group primary care providers in larger primary care centres (Sweden, Finland, parts of the United Kingdom, the Netherlands), although concerns have been raised that this strategy reduces continuity of care and may be less cost-effective than individual general practitioners (see below). Some countries have sought to take this reconfiguration even further, hoping to transform the rapidly growing constellation of chronic and long-term care services (particularly home care), within primary health care and to create a second, core group of services equivalent to the traditional core group of hospital-based services (e.g. Norway and Denmark). This effort to create, in effect, a bipolar structure of power within the delivery system has so far been difficult to achieve.

Population ageing and the increasing burden of chronic disease have combined to push policy-makers to explore a large number of additional strategies (Nolte and McKee 2008). The central objective in these reforms has been to promote seamless packages of care for chronically ill people in the most clinically appropriate and cost-effective setting. These include networks based in primary care and nurse-led strategies, particularly in countries with strong primary care traditions such as the Netherlands, Sweden and the United Kingdom; explicit mechanisms to coordinate providers such as 'health networks' in France or 'chains of care' in Sweden; and disease management programmes (Germany, the Netherlands); and self-care (Denmark, England) (Nolte and McKee 2008). These are often facilitated by strategies to adapt skill mix, foster multidisciplinary teams and support audit and quality monitoring. Reforms in financing and in incentive schemes have been equally key in ensuring care is fully integrated.

There has also been a trend towards substitution of services, with responsibilities being reassigned across tertiary, secondary and primary care boundaries and the health and social care interface. There has been more emphasis on delivering care in the most cost-effective location supported by the most appropriate mix of skills and technologies (Boerma 2003). In particular, there has been a transfer of inpatient care to other settings, illustrated by the growth of day surgery (McKee and Healy 2002). A survey of 19 countries revealed very high rates of day surgery for some procedures such as hernia repairs and cataract removals in Denmark, Sweden and Norway (along with the United States and Canada), with much lower rates in Portugal, France, Scotland and Germany (Castoro et al. 2007), although caution is required in interpreting the data because of differing definitions. There has been a visible decline in the number of hospital beds per capita across the region, reflecting two policy objectives: the shifting of inpatient care to ambulatory settings, and the shifting of psychiatric care from institutions to the community. The decline has been most pronounced in the Commonwealth of Independent States (CIS), where hospital capacity has traditionally been much higher than in the west, falling from 1077 to 856 beds per 100,000 population between 1996 and 2005 (representing a 20% decline), although there is still much greater supply than in the EU (690 to 580 beds, or 16% decline in the same period) (WHO Regional Office for Europe 2007).

Restructuring publicly operated providers

Health care providers are introducing a large number of innovative management strategies (often called New Public Management) in an effort to shift the operation of health facilities from a passive 'administration' model to a more hands-on 'management' approach to daily operating decisions (Pollitt 2000). One of the most widely adopted new public management models has been to restructure publicly owned hospitals into semi-independently managed public firms (Estonia, Norway, United Kingdom, Portugal; new hospitals in Andalucia in Spain; university hospitals in Veneto in Italy), giving each institution its own semi-autonomous management (often with its own separate Board of Trustees), yet retaining public ownership and with it public accountability for the institution's overall performance (Saltman, Durán and Dubois in press).

A wide range of other New Public Management strategies also have been adopted in a number of countries. One popular approach has been to contract out management of primary health centres to private not-profit-making and profit-making firms (Sweden, Finland). A second type of initiative sought to give patients a publicly funded fixed budget with which to hire and pay for providers for chronic (United Kingdom) and home care (the Netherlands, United Kingdom) services (Smits and Janssen 2008). Disease management programmes have been adopted in some social health insurance systems (Germany) to overcome structural barriers created by existing payment systems.

Many countries have also sought to enhance patient choice (Chapter 8). In tax-based systems, choice typically has been introduced among providers on the production side (Sweden, Denmark, Norway). The United Kingdom has introduced some patient choice of both private and public hospitals, funded by the National Health Service (NHS). In countries with social health insurance, new choice arrangements have focused on selecting sickness funds (Germany, Switzerland) or 'insurance companies' (Netherlands, Czech Republic). It is important to note, however, that these insurer choices have been introduced within a tightly regulated environment. Experience in several CCEEs has demonstrated that choice of insurer needs to be heavily regulated by the state if adverse effects upon the macroeconomy and solidarity are to be avoided.

In addition to increased choice, a wide range of measures have been put in place seeking to empower the patient, including patient rights legislation, formal representation on the boards of purchaser and provider organizations, introduction of ombudsman services and increased participation of patients in decision-making about their own care. The last is particularly relevant in the context of chronic diseases as patient participation and self-management have been shown to improve outcomes in certain circumstances. However, this requires health literacy, active patient involvement in treatment decisions and education of patients to play an active role (Askham, Coulter and Parsons 2008).

All these measures reflect a changing view of public and private sectors in European health systems. Traditional hard boundaries have increasingly melted (Saltman 2003) and the willingness to combine various forms of public and private actors within a publicly accountable market structure is now accepted in many countries.

Enhancing quality of care

Across Europe, countries have put in place a series of quality initiatives ranging from the broad system level to the clinical setting. These include national legislation and policies on quality of care, comprehensive patient safety strategies and registration and licensing for new technologies and pharmaceuticals; training programmes on quality; accreditation of providers; and clinical guidelines, information systems and quality assurance methods at clinical level (Legido-Quigley, McKee and Nolte 2008; Legido-Quigley et al. 2008). In some western European counties, recognition of the importance of systematic quality improvement efforts has led to the establishment of comprehensive strategies. For example the Danish Society for Quality in the Health Care System was set up in 1991, and in 1992 the National Board of Health established a national council, which published the national strategy for quality improvement in 1993 (Knudsen, Fugleholm and Kjærgaard 2004). In Norway, government policy and provisions for quality improvement work are laid down in a series of documents, including the annual state budgets for the Ministry of Health and Care Services and the Ministry of Labour and Social Affairs. In Sweden, a series of initiatives to improve quality have been developed at the national, municipal and county council level, including national guidelines for care and treatment; information technology-based and appropriate care documentation; national quality indicators comparing medical outcomes in the health care system, patient experiences, access and costs; and support for systematic quality work (Nordic Council of Ministers 2007). In the English NHS, provider organizations have a statutory duty to ensure quality as part of the clinical governance framework; national standards of care exist for many major conditions and for a large number of health technologies, and all doctors are subject to annual appraisals.

The extent to which legislation addressing quality of health care has been enacted and implemented varies across countries (Merkur, Mossialos and Lear 2008). Among member states of the EU, Cyprus, Greece, Latvia, Luxembourg, Malta, Portugal, Poland and Slovakia have chosen to adopt local initiatives and rely on more voluntary quality assurance mechanisms. Some countries recently adopted quality of care laws, including the Czech Republic, Estonia, Hungary, Ireland, Lithuania and Slovenia. Meanwhile, countries with a long-standing tradition of quality legislation and national strategies are found in western

Europe, such as in Belgium, France, Finland, Germany, Italy, Spain and Sweden, with Denmark, the Netherlands, and the United Kingdom making major system changes and introducing strong quality regulatory mechanisms.

Patient safety is increasingly recognized as integral to ensuring quality, and has recently being prioritized in Europe, where only a few countries (e.g. the United Kingdom and Denmark) have formal systems in place. Clinical practice guidelines represent one instrument that can be used to improve quality, reduce disparities in clinical practice and improve patient safety (Walley and Mossialos 2004). While some countries already have such systems in place, such as the Czech Republic, Finland, France, Spain, the Netherlands and the United Kingdom, others are beginning to introduce guidelines (e.g. Austria, Belgium, Cyprus, Estonia, Latvia and Poland).

Assessing health technologies

Many countries have promoted the specific assessment of pharmaceuticals and other medical technologies with the aim of avoiding inefficacious or iatrogenic interventions and achieving value for money. Health technology assessment (HTA) tends to consider criteria of safety, efficacy, cost and cost-effectiveness as well as social, organizational, legal and ethical implications (Velasco-Garrido and Busse 2005). Formal HTA agencies have been established across Europe from (in sequence) France, Sweden and the Netherlands in the 1980s; Austria, Spain, Finland, Latvia, the United Kingdom, Denmark and Germany in the 1990s; and Hungary and Belgium (2001–2003) (Velasco-Garrido and Busse 2005).

Agencies responsible for HTA can play an advisory or regulatory role in the decision-making process (Zentner, Valasco-Garrido and Busse 2005) although all have the potential to bring together commitment to quality and efficiency and to enhance health system sustainability. While HTA programmes have generally improved transparency in decision-making processes through mechanisms such as independent systematic reviews and stakeholder involvement, an explicitly defined benefits package based on robust evidence of cost-effectiveness has not yet been achieved in any country (Sorenson, Drummond and Kanavos 2008). One country that has been relatively advanced in these attempts has been Israel, where a broadly representative council makes decisions about the services included in the social health insurance system (Rosen 2003). Barriers to more effective use of HTA include resource constraints and limited technical expertise, lack of transparency in the criteria for inclusion/exclusion of interventions and lack of political will to enforce decisions.

Strengthening public health, prevention and health promotion

Three broad approaches can be seen in policies to reform public health delivery: integrating population health interventions into primary care; reforming public health services, particularly in parts of eastern Europe; and establishing new organizational structures to deliver public health programmes.

General practitioners spend a considerable amount of their time delivering primary prevention, including health advice, screening and vaccinations (Pelletier-Fleury et al. 2007). In this way, primary health care has taken on an increasing role in cost-effective public health interventions such as systematic screening for hypertension, cholesterol and a range of cancers and the provision of health advice on risks, including diet, alcohol and smoking. An important aspect of this process has been a shift of vertical health programmes (such as immunization or management of tuberculosis or sexually transmitted diseases) into horizontally integrated primary care structures. This responds to increasing evidence that integration increases efficiency and improves outcomes in areas like HIV, mental health and certain communicable diseases. Despite the management advantages, however, this approach is not without problems, nor is it applicable across all health programmes or in all situations (Atun, Bennett and Durán 2008; Figueras et al. 2008a).

An important reform strategy is the expansion of public health services. Elements of this strategy are the reform of the sanitary–epidemiology (sanepid) services in the CCEEs and CIS (Gotsadze et al. 2010), the establishment of new organizational settings for the delivery of public health services in all parts of Europe and the partial absorption of public health services in primary health care settings.

In most CCEEs and the CIS, the inadequacy of public health services was the motivation for this strategy. In these countries, the major provider of public health services was the sanepid services, products of the Soviet era. These had produced tangible achievements through their vaccination programmes and communicable disease control. However, they were not concerned with the social determinants of health. As a consequence, health promotion was underdeveloped or almost non-existent. Sanepid services were also relatively ineffective in combating environmental pollution, occupational disease and noncommunicable disease because the capacity to impose changes on state-owned manufacturing and agricultural industry was very limited (MacArthur and Shevkun 2002; Bobak et al. 2004). Expansion of public health services is an important strategy for many countries in the western part of Europe too, where often public health services have not received the same attention as health care services.

A key element of the reform strategy in CCEEs and the CIS has been the revision of public health laws. Some countries have abolished their sanepid services altogether and introduced new organizational structures. An example is Kazakhstan, which established a national centre for healthy lifestyles in 1997. In parallel, an intersectoral health promotion council was established (Kulzhanov and Rechel 2007). Similar approaches are now being considered in Kyrgyzstan, Tajikistan and Uzbekistan, although with limited success given financial constraints (Ahmedov et al. 2007; Kulzhanov and Rechel 2007).

Social health insurance systems in western Europe are also expanding their public health services in light of a perceived neglect of health promotion. Some countries like Austria and Switzerland (Organisation for Economic Co-operation and Development 2006) have established new health foundations to strengthen health promotion. France and Germany are revising their existing structures for health promotion (L'Assemblée nationale, Sénat Le Président de la République

2004). New organizational settings, however, can pose new challenges. Personal and population-based health services are often intrinsically connected.

Resource generation: appropriate level and mix of inputs

A second major area of reform activity has been resource generation. Shortages of staff (particularly primary care physicians and higher-level nurses) in many parts of western Europe contrast with the inherited oversupply of physicians and beds in many countries in eastern Europe. Capital for renovating existing institutions, purchasing new medical equipment and for building new hospital facilities is a critical element of the pursuit of quality and safety (McKee and Healy 2002).

Improving performance of the health care workforce

Challenges facing the health care workforce in Europe reflect the increasing pace of change in the delivery and organization of health care, such as changing patterns of disease and demographic changes, diffusion of new and sophisticated technologies, increasingly informed and demanding patients, growing demands for evidence-based medicine and broader economic conditions and legislative changes (e.g. the EU Working Time Directive) (Dubois, McKee and Nolte 2006a). The health workforce itself is also changing, with a growing proportion of female doctors and a blurring of boundaries between categories of workers. Reflecting their divergent situations, policy-makers have sought a variety of approaches through which to address the efficiency and effectiveness of resource utilization in their health systems.

There is substantial variation in the supply of physicians and nurses per capita across Europe, although as always caution is required in interpreting the data. The highest density of physicians is seen in Greece and Georgia, with almost 500 physicians per 100,000 population. High density also exists in Belgium, Belarus and the Russian Federation (over 400 per 100,000), with the lowest density in Albania, Bosnia, Montenegro, Tajikistan, Turkey and Romania, along with the United Kingdom (under 200 per 100,000). The supply of nurses varies widely across the region, with under 400 per 100,000 population in Turkey, Romania, Greece and Albania and between 1000 and 1500 per 100,000 in Belgium, the Netherlands, Norway, Ireland, Sweden, Belarus and Uzbekistan (WHO Regional Office for Europe 2007). Variations in supply may reflect different organizational arrangements for ambulatory care. For example, more nurses are needed in some countries because they are the first point of contact, as in the Netherlands with the greatest nursing supply, while in others, patients visit general medical practitioners or can access specialists directly (Ettelt et al. 2006).

In western Europe, there appears to be a declining trend in physicians who are generalists, partly reflecting the increasing complexity of medical treatments (Simoens and Hurst 2006) and financial factors. Consequently, some countries have stepped up measures to train additional numbers of primary care physicians (Sweden, Finland). Some have also accelerated efforts to train more nurses (e.g. the Netherlands) and/or to retain nurses who were thinking about leaving or re-attract those who had already left the sector.

Planning how many physicians and in what specialties will be needed is a complex and enduring policy challenge. One of the most widely used tools to manage supply is to limit medical school admissions. Among western European countries, Austria, Germany, Switzerland and, to some extent, Belgium and Greece do not place a restriction on the number of admissions to medical schools (Simoens and Hurst 2006). It has been suggested that the level and growth rate of physician density over time has been higher in those countries that do not, or have only recently, controlled intake to medical schools (Simoens and Hurst 2006). For example, from 1990 to 2005, the annual number of medical students graduating in France, Germany, Italy, Japan, Spain and Switzerland declined. But the lower numbers of physicians also reflect broader cost-containment measures introduced by many countries during the 1980s and 1990s. Because of the long-term implications of reducing medical school admissions, alongside the coming retirement of the post-First World War cohort of doctors, countries may find that they will have to depend to an even greater extent than at present on foreign-trained doctors.

The geographical distribution of physicians within a country is another important policy issue. Many countries have introduced measures to attract physicians to rural and deprived urban areas. In Greece, newly qualified doctors are required to undertake two years of practice in rural areas. In the United Kingdom, the general practitioner vocational training schemes encourage an equitable distribution of trainees. Norway and Sweden locate medical schools in sparsely populated parts of the country to attract students from those regions. Financial incentives related to training, such as offering scholarships to medical students who commit themselves to practise in areas that are poorly served, as seen in Norway, are also used. Regulatory mechanisms to improve geographical equity in physician supply, such as setting a threshold for the number of physicians contracted by a regional insurance fund, exist in Austria and Germany. Financial incentives linked to the payment mechanism to attract physicians to poorly served areas are used in the United Kingdom and have proved to be effective, although possibly more costly (Simoens and Hurst 2006).

In CCEEs, programmes have included efforts to transform substantial numbers of polyclinic specialists into general practitioners – an effort which began in the mid 1990s in countries like Estonia and Hungary and which is ongoing in countries further south and east. Meanwhile, in western Europe, the contrary is seen, with increasing attention paid to developing specialized polyclinics to substitute for independent general practice facilities, for example in Germany and the United Kingdom.

Training and recertification of health care professionals has been a topic of debate across the region. A growing number of countries now encourage continuing education programmes as part of a regular physician recertification process (Merkur et al. 2008). An extremely ambitious programme in the United Kingdom has faced major problems of implementation. National policy-makers have also introduced pilot schemes to help to develop a range of different physician substitutes and care extenders (particularly nurse practitioners and physician assistants). Training is increasingly addressing management and leadership skills, since these are needed by clinicians in positions of managerial and budgetary responsibility.

A high-performing workforce depends on the regulatory and financial incentive structures in the system (Maynard 2006) in addition to the working conditions to foster a healthy motivated workforce (Gunnarsdóttir and Rafferty 2006). With regards to the former, countries are introducing new models of regulation; for example, the United Kingdom introduced a costly system of regulation, inspection, target setting and audit for health and social care facilities, including new organizations mandated to establish evidence-based standards of practice (National Institute for Health and Clinical Excellence) and performance audits (Health Care Commission). Also, countries are introducing more blended payment systems and attempting to better link payment with performance.

Other efforts at improving value for money in the delivery of care have led to changes in professional boundaries and introduction of skill-substitution policies (Dubois, McKee and Nolte 2006b). An example is the creation of nurse-led clinics to manage chronic diseases. Substituting one type of provider for another, such as nurses instead of physicians as the first point of contact, is increasingly being seen as a way to improve patient satisfaction and quality, and has been shown to achieve this in certain circumstances. These changes in professional roles may be one way to ensure a more flexible and cost-effective delivery system, although there needs to be careful attention to ensure effectiveness is achieved, training and educational supports are in place and in some cases regulatory barriers are removed.

Most western European countries have been forced to recruit physicians and nurses from other EU countries (Polish physicians to Sweden; Danish physicians to Norway; Swedish nurses to Norway) and beyond (general practitioners from southeast Asia and Africa in the United Kingdom).

Increasing international recruitment of health care personnel can seem attractive to policy-makers (Buchan 2006) but it poses challenges both to the countries that lose their workers and to those that rely on foreign workers, in terms of language and other obstacles to adaptation into the new system. Reflecting the widespread use of English in developing countries, the United Kingdom is one of the countries relying most on migrant health professionals, though mainly from outside the EU (e.g. South Africa and India): approximately one-third of the 70,000 NHS hospital medical staff were from other countries in 2002; in 2003, more than two-thirds of the 15,000 new full medical registrants were from outside the United Kingdom (Buchan 2006). Poland is one of the countries that has experienced the most out-migration, though the level seems to be less than feared at the time of EU accession. Since 1995, 16,000 physicians left the country to work abroad, and currently about 40% of first-year nursing students are thinking of working abroad. There is a need to develop better information bases to monitor flows of staff, including those migrating as health workers and those moving into other forms of employment. Managed migration will become increasingly important in future because of demographic changes and continued EU enlargement. This could take the form of introducing educational and training supports, developing bilateral agreements between governments and/or employers in different countries and considering the possibility of arranging some sort of compensation for source countries (Buchan 2006).

Strengthening the public health workforce

The effective delivery of public health services requires an adequate workforce in terms of both skills and numbers. Many countries in Europe have been struggling to adjust to this challenge. Given the rapid development of knowledge on the effectiveness of public health interventions, it has become apparent that there is a lack of both scientists and practitioners in many countries. Different approaches in strengthening the workforce in terms of numbers and qualifications can be observed throughout Europe. Some countries, such as Hungary and Kazakhstan, have established new schools of public health. Between 1989 and 1995, Germany established several postgraduate courses. France reconfigured its public health training as part of its public health reform in 2004. Estonia introduced modern health promotion in the curriculum of medical and nursing training and initiated public health training for civil servants and teaching staff (Polluste, Mannik and Axelsson 2005). Croatia employed a modular training programme in order to compensate a lack of competence in public health, particularly in health management and strategy development, but also in health surveillance and prevention (Sogoric et al. 2005). The effectiveness of multifaceted programmes that include training and dialogue on various levels and with different professions has been demonstrated in the Russian Federation (Jenkins et al. 2007). There are now well-established links among public health schools, universities and public health associations across Europe (Gulis et al. 2005).

Paying for capital structure

Innovative policy programmes have been introduced to create new models of ownership of public hospitals (foundation hospitals in United Kingdom, Spain and Portugal) and also private finance for building turnkey public hospitals (private finance initiative in United Kingdom). There have been concerns raised that this strategy, while substituting for expensive publicly raised capital, can still lead to higher total expenditures on interest and rent over the longer (often 30 year) term. There are growing concerns that these models will tie public authorities into physical structures that may be less than optimal for meeting service requirements in the future (McKee, Edwards and Atun 2006).

There also have been major programmes, initially in CCEEs and continuing in CIS countries and funded by the European Investment Bank and the World Bank and several bilateral donor agencies, to build new hospitals, to renovate existing facilities and to re-equip hospitals to make them more clinically efficient and effective. While the quality of the capital stock in CCEEs and the Baltic countries has improved dramatically since 1990, there remain a substantial number of challenges. At the same time, there is growing recognition of the need for innovation in hospital design to take account of new models of health care (Rechel et al. 2010).

Focusing on pharmaceuticals

Differing patterns of pharmaceutical expenditure growth can be seen in most countries in recent decades. Measured as the proportion of total health spending derived from pharmaceuticals, notable increases during the period 1996 to 2005 can be seen in Estonia (17 to 27% of total health spending), Serbia (12 to 22%), Czech Republic (25 to 30%), the Netherlands (11 to 14%) and Spain (20 to 23%), although there was a decline over this period in some countries such as Italy and Portugal, where pharmaceutical spending was already above 20% of total health expenditure (WHO Regional Office for Europe 2007).

One of the primary mechanisms governments used to control pharmaceutical expenditure is price regulation, including price control, profit control, international price comparisons and reference pricing (Mrazek and Mossialos 2004). Price fixing is based on what is determined to be a 'reasonable' price for the product based on affordability and effectiveness. Setting a maximum price can be done through negotiated prices, price caps and price comparisons with other countries; the least transparent of these approaches is negotiation between industry and government. International price comparisons are used in the majority of countries, including CCEEs and all countries in western Europe except Germany and the United Kingdom.

Reference pricing, a form of indirect price control, refers to setting a maximum reimbursement level that the third-party payer, whether government or insurance fund, pays. The reference price can be defined in different ways, such as the lowest priced generic equivalent available on the market (as in Denmark, Italy and Portugal), the average or median price of drugs with similar pharmacotherapeutic effects (as in Germany and the Netherlands) or at a proportion lower than the price of the original branded drug (as in Belgium, fixed at 26% lower) (Mrazek and Mossialos 2004). Reference pricing is also widely used in CCEEs, including the Czech Republic, Estonia, Hungary, Lithuania, Poland, Romania and Slovakia. Reference pricing can also be linked to reimbursement decisions by setting a maximum level of reimbursement by the payer beyond which the patient must bear any additional cost. Evidence suggests, however, that cost savings through reference price systems have generally been only short term (Mossialos, Brogan and Walley 2006), and as noted above pharmaceutical costs continue to rise as a proportion of total health spending in most countries.

Profit control as a method of limiting spending is currently unique to the United Kingdom, where free pricing exists at the time of drug launch but later profits are clawed back by the government (the maximum allowable profit is set at a 21% rate of return on capital). Because expenditure depends on a combination of price and volume, direct price regulation schemes may not be effective in controlling expenditure since savings could be offset by volume increases. Furthermore, price control systems currently do not provide incentives to reward therapeutic value of a drug and clinical gains. While the profit-control system in the United Kingdom may not have been successful in containing costs, it does appear to encourage innovation (Mossialos, Brogan and Walley 2006).

Decisions about whether and at what level to reimburse the cost of drugs to the insurance beneficiaries depend both on negotiations between the pharmaceutical company and the payer and policy decisions regarding cost-sharing arrangements. Increasingly, economic evaluation is being used to make reimbursement decisions, for example in Finland and the United Kingdom. However, there are numerous challenges involved, such as deciding what costs and consequences to include in the analyses, how to ensure consistent application of guidelines, limited generalizability of the results because of context-specific factors, and the extensive resources needed to undertake analyses. Many countries are now including economic concepts in applying for reimbursement listing; however, the extent to which this information is used by payers is not always clear. In Finland, a product's price and reimbursement are explicitly linked to the results of economic evaluation, but in many other countries (Denmark, Switzerland, Sweden, the Netherlands, Italy, Portugal, Norway, England and Wales, and the Baltic States), economic evidence is considered to some extent. In Germany and France, cost-effectiveness analyses are used to inform decisions about reimbursement, but not prices (although it is becoming more important for pricing in France).

Other possible pricing mechanisms to contain costs include the Ramsay method – that prices should differ across market segments inversely with their demand elasticities – or that governments should purchase patents and releasing them for public use through auction. More importantly, to contain pharmaceutical costs while encouraging innovation and best value, the integration of pricing and reimbursement activities seems to be advantageous, as increasingly seen in some countries such as Belgium, the Netherlands and Sweden (Mossialos, Brogan and Walley 2006).

Policies to promote generic drugs are prevalent in Europe, with most countries choosing a combination of approaches. Financial incentives for pharmacists, such as higher margins or additional payments, may provide an incentive to dispense a lower-cost generic equivalent (e.g. in France, the Netherlands, Norway, Spain and the United Kingdom). Similarly, in Romania and Estonia, pharmacists are required to dispense the least-cost multisourced product. However, this policy is contingent on pharmacists being authorized to make changes to a physician's prescription. In some countries, physicians are mandated or encouraged to prescribe by generic name, as in Finland, France, Germany, Ireland, Italy, Luxembourg, the Netherlands, Portugal, some regions in Spain, and the United Kingdom. Since generic substitution is only permitted in some countries (e.g. Denmark, Finland, France, Norway, Spain; with the physician's consent in Poland; and only if the original brand is not available in the Czech Republic), financial incentives are instead placed on patients in the form of reference pricing (as mentioned above). These measures have contributed to the growing share of the pharmaceutical market held by generics, but it is less clear to what extent they have slowed overall expenditure growth.

In containing pharmaceutical costs, much depends on whether physicians are given the appropriate incentives to prescribe generics and aim for best value for money. Recent years have seen a growth in incentives for physicians, such as individual, practice or collective prescribing budgets in the United Kingdom and Germany, or prescribing guidelines in France. Evidence of the impact of these different types of incentive is not conclusive. Their effectiveness relies on both adequate information systems to track the guidelines and also explicit quality assurance mechanisms (Mossialos, Walley and Rudisill 2005).

Financing (collection and pooling): ensuring sustainability and solidarity

How health systems raise the funds they need to operate and the structure of the pooling arrangements they adopt to share risk are crucial to the ability of these systems to meet both their clinical and their social responsibilities (Mossialos et al. 2002). Efforts to reconfigure funding can be found equally in systems with non-competitive single source tax-based funding as in social health insurance systems, and in both western European countries and CCEEs.

Spending on health varies widely across countries, with higher spending as a proportion of GDP generally found in richer countries. Since the mid 1990s, expenditure on health as a proportion of GDP has risen in most countries, with some exceptions such as Estonia, Finland, Lithuania, Azerbaijan, Croatia, the Russian Federation and Uzbekistan (WHO Regional Office for Europe 2007). Taking a longer view, among western European countries where data on expenditure are available for more years, the period of most rapid growth for most countries appears to be the 1970s. Over the three decades health care expenditure as a proportion of GDP more than doubled in several countries, with growth by only a third in Finland, the Netherlands and Sweden (Organisation for Economic Co-operation and Development 2007; Thomson, Foubister and Mossialos 2008). Table 9.1 shows the average expenditure as a proportion of GDP for the following country-groupings: WHO European Region, the EU, the western European countries that were EU Member States before May 2004 (EU15), the EU Member States since enlargement (2004 (EU25) or 2007 (EU27)) and CIS.

Funding health services

European health care systems rely on a mix of contribution mechanisms to finance health care, with the majority providing universal (or near universal) statutory health coverage. In most countries, the majority of expenditure on health (as a proportion of GDP) is generated publicly. Since 1998 the trend has been towards a modest increase in the public share of expenditure on average, although a decline was seen in several countries: Andorra, Belarus, Bulgaria, Croatia, Czech Republic, Estonia, France, Germany, Hungary, Lithuania, Luxembourg, Moldova, Slovakia, Slovenia, Sweden and the former Yugoslav

Table 9.1 Total health expenditure as a proportion of gross domestic product in the European Region, European Union and the Commonwealth of Independent States, 1998–2008

	1998	2000	2002	2004	2006	2008	Percentage change 1998–2008 %	Percentage point change 1998–2008 %
European Region	7.2	7.0	7.5	7.5	7.5	7.6	5.6	0.4
EU	7.9	8.1	8.5	8.8	8.9	9.0	13.9	1.1
EU 15	8.6	8.7	9.1	9.4	9.5	9.7	12.8	1.1
EU 25/27	5.8	5.9	6.5	6.4	6.3	6.4	10.3	0.6
CIS	6.5	5.5	5.8	5.4	5.5	5.4	−16.9	−1.1

Source: WHO Regional Office for Europe 2011

Republic of Macedonia (Table 9.2 shows average public sector contributions to total expenditure for the five country groupings).

The most common funding mechanisms are general taxation and dedicated taxation (usually in the form of payroll taxes for compulsory contributory-based 'social' health insurance), although out-of-pocket payments represent an important financing mechanism in many countries (notably, Bulgaria, Cyprus, Greece, Latvia, and most of the countries in the former USSR) (Fig. 9.1).[1] Decisions about health care funding are inevitably political as they involve redistribution of resources. Hence, developments reflect the prevailing political complexion of governments. Some mechanisms being explored at present include diversifying contribution mechanism to finance health care, shifting the burden from collective financing to the individual, reforming the mechanisms used to pool funds, extending insurance competition and extending or reorganizing the funding of long-term care.

Table 9.2 Public sector expenditure as a percentage (%) of total health expenditure, 1998–2008

	1998	2000	2002	2004	2006	2008	Percentage change 1998–2008 %	Percentage point change 1998–2008 %
European Region	68.4	66.6	67.5	68.1	69.0	70.0	2.3	1.6
EU	74.5	74.9	75.1	75.0	76.1	76.6	2.8	2.1
EU 15	75.7	75.9	76.0	76.1	77.2	77.5	2.4	1.8
EU 25/27	70.2	71.2	71.6	70.9	72.1	73.0	4.0	2.8
CIS	57.4	53.4	53.9	55.4	57.2	58.8	2.4	1.4

Source: WHO Regional Office for Europe 2011

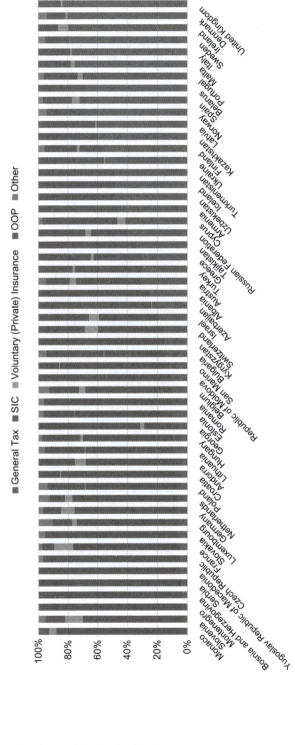

Legend: ■ General Tax ■ SIC ■ Voluntary (Private) Insurance ■ OOP ■ Other

Figure 9.1 Health financing mix by expenditure agent in European countries, 2009

Source: World Health Organization 2011

Notes: SIC is social insurance contributions, OOP is out-of-pocket payments. For countries in western Europe, SIC refers to all funds channelled through health insurance funds, which may include substantial amounts of tax revenue. For all other countries, SIC refers specifically to dedicated taxes (earmarked payroll or earmarked income tax revenues for health insurance), while tax revenue includes only general taxes.

Diversifying contribution mechanism to finance health care

In response to rising cost pressures, national policy-makers have adopted a wide range of sometimes contradictory initiatives. One major set of initiatives has sought to diversify contribution mechanisms to finance care in publicly operated health systems. By broadening the contribution mechanisms, policy-makers have tried to reduce their reliance on highly visible and tightly constrained income taxes, and to tap new sources that can provide additional revenues. Some have sought to broaden public funding, for example shifting the burden to regional governments (as in Italy, Sweden, Finland and Spain). In some western European countries such as France, Germany and the Netherlands, there have been efforts to broaden revenue bases linked to employment (see below). This contrasts with the experience in the CCEEs in the 1990s, where there was a shift away from tax financing to employment-related insurance contributions. Other measures have sought to increase private contribution mechanisms, both collective in the form of private insurance and individual, with increased cost-sharing.

Shifting the burden from collective financing to the individual

Some countries have sought to shift the burden from collective financing to the individual, whether through encouragement of private, risk-related voluntary insurance, as in the CCEE (though the private market remains limited) and France and Slovenia (indirectly through complementary insurance covering statutory cost-sharing). Elsewhere, the cost has been shifted directly to those receiving care, through increased co-payments and deductibles and no-claim bonuses. Cost sharing was introduced in all CCEEs as a means of raising revenue following independence, and more recently was extended in several countries, such as Austria, the Czech Republic, Estonia, France, Germany, Hungary, the Netherlands, Portugal and Romania. An increase in private funding in CCEEs can be seen since the mid 1990s, which has been almost wholly driven by an increase in out-of-pocket payments.

Nearly all of the CIS countries experienced a severe economic and fiscal contraction in the early 1990s, which translated into substantial declines in government spending on health, and a consequent rise in out-of-pocket spending. This was driven more by the wider economic context than explicit policy choices, and in many cases was an attempt to formalize the widespread informal payments in many countries (Lewis 2002; Vagac and Haulikova 2003). In 2004 in several countries (Georgia, Azerbaijan, Tajikistan, Armenia, Kyrgyzstan, Albania and Uzbekistan), out-of-pocket spending constituted over half of total health spending (Sheiman et al. 2010).

Reforming the pooling of funds

Several countries have changed responsibilities for pooling funds. In some cases, this has taken place within 'budgetary' systems of universal population-based entitlement, for example in Italy (1997–2001), Finland (1990s), Spain (2001) and Sweden (1980s and 1990s), where responsibility for pooling (and purchasing) health care was decentralized from the national level to the regions, and, conversely, in Denmark (2007), where the shift was from regional to national level.

Also within the public sector, there was a shift from a reliance on general tax revenues and universal, population-based entitlement to a reliance on dedicated (usually payroll) tax funding and contribution-based entitlement in most of the CCEE. Here there were important differences in motivation and historical experience between (i) the CIS countries, (ii) the countries that emerged from Yugoslavia, and (iii) the other central European and Baltic countries. Beginning with the last, most countries introduced social health insurance arrangements that marked, at least in symbolic form, a return to the systems in place in the pre-Communist era. This began with Hungary in 1990, Estonia in 1992, the Czech Republic in 1993, Slovakia in 1994, Lithuania in 1997, and most recently Bulgaria, Poland and Romania in 1999. The successor states to Yugoslavia inherited a highly decentralized system of social health insurance that was actually introduced in 1948 (Davis 2010). Most of these countries switched to a centralized single insurance fund approach early in the 1990s (the former Yugoslav Republic of Macedonia in 1991, Serbia and Montenegro – each with its own fund – in 1992, and Croatia and Slovenia in 1993). Pooling in Bosnia and Herzegovina remains decentralized, reflecting the failure to reach agreement among the communities involved, with 13 cantonal funds for 3.9 million people. By way of contrast, only 5 of the 12 CIS countries introduced some form of compulsory health insurance, including the Russian Federation in 1993, Georgia in 1995, Kazakhstan in 1996, Kyrgyzstan in 1997 and the Republic of Moldova in 2004. Georgia and Kazakhstan abandoned their efforts to introduce social health insurance, although they kept some features rather than simply reverting to the previous Soviet-era model (Kutzin et al. 2010).

Some countries that introduced new insurance funds used them to reduce fragmentation of pooling. The CIS countries inherited highly fragmented and decentralized health systems, with each administrative level of government (central/republican, provincial/oblast, district/city/rayon, and even in villages in some cases) having its own vertically integrated financing (pooling and purchasing) and delivery system. In urban areas, these systems overlapped, leading to duplication of infrastructure for the local population (e.g. oblast capitals would have separate city and oblast children's hospitals, maternity hospitals, tuberculosis hospitals, etc.). In Kyrgyzstan in 2001, the Mandatory Health Insurance Fund (MHIF) was used as the agent to change this system. Over a four-year period, general budget revenues from local (rayon and oblast) governments were pooled in the oblast department of the MHIF, and in turn providers were separated administratively from the MHIF and paid on the basis of outputs (case-based payment for hospitals) and population need (capitation for primary care). This eliminated the fragmentation that existed within oblasts, and in 2006 the locus of pooling was shifted from oblast to national level. This centralization of pooling, combined with output- and population-based payment methods, meant that differences between oblasts in the level of government health spending per capita were reduced in 2006 compared with 2005 (Kutzin et al. 2010). Similarly in the Republic of Moldova in 2004, nationwide implementation of a compulsory health insurance fund managing a single national pool of funds from a prior system in which pooling was decentralized to rayon level led to improved equity in government health spending across rayons following the reform (Shishkin, Kacevicius and Ciocanu 2008).

The shift from collecting and pooling funds at national level to social insurance funds has brought about new challenges, particularly if there are weak collection systems, as is the case in some countries. For example, in Hungary, Estonia and Romania difficulties enforcing collections led to a shift in responsibility for collecting revenue from the insurance funds (in Romania for the employed but not self-employed people) to the central government tax agency in 1998, 1999 and 2002, respectively. In Hungary, an online system was also introduced to verify that the users of health services had paid their contributions (Thomson, Foubister and Mossialos 2008). However, in some countries, such as Romania and Bulgaria, difficulties in obtaining identity documents and registering with the insurance scheme have systematically discriminated against the already severely disadvantaged Roma population.

Extending insurance competition

Other countries have sought to create or extend competition between funds managing compulsory social insurance revenues (including non-profit-making and profit-making insurers) with one or several of the following aims: to improve responsiveness to consumers, to improve equity in contributions or entitlements (by introducing choice and risk adjustment in systems in which people were formerly assigned to funds on the basis of occupation or other criteria), and in the hope of creating create incentives for improved purchasing and greater efficiency and quality in service delivery (Czech Republic, Germany, the Netherlands and Slovakia in the 1990s, and Switzerland in the early 2000s). However, this approach faces many obvious challenges, in particular the scope for risk selection, and poses serious threats to equity. Evidence suggests that these reforms have not achieved their aims; for example, only short-term convergence of contribution rates was seen in Germany (Gresz et al. 2002; Schut, Gresz and Wasem 2003), and in Germany and the Netherlands it appears that younger, healthier and better-educated people are more likely than others to change fund (Zok 1999; Gresz et al. 2002). Moreover, while some types of risk adjustment mechanism are in place in these countries to compensate health insurance funds for high risk members, they can be technically and politically challenging and incur high transaction costs (van de Ven et al. 2007).

The Netherlands has developed a complex risk adjustment model that operates at both the level of the individual subscriber and at the level of the entire fund vis-à-vis the national funding pool. The individual-level adjustment has been instrumental in making elderly and/or chronically ill individuals attractive to commercial insurers on the competitive market (Groenewegen and de Jong 2007), while the fund-level adjustment is still less than 50% of total expenditures and is subject to continual change in the risk level (van Ginnekin, Busse and Gericke 2008). Germany instituted a risk-adjustment process at the fund level for older people in 1989, which was subsequently expanded to include disabled people and also patients enrolled in disease management programmes (Busse 2001).

Another notable example is the Czech reform introduced in 2003 and intended to progressively increase (over a three-year period) the scope of redistribution from 60% of health insurance contributions to 100% of these contributions, reducing differences in conditions for people enrolled in different funds and also reducing the private benefits of risk selection behaviour by insurers.

Funding long-term care

One area where considerable reform has been underway has been in the funding of long-term care. Dedicated funding arrangements tied to separate social insurance funds were established in Austria (1993), Germany (1995) and France (2002). These have now been joined by reformed public funding arrangements in Sweden (1993) while other tax-funded countries have recently extended basic entitlements to long-term care funded through taxation in Luxembourg (1998), Scotland (2002) and Spain (2006–2007). In Sweden, by comparison, efforts have been made by municipal governments to cover higher long-term care and home care costs by increasing co-payments from service recipients.

A number of countries have responded to the particular challenges of long-term care with a range of innovative payment strategies (Saltman, Dubois and Chawla 2006). One example, used in Germany, is funding previously unpaid members of family and/or neighbours who are caring for a frail elderly person to keep them in their own homes as long as possible (thus avoiding the construction and operating costs of institutional facilities). Sweden and Finland, for similar reasons, allow informal carers to receive pension credits from the national pension system. Several countries have dedicated funds for respite care, as well as training and telephone advice on caring issues.

Funding public health

Strengthening the financing function for public health services is an important reform strategy for improving health system performance. The elements of this reform strategy are scaling up investment for health, determining levels of funding, using pooled budgets and introducing new mechanisms for collecting funds.

Spending on public health is very difficult to measure reliably. The available data suggest that in western Europe, despite increased political rhetoric, there has been an increase in funding only in some countries, for example Austria (from 1.6% total health spending in 1995 to 2% in 2005), and the Netherlands (from 3.5% to 4.7%) (Organisation for Economic Co-operation and Development 2007). Funding levels are very low in most countries, with public health and prevention accounting for about 0.7% in Italy, to 4.7% in the Netherlands and 3.9% in Finland. Spending on prevention includes a wide range of programmes, such as vaccination programmes and public health campaigns on alcohol abuse and smoking. It is important to exercise caution when interpreting public health expenditure data: some public health programmes may not be accounted for, such as those undertaken by general practitioners; public health activities may be coordinated or funded by other ministries, such as social and environmental ministries; and costs for some activities, in particular occupational health programmes, may be undertaken in the private sector.

The expansion of public health services requires scaling up of investment. The influential Wanless Report commissioned by the United Kingdom Treasury made the case for substantially increasing expenditure on public health to meet future societal and demographic challenges (Wanless 2002). Countries such as Austria, Germany (Wanek 2008), France (L'Assemblée nationale, Sénat Le Président de la République 2004), Switzerland (Institute of Microeconomics and Public Finance 2007) and Finland (Vuorenkoski 2007) have formulated similar intentions and commitments. It has been questioned whether these commitments to scale up investment in public health services will translate into real increases in funding (Martin 2006; Wanek 2008), particularly since many countries are introducing severe austerity measures.

Decisions on the level of investment in each country are essentially political, hopefully informed by scrutiny of expenditure for existing services (Fachkommission 2006) and decisions on the balance between different types of service (de Bekker-Grob et al. 2007).

Pooling budgets is another strategy to improve health system performance. The United Kingdom and Sweden have experimented with pooled budgets for integrated health and welfare services, facilitating collaboration by different services, programmes and professions (Hultberg, Lonnroth and Allebeck 2003; Hultberg et al. 2005). The pooled budgets may also help to scale up investment in health.

Countries have also introduced new mechanisms to collect funds for public health. For example, every insured person in Switzerland pays an annual contribution of SFr. 2.40 for health promotion that is collected by the social health insurance companies and pooled by the federal health promotion agency Health Promotion Switzerland (Fachkommission 2006). Estonia has introduced a similar mechanism (Bayarsaikhan and Muiser 2007).

Financing (purchasing): ensuring allocative (health gain) and technical efficiency

A second critical dimension of financing is the process of allocating pooled revenues to health service providers, or purchasing health care. This can be achieved through a wide variety of different mechanisms (budgets, contracts, reimbursement formulae), each of which brings a different package of incentives to bear on the performance of health professionals and institutions.

Strategic purchasing to improve performance

A few countries made some tentative moves towards some form of strategic purchasing model (defined as linking the allocation to providers to *information* on provider performance or the needs of the population they serve) from the early 1990s onwards. A separation of purchaser and provider functions in theory should make it possible to focus resources on priority areas, giving purchasers a potential lever to improve provider performance. Following the 'internal market' in the United Kingdom NHS introduced in 1991, Italy, Portugal and some regions in Spain and Sweden also introduced purchaser–provider splits. A variety of different mechanisms are available, beginning from health needs assessment and the use of contracts, which may include quality monitoring and performance-based payment systems. Each brings a different package of incentives (often financial) to bear on the performance of health professionals and institutions.

There has also been considerable interest in the perceived money-saving potential of selective contracting mechanisms, particularly in social health insurance systems where patients have traditionally had the right to see any doctor or hospital they want. However, the restrictions required by selective contracting run directly counter to the growing desire for greater patient choice of provider, a trend that has continued to strengthen in tax-funded health systems.

Purchasing mechanisms can also link the flow of funds to compliance with a range of performance measurement instruments. In the United Kingdom in 2003, higher pay for general practitioners was tied to participation in performance monitoring. In 2006, the Netherlands adopted a complex new system of pooling and purchasing for health care services (Groenewegen and de Jong 2007; van Ginnekin, Busse and Gericke 2008). Individuals, responsible out of pocket (with public subsidies for low income) for 50% of their health contributions (the 'nominal premium'), can join a wide range of existing (employer, patient associations) and newly created (online voluntary groupings) 'collectives' through which to pool funds and negotiate coverage levels and benefits with the new hybrid 'health insurers'. At the same time, the other 50% of their health premium, collected from workers' salaries but then reimbursed by employers, are brought together in a state-run national pool and allocated to these same hybrid insurers on a prospective, individual form of risk assessment. It is as yet unclear the extent to which this complex system can meet the efficiency and cost-control objectives of its designers. One key problem is that the individual mandate basis upon which this model is based has so far resulted in 240,000 adults not purchasing health insurance.

Performance-based payment: hospitals

An increasing number of countries have experimented with mechanisms to improve the efficiency and transparency of hospital services. Most European health systems have in place a hospital payment system based on global budgets, although increasingly case-based payments (often referred to as diagnosis-related groups) – a fixed fee for service that is risk adjusted by case mix complexity – are being introduced to define the budgets or as a form of payment. While (hard) budgets have the potential to contain costs, case-based payments bring incentives to increase activity and also increase transparency in typically opaque hospital accounting systems.

Although the specific goals of introducing case-based payments in hospital care vary across countries, with some aiming to increase activity and lower waiting times and others seeking to control costs and improve transparency in financing, all broadly aim to create incentives for greater provider efficiency. There are also variations in the design of the hospital case-based payment systems; for example, the broader *Diagnose Behandel Combinatie* in the Netherlands includes payment for both specialist physicians and hospitals in one package. There are inevitably risks of premature discharge along with increasing readmission rates, so careful monitoring is required. Results of a recent review suggest that diagnosis-related groups have the advantage of increasing activity, generating information on hospital costs and case mix along with encouraging cost control per diagnosis, although these can potentially be undermined by incentives for cream skimming, up-coding, cost shifting and quality skimping (Busse, Schreyögg and Smith 2006).

Performance-based payment: physicians

Across Europe, the main approaches for paying providers are salary, capitation and fee for service. In the public sector, most primary and outpatient care doctors are paid on a salaried or capitation basis, or a combination of the two. In primary care, capitation payments are predominantly used in Croatia, the United Kingdom, Estonia, Hungary, Italy, Kazakhstan, Kyrgyzstan, Lithuania, the Netherlands, Poland, Romania and Slovakia, and are being piloted in the Russian Federation, and Serbia and Montenegro. Fee-for-service payments prevail in Austria, Belgium, France, Germany, Luxembourg and Switzerland. This method of payment is also the norm for privately delivered primary and outpatient care. For hospital doctors, however, salary payment is the most common method, with the exception of Belgium and Switzerland. Fee-for-service systems have an incentive to increase activity, while salary and capitation methods may control costs but have incentives to decrease activity and shift patients' costs onto other providers. Several studies have found evidence for payment method having effects on physician behaviour (Chaix-Couturier et al. 2000; Gosden, Forland and Kristiansen 2000); therefore, countries are increasingly experimenting with blended, or mixed, payment schemes that include elements of the different methods to maximize the positive and moderate the negative incentives.

In some countries, particularly in CCEE, there has been a move away from payment of primary care providers by salary towards fee for services or payment based on capitation; in other countries, for example many in western Europe, there has been an extension of fee-for-service payments in addition to capitation to increase the provision of preventive care and reward good performance.

Purchasing mechanisms may be able to offset the effects of perverse incentives by careful linkage of funds to compliance with quality indicators. Provider contracts are, in a few countries, being tied to quality indicators, which may include meeting quality standards, following quality assurance procedures or achieving defined outcomes. In the same way, some countries are moving towards performance-based payment systems for professionals, with explicit financial incentives to reward certain behaviours and outcomes. The payment system for English general practitioners brings higher rewards to those achieving certain quality targets. However, as with all types of performance-related pay, it also has problems. In this case, it was found that most general practitioners already met the targets (White 2006), so that the budget was exceeded, leading to subsequent failure to increase fees with inflation and resulting reduced morale.

Strengthening stewardship

Stewardship and governance sit at the heart not just of health reform strategies but of health policy-making in general. They signal the obligation of governments to ensure that policy decisions are carefully thought through, that the implications for differing constituencies are adequately balanced and that the overall outcome within the health system is both optimal and fair.

The concept of stewardship was first applied to health systems in *The World Health Report 2000* (World Health Organization 2000). At that time, it was a new way to conceptualize health system governance, drawing upon previous concepts of a good steward taken from religious and environmental organizations (Saltman and Ferroussier-Davis 2000). Stewardship, in a key departure from previous governance approaches, entails a focus on steering health systems at a strategic level – rather than directly managing or operating important organizational units. Instead of dealing with day-to-day operational issues, stewardship sets out goals and objectives to be achieved and stipulates the rules under which those goals are to be reached. Moreover, a good steward seeks strategies to pursue those objectives that can achieve efficient as well as equitable outcomes. In many ways, stewardship involves establishing the clinical, legal, financial and managerial 'rules of the game', the basis on which the overall health system takes form and acts. In this sense, stewardship and governance are where the other three functions – service delivery, resource generation, and financing – are brought together to generate the desired health system structure and outcome.

The concept of stewardship touches on nearly all aspects of service delivery: staffing, training, management, patient safety, quality of care and equity of both access and of outcome, as well as on more structural issues such as the financing arrangements and the ownership of providers. It also applies directly to expanding activities in public health, health promotion, disease prevention and population health. This section will focus on three central elements of effective stewardship: regulating health services delivery, decentralization of organizational structure, and public health and health promotion.

Regulating the delivery of health services

The regulatory environment for health services has become more complex since the mid 1980s as the role of the state has changed to accommodate a variety of structural developments in health systems. A key factor in this shift has been the melting of organizational and political boundaries between public and private actors in the health sector, particularly among providers (Saltman 2003). A second, accompanying element has been the increasingly complex mix of market and state mechanisms and incentives, again primarily among providers but also in some countries in financing (for example the Netherlands, with the emergence of 'health insurers'). Both structural shifts have required governments to rethink how they regulate health sector actors, and to reconsider the tools they utilize to do so.

Moreover, they have had to do so in a complicated environment that includes other regional and local governments, often as well as traditional self-regulatory roles for professional associations (Saltman, Busse and Mossialos 2002). In a useful summary of the characteristics of different regulatory actors, Baldwin and Cave (1999) noted some of the different capabilities that go into this regulatory mix: self-regulators tend to be strong on specialist knowledge but weak on accountability to the public; local authorities strong on local democratic accountability, weak on coordination; parliament strong on democratic authority, weak on sustained scrutiny; courts and tribunals strong on fairness, weak on planning; central departments strong on coordination with the government, weak on neutrality; agencies strong on expertise and combining functions, weak on neutrality; and directors general strong on specialization and identification of responsibility, weak on spreading discretionary powers. The stewardship role of national governments obligates them to harness these different characteristics to a regulatory regime that can optimize the ability of the overall system to reach the objectives that the state has set for it.

Recent regulatory initiatives in European health systems have sought to balance reform-driven efforts to stimulate greater entrepreneurialism with legislatively mandated requirements to maintain existing social and economic policy objectives. Policy-makers have had to accommodate the differing rationales and expectations that various health sector actors bring to the regulatory process, seeking strategies and tools with which to establish effective yet not overly restrictive frameworks to steer institutional decision-making.

This need to balance the shifting public–private mix of actors along with the rights and interests of multiple decision-making institutions has generated four different categories of regulatory initiatives (Saltman and Busse 2002). The first, regulation that stimulates entrepreneurial opportunities, needs to be differentiated from a second, regulation that promotes competition but restricts the entrepreneurial freedom of individual actors. This differentiation is, however, not as clear cut as it may initially appear. A considerable degree of regulation restricts individual entrepreneurs in the short term in order to facilitate sustainable competitive markets in the long term. Pro-competitive regulation can, therefore, either stimulate or restrict short-term entrepreneurial behaviour. A third category of regulation restricts entrepreneurial decisions as a way to safeguard the social and economic policy objectives discussed above. A fourth category concerns regulation restricting entrepreneurial freedom that cannot be directly associated with specific social and economic policy objectives.

These four categories provide a conceptual template with which governments have sought to steer the activities and behaviour of health sector actors towards the desired objectives. While some governments have been notably successful in this new regulatory environment (the Netherlands and Switzerland), others have found it difficult to accommodate the varying interests involved. Powerful providers and/or interest groups have sought to twist the regulatory process to their own short-term advantage (known as 'regulatory capture'). This process has been particularly complicated in a number of CCEEs and the CIS, reflecting a lack of experience with state regulation of independent non-state entities. One particular problem in these countries has been the somewhat counter-intuitive importance of preceding needed deregulation of overly intrusive directives with the establishment of a new, less-intrusive but nonetheless effective regulatory regimen – in short, the need for a good steward to re-regulate before de-regulating.

Decentralizing organizational structures

The logic of decentralization is based on an intrinsically powerful idea (Saltman, Bankauskaite and Vrangbæk 2007). It is, simply stated, that smaller organizations, properly structured and steered, are inherently more agile and accountable than are larger organizations. In a world where large organizations control wide swaths of both public and private sector activity, the possibility of establishing more locally operated, locally responsible institutions holds out great attraction as an inherently more democratic and also more economically efficient approach. Given these potential outcomes, decentralization has been viewed in many countries in Europe as a necessary and logical element of wise stewardship of a health care system.

However, when probed more deeply, this single, seemingly simple charac-ter of decentralization opens up a broad array of concepts, objectives and con-sequences. Europe contains a large number of political, economic, organizational and legal variants of decentralization, each supported by its own specific logic. Decentralized bodies range from otherwise distinct countries containing millions of people and with their own health, education and legal systems (such as Scotland, Wales and Northern Ireland within the United Kingdom) to tiny hamlets with only several hundred residents (Finland, Norway). Moreover, the health-related powers of these decentralized bodies run from nearly independent decision-making (regions in Spain) to serving as little more than administrative paper processors for the national government (provinces in Finland). The decentralized bodies themselves may be publicly operated institutions (tax-funded countries), not-profit-making private bodies (sickness funds in social health insurance countries), or profit-making companies listed on the stock exchange (insurers in Switzerland).

A central issue is whether decentralized units are primarily political entities (run according to democratic rules), administrative entities (run according to managerial precepts) or fiscal entities (run primarily as financial bodies) (Saltman and Bankauskaite 2006). Further, as administrative and/or fiscal entities, it is unclear whether decentralized units are more efficient than centralized units (as some economists suggest) or less efficient (as other economists contend). Regarding the ability to accommodate key aspects of modern systems, it is unclear whether decentralized units are more sensitive to equity issues (the democratic argument) or less sensitive (the tyranny of the majority argument).

Recently, there are a small but growing number of countries that appear to be retreating from key tenets of decentralization and are, instead, recentralizing important health system functions (Saltman 2008). In 2002, Norway recentralized operating authority from 19 elected county councils into state hands, then allocated it to six new, appointed regional boards. Moreover, health sector financing in Norway has remained a national not a regional responsibility. Similarly, the Danish National Government in 2006 recentralized both operating and financing responsibility away from its 14 elected county councils, dismantling these bodies to give operating authority to five new regional entities, while making the financing of health care an exclusive function of the state. Elements of recentralization also have played a prominent role in recent health care reforms in Ireland, Poland and Germany, as well as in recent funding criteria introduced in Italy. Moreover, as noted above, the centralization of pooling in countries like the Republic of Moldova is seen to have improved the degree of equity in the health system.

This recent upsurge in countries that are, in effect, reversing trend and beginning to recentralize key functions within their health systems raises important questions about the overall strategy of decentralization in the health sector. To what extent is the primacy of the local democracy argument now being supplanted by an economic efficiency argument? How in this context does one understand the upsurge in discussion about and, to a lesser degree, adoption in European health systems of a greater role for private sector actors? Further, and somewhat contentiously, will countries that remain assiduously committed to decentralization, for example Spain (Bohigas 2008), find in the future that they too will have to reassess their basic governance assumptions?

In response to these developments, it is become apparent that decentralization is not a 'magic bullet' capable of solving all structural and policy dilemmas at a single stroke. There is no set model, no perfect or permanent solution that all countries should seek to adopt. Rather, there are multiple models of configuration, each developed to fit the particular context and circumstances of an individual country (Saltman, Bankauskaite and Vrangbæk 2007). Typically, health systems in which some areas are decentralized will have other areas that have been centrally controlled or may be recentralized. Consequently, the key questions for policy-makers continue to lie in the mix of decentralization and recentralization strategies in a given system and the balance between those strategies.

Public health and health promotion

Stewardship in public health is evident by the national public health strategies and accompanying goals that have been developed in many countries. The strategies differ, reflecting the national context and political choices, but they also have much in common, for example the widespread emphasis on tackling inequalities in health. Comprehensive policies to reduce social inequalities in health can be seen in England, Sweden, Finland and, at a local level, in the Netherlands (Judge et al. 2006). The concept of health strategies has echoes at international level. In the EU, following the Maastricht Treaty in 1992, eight priority areas were identified for community action programmes based on the burden of the disease, its socioeconomic impact, the degree to which it is amenable to preventive action and whether the programmes would be valuable and complementary to current practice in the Member States (Merkel and Hübel 1999). These priority areas were identified as health promotion, cancer, AIDS, drug dependence, health monitoring, injuries, rare diseases and pollution-related diseases. The EU's multi-annual public health programme running from 2003 to 2008 sought to improve information and knowledge for the development of public health, to enhance the capability of responding rapidly and in a coordinated fashion to threats to health, and to promote health and prevent disease through addressing health determinants across all policies and activities. The programme's implementation is overseen by the European Commission's Public Health Executive Agency.

However, no country has a systematic procedure for making decisions affecting public health, or setting priorities among different public health interventions. One exception may be in the United Kingdom, with the recent inclusion of public health intervention cost-effectiveness evaluation in the remit of the National Institute of Health and Clinical Excellence. The methodology used for making decisions and setting priorities in public health typically relate to population health status, epidemiological data, burden of disease and, at times, scope for prevention. Also important in this process, but less documented, are political negotiations, pressure from interest groups and informal processes (Allin et al. 2004).

Health in All Policies (HiAP) is a key strategy for strengthening the stewardship function for public health in order to improve health system performance. Key elements of this strategy are health impact assessment (HIA), intersectoral mechanisms and intersectoral health targets.

The HiAP approach has been widely endorsed by ministries of health over recent years. The strategy was included in the WHO *Health for All* policy (WHO Regional Office for Europe 2005), a Council conclusion on HiAP was endorsed by EU Member States under the Finnish Presidency (Council of the European Union 2006) and HiAP has become one of the principles of the new EU health strategy (Commission of the European Communities 2007). Finally, Member States of the EU, together with WHO and the European Commission, endorsed a declaration to implement HiAP in their countries (Ministries of Health of the 27 EU Member States 2007).

The HiAP aims at improving the health of the population by tackling the determinants of health (Dahlgren and Whitehead 2000). Among them are transport, housing, the environment, education, fiscal policies, tax policy and economic policy. These determinants are outside the remit of the Ministry responsible for health (Wismar et al. 2006a). It is, therefore, a key stewardship task to reach out to engage in dialogue and collaborate with other ministries and sectors.

A key HiAP mechanism is HIA. This is a decision support tool that helps to inform decision-makers on the health consequences of pending decisions and their alternatives (Kemm 2007). It has been employed in different countries and on different political administrative levels. In the past it has been quite frequently used in the United Kingdom, Finland and the Netherlands. It can be applied to policies, programmes and projects (Blau et al. 2006). Lithuania is among the first countries to make HIA legally mandatory (Striçka, Zurlyte and Grabauskas 2006). The influence of HIA on decisions may vary, but there is ample evidence that it can be substantial (Wismar et al. 2007). In addition, economic evaluation conducted in England and Wales has concluded that the benefits of HIA outweigh the costs (O'Reilly et al. 2006). The remaining challenge, however, is demonstrating to stakeholders of other sectors the advantage of using HIA systematically and to find context adequate implementations strategies.

There are other mechanisms that have also been shown to be very useful. The Finnish Ministry of Social Affairs and Health employed bilateral policy dialogues and health policy reporting between ministries to strengthen intersectoral cooperation on the determinants of health (Ståhl et al. 2006). There are numerous other mechanisms that facilitate HiAP, although they are all context dependent and have not been subject to systematic or comparative analysis. Among these mechanisms are intersectoral committees, interservice groups, public health expert panels, consensus conferences, formal consultations in drafting legislation and public referenda (Ritsatakis and Järvisalo 2006).

Using intersectoral health targets to strengthen stewardship is another important element of the reform strategy. Targets have the capacity to support dialogue, inform allocation of resources and influence management and behaviour of organizations and individuals. They are an important mechanism to determine achievement levels for performance measurement. Health targets are a common stewardship mechanism in health policy formulation throughout Europe (van de Water and van Herten 1998; Welteke, Menke and Brand 2000; Busse and Wismar 2002; Wismar and Busse 2002; Claveranne and Teil 2003). The most recent and most comprehensive mapping exercise showed that most countries are formulating comprehensive health policies using health targets (WHO Regional Office for Europe 2005).

Health targets are, however, a demanding tool since the definition and monitoring requires sophisticated technical skills, political influence and an adequate infrastructure. Experiences from England (Smith 2008), Germany (Wismar, Philippi and Klus 2008), Hungary (Vokó and Ádány 2008) and Catalonia, Spain (Tresserras and Brugulat 2008) show how much initiative and energy it takes to develop meaningful health targets and how important is the development of adequate health intelligence. A case study on the health targets of the Belgian region of Flanders shows that health targets can deliver results even without committing additional funding or exerting influence. But this is an exception. In general, evidence shows that health targets will produce few effects unless they are embedded in adequate accountability frameworks and supported by suitable health intelligence (Wismar et al. 2006b, 2008).

Conclusions

Viewed overall, the review of health systems in this chapter would appear to support two key observations about current developments within European health care systems. The first is that health reform has become a complex, multifaceted process, encompassing a wide range of measures in the six areas of reform discussed in the Introduction. In this context, pursuing health reform becomes a demanding exercise, which needs to be pursued in a systematic, coordinated manner if it is to be effective. In this regard, the rapidly growing sophistication of information technology systems has become central to the capacity of national policy-makers to generate and evaluate the data needed to pursue this complex reform exercise.

The second observation is that the process of health system reform across Europe has made significant progress since its beginnings in the late 1980s and early 1990s. Reform programmes in many countries have developed considerably in empirical knowledge and in organizational focus. Most importantly, as this review has highlighted, incremental improvements in health system activities and outcomes have been achieved in a substantial number of policy areas.

Most of the key objectives for health system development, including the importance of population-based public health measures, are now widely accepted among European health policy-makers. Along each of the four functional axes detailed above – finance, resource generation, delivery of population-based and personal health services, and governance and stewardship – the assessments presented in this chapter point towards specific positive steps and towards incrementally improved outcomes. Further policy developments are underway that can be expected to improve the organizational and institutional as well as the health outcome and health status dimensions of European health systems. This is not to argue that there is not a great deal more reform work to do. Nor is it to claim that spirited debate about how best to achieve the next stages of advancement is not necessary – the complexities of the reform process as detailed in this chapter clearly suggest that continued discussion on how to move forward is essential.

Despite the work that remains to be done, however, the momentum and direction of the reform process across Europe appears to be in a positive and potentially transformative structural and organizational direction.

Acknowledgements

Several sections of this chapter benefited from points raised in Figueras et al. (2008b), a background document for WHO Regional Office for Europe's Tallinn Ministerial Conference in 2008. The chapter greatly benefited from comments made by participants at the author's workshop on 6–7 March 2008 in Brussels. Particular thanks go to Josep Figueras and Martin McKee for extensive comments on earlier versions.

Endnote

1. It is important to note that the general tax component of public expenditure is not always evident because of the way in which data are collected. The WHO and OECD expenditure data classify all funds channelled through social insurance funds as social insurance contributions in spite of the often substantial amounts of tax-based funds

that are allocated to insurance funds to subsidize for those who do not contribute or as a policy of mixed finance; this leads to overestimations of the level of social insurance contributions in all countries where there are transfers from general revenues to compulsory insurance funds. The magnitude of the overestimation is in proportion to the share of compulsory insurance revenues coming from such transfers. In Latvia, for example, all revenues managed by the State Compulsory Health Insurance Agency come from general revenue transfers (Tragakes et al. 2008), while in the Republic of Moldova in 2005, about 65% of compulsory insurance revenues came from such transfers (Shishkin, Kacevicius and Ciocanu 2008).

References

Ahmedov, M., Azimov, R., Alimova, V. and Rechel, B. (2007) Uzbekistan: health system review. Health Systems in Transition, 9(3): 1–210. Copenhagen: WHO Regional Office for Europe on behalf of the European Observatory on Health Systems and Policies.

Allin, S., Mossialos, E., McKee, M. and Holland, W.W. (2004) *Making Decisions on Public Health: A Review of Eight Countries*. Copenhagen: WHO Regional Office for Europe on behalf of the European Observatory on Health Systems and Policies.

Askham, J., Coulter, A. and Parsons, S. (2008) *Where Are the Patients in Decision-making about Their Own Care?* Copenhagen: WHO Regional Office for Europe on behalf of the European Observatory on Health Systems and Policies (HEN-OBS Joint Policy Brief No. 3).

Atun, R.A., Bennett, S. and Durán, A. (2008) When Do Vertical (Stand-Alone) Programmes have a Place in Health Systems? Copenhagen: WHO Regional Office for Europe on behalf of the European Observatory on Health Systems and Policies (HEN-OBS Joint Policy Brief No. 5).

Baldwin, R. and Cave, M. (1999) *Understanding Regulation: Theory, Strategy and Practice*. Oxford: Oxford University Press.

Bayarsaikhan, D. and Muiser, J. (2007) *Financing Health Promotion*. Geneva: World Health Organization (discussion paper number 4 – 2007).

Blau, J., Ernst, K., Wismar, M., et al. (2006) The use of health impact assessment across Europe, in T. Ståhl, M. Wismar, E. Ollia, E. Lahtinen and K. Leppo (eds.) *Health in All Policies: Prospects and Potentials*. Helsinki: Ministry of Social Affairs and Health: 209–30.

Bobak, M., McCarthy, M., Perlman, F. and Marmot, M. (2004) Modernizing public health, in J. Figueras, M. McKee, J. Cain, and S. Lessof (eds.) *Health Systems in Transition: Learning from Experience*. Copenhagen: WHO Regional Office for Europe on behalf of the European Observatory on Health Systems and Policies: 135–52.

Boerma, W.G.W. (2003) *Profiles of General Practice in Europe. An International Study of Variation in the Tasks of General Practitioners*. Utrecht: NIVEL.

Bohigas, L. (2008) Comment on decentralization, re-centralization and health policy in Europe. *European Journal of Public Health*, 18(3): 220.

Buchan, J. (2006) Migration of health workers in Europe: policy problem or policy solution? in C.-A. Dubois, M. McKee and E. Nolte (eds.) *Human Resources for Health in Europe*. Copenhagen: WHO Regional Office for Europe on behalf of the European Observatory on Health Systems and Policies: 41–62.

Busse, R. (2001) Risk structure compensation in Germany's statutory health insurance. *European Journal of Public Health*, 11(2): 174–7.

Busse, R. and Wismar, M. (2002) Health target programmes and health care services: any link? A conceptual and comparative study (part 1) *Health Policy*, 59: 209–21.

Busse, R., Schreyögg, J. and Smith, P.C. (2006) Editorial: hospital case payment systems in Europe. *Health Care Management Science*, 9: 211–13.

Castoro, C., Bertinato, L., Drace, C.A. and McKee, M. (2007) *Day Surgery: Making it Happen*. Copenhagen: WHO Regional Office for Europe on behalf of the European Observatory on Health Systems and Policies.

Chaix-Couturier, C., Durand-Zaleski, I., Jolly, D. and Durieux, P. (2000) Effects of financial incentives on medical practice: results from a systematic review of the literature and methodological issues. *International Journal for Quality in Health Care*, 12(2): 133–42.

Claveranne, J.-P. and Teil, A. (2003a) *Les Modalités de Définition des Objectifs et Stratégies de Santé. Description et Analyse de Dispositifs des Pays de l'Union Européenne et d'Amerique du Nord*, Vols. I and II: *Descriptions Verticales*. Lyon: GRAPHOS-CNRS.

Commission of the European Communities (2007) *Together for Health: A Strategic Approach for the EU 2008–2013* (White Paper COM(2007) 630 Final). Brussels: European Commission.

Council of the European Union (2006) *Council Conclusions on Health in All Policies (HiAP) (EPSCO)*. Brussels: Council of the European Union.

Dahlgren, G. and Whitehead, M. (2000) *Policies and Strategies to Promote Equity in Health*. Copenhagen: WHO Regional Office for Europe.

Davis, C. (2010) Understanding the legacy: health financing systems in the USSR and Central and Eastern Europe prior to transition, in J. Kutzin, C. Cashin and M. Jakab (eds.) *Implementing Health Financing Reform: Lessons from Countries in Transition*. Copenhagen: WHO Regional Office for Europe on behalf of the European Observatory on Health Systems and Policies: 25–63.

de Bekker-Grob, E.W., Polder, J.J., Mackenbach, J.P. and Meerding, W.J. (2007) Towards a comprehensive estimate of national spending on prevention. *BMC Public Health*, 7: 252.

Dowling, B. and Glendinning, C. (eds.) (2003) *The New Primary Care: Modern, Dependable, Successful?* Maidenhead: Open University Press.

Dubois, C.-A., McKee, M. and Nolte, E. (eds.) (2006a) *Human Resources for Health in Europe*. Maidenhead: Open University Press.

Dubois, C.-A., McKee, M. and Nolte, E. (2006b) Human resources for health in Europe, in C.-A. Dubois, M. McKee and E. Nolte (eds.) *Human Resources for Health in Europe*. Maidenhead: Open University Press: 1–14.

Ettelt, S., Nolte, E., Mays, N., Thomson, S. and McKee, M. and the International Healthcare Comparisons Network (2006) *Health Care Outside Hospital: Accessing Generalist and Specialist Care in Eight Countries*. Copenhagen: WHO Regional Office for Europe on behalf of the European Observatory on Health Systems and Policies.

Fachkommission (2006) *Prävention und Gesundheitsförderung. Zukunft von Prävention und Gesundheitsförderung in der Schweiz*. Bern: Bundesamt für Gesundheit.

Figueras, J., McKee, M., Lessof, S., Durán, A. and Menabde, N. (2008a) *Health System, Health and Wealth: Assessing the Case for Investing in Health Systems,* background document. Copenhagen: WHO Regional Office for Europe on behalf of the European Observatory on Health Systems and Policies.

Figueras, J., McKee, M., Kutzin, J. and Menabde, N. (2008b) *Summary for the WHO Regional Office for Europe's Tallinn Ministerial Conference, 25–27 June 2008*, background document. Copenhagen: WHO Regional Office for Europe.

Gosden, T., Forland, F. and Kristiansen, I.S. (2000) Capitation, salary, fee-for-service and mixed system of payment: effects on behaviour of primary care physicians. *Cochrane Database of Systematic Reviews*, (3): CD002215.

Gotsadze, G., Chikovani, I., Goguadze, K., Balabanova, D. and McKee, M. (2010) Reforming Sanitary-Epidemiological Service in central and eastern Europe and the former Soviet Union: an exploratory study. *BMC Health Service Research*, 10: 440.

Gresz, S., Groenewegen, P., Kerssens, J., Braun, B. and Wasem, J. (2002) Free choice of sickness fund in regulated competition: evidence from Germany and the Netherlands. *Health Policy*, 60(3): 235–54.

Groenewegen, P.P. and de Jong, J.D. (2007) Dutch health insurance reform: the new role of collectives. *Eurohealth*, 13(2): 10–13.

Gulis, G., Korcova, J., Letanovsky, P. and Marcinkova, D. (2005) Transition and public health in the Slovak Republic. *British Medical Journal*, 331: 213–15.

Gunnarsdóttir, S. and Rafferty, A.M. (2006) Enhancing working conditions, in C.-A. Dubois, M. McKee and E. Nolte (eds.) *Human Resources for Health in Europe*. Maidenhead Open University Press: 155–72.

Hultberg, E.L., Glendinning, C., Allebeck, P. and Lonnroth, K. (2005) Using pooled budgets to integrate health andwelfare services: a comparison of experiments in England and Sweden. *Health and Social Care in the Community*, 13: 531–41.

Hultberg, E.L., Lonnroth, K. and Allebeck, P. (2003) Co-financing as a means to improve collaboration between primary health care, social insurance and social service in Sweden. A qualitative study of collaboration experiences among rehabilitation partners. *Health Policy*, 64: 143–52.

Institute of Microeconomics and Public Finance (2007) Switzerland: law on prevention to provide transparency and equality, in R. Busse and S. Schlette (eds.) *Health Policy Developments 7/8*. Gütersloh: Bertelsmann Stiftung: 205–6.

Jenkins, R., Lancashire, S., McDaid, D. et al. (2007) Mental health reform in the Russian Federation: an integrated approach to achieve social inclusion and recovery. *Bulletin of the World Health Organization*, 85: 858–66.

Judge, K., Platt, S., Costongs, C. and Jurczak, K. (2006) *Health Inequalities: A Challenge for Europe*. London: The Stationery Office.

Kemm, J. (2007) What is HIA and why might it be useful? in M. Wismar, J., Blau, K. Ernst and J. Figueras (eds.) *The Effectiveness of Health Impact Assessment: Scope and Limitations of Supporting Decision-making in Europe*. Copenhagen: WHO Regional Office for Europe: 3–14.

Knudsen, J.L., Fugleholm, A.M. and Kjærgaard, J. (2004) Kvalitetsvurdering i Sundhedsvæsenet 1 Beslutningen om Den Danske Kvalitetsmodel [Quality control in the national health service. 1 The decision to develop a Danish quality model]. *Ugeskrift for Læger*, 166: 1779–83.

Kulzhanov, M. and Rechel, B. (2007) Kazakhstan: health system review. *Health Systems in Transition*, 9(7): 1–158.

Kutzin, J., Shishkin, S., Bryndová, L., Schneider, P. and Hrobon, P. (2010) Reforms in the pooling of funds, in J. Kutzin, C. Cashin and M. Jakab (eds.) *Implementing Health Financing Reform: Lessons from Countries in Transition*. Copenhagen: WHO Regional Office for Europe on behalf of the European Observatory on Health Systems and Policies: 119–53.

L'Assemblée nationale, Sénat Le Président de la République. (2004). *Loi no. 2004–806 du 9 août 2004 relative à la politique de santé publique (1)* Paris: Legisfrance, http://www.legifrance.gouv.fr/affichTexte.do?cidTexte-JORFTEX000000787078&dateTexte=/ (accessed 9 September 2010).

Legido-Quigley, H., McKee, M. and Nolte, E. (2008a) *Assuring the Quality of Health Care in the European Union: A Case for Action*. Copenhagen: WHO Regional Office for Europe on behalf of the European Observatory on Health Systems and Policies.

Legido-Quigley, H., McKee, M., Walshe, K., Suñol, R., Nolte, E. and Klazinga, N. (2008b) How can quality of health care be safeguarded across the European Union? *British Medical Journal*, 336: 920–3.

Lewis, M. (2002) Informal health payments in central and eastern Europe and the former Soviet Union: issues, trends and policy implications, in E. Mossialos, A. Dixon, J.

Figueras and J. Kutzin (eds.) *Funding Health Care: Options for Europe*. Buckingham: Open University Press: 184–205.

MacArthur, I. and Shevkun, E. (2002) Restructuring public health services, in M. McKee, J. Healy and J. Falkingham (eds.) *Health Care in Central Asia*. Buckingham: Open University Press: 165–78.

Martin, D. (2006) Wanless: public health reform has fallen victim to pay rises. *Health Services Journal*, 116: 5.

Maynard, A. (2006) Incentives in health care: the shift in emphasis from the implicit to the explicit, in C.-A. Dubois, M. McKee and E. Nolte (eds.) *Human Resources for Health in Europe*. Maidenhead: Open University Press: 140–54.

McKee, M. and Healy, J. (2002) *Hospitals in a Changing Europe*. Buckingham: Open University Press.

McKee, M., Edwards, N. and Atun, R. (2006) Public–private partnerships for hospitals. *Bulletin of the World Health Organization*, 84: 890–6.

Merkel, B. and Hübel, M. (1999) Public health in the European community, in W.W. Holland and E. Mossialos (eds.) *Public Health Policies in the European Union*. Aldershot: Ashgate: 49–67.

Merkur, M., Mossialos, E. and Lear, J. (2008) *Quality in Health Care Systems: With an Emphasis on Policy Options for Austria*. Vienna: Main Association of Austrian Social Insurance Institutions, http://www.hauptverband.at/portal27/portal/hvbportal/channel_content/cmsWindow?action=2&p_menuid=67679&p_tabid=5&p_ubid=142302 (accessed 15 September 2010).

Merkur, S., Mossialos, E., Long, M. and McKee, M. (2008) Physician revalidation in Europe. *Clinical Medicine*, 8: 371–6.

Ministries of Health of the 27 EU Member States (2007) *Declaration on Health in All Policies*. Rome: European Commission.

Mossialos, E., Brogan, D. and Walley, T. (2006) Pharmaceutical pricing in Europe: weighing up the options. *International Social Security Review*, 59(3): 3–25.

Mossialos, E., Walley, T. and Rudisill, C. (2005) Provider incentives and prescribing in Europe. *Expert Review of Pharmacoeconomics and Outcomes Research*, 5(1): 81–93.

Mossialos, E., Dixon, A., Figueras, J. and Kutzin, J. (eds.) (2002) *Funding Health Care: Options for Europe*. Buckingham: Open University Press.

Mrazek, M. and Mossialos, E. (2004) Regulating pharmaceutical prices in the European Union, in E. Mossialos, M. Mrazek and T. Walley (eds.) *Regulating Pharmaceuticals in Europe: Striving for Efficiency, Equity and Quality*. Maidenhead: Open University Press: 114–29.

Nolte, E. and McKee, M. (eds.) (2008) *Caring for People with Chronic Conditions: A Health System Perspective*. Maidenhead: Open University Press.

Nordic Council of Ministers (2007) Kvalitetsmåling i sundhedsvæsenet i Norden [Quality measuring in the Nordic health care system]. *TemaNord* 519.

O'Reilly, J., Trueman, P., Redmond, S., Yunni, Y. and Wright, D. (2006) *Cost Benefit Analysis of Health Impact Assessment*. London: The Stationery Office.

Organisation for Economic Co-operation and Development (2006) *Reviews of Health Systems: Switzerland*. Paris: Organisation for Economic Co-operation and Development.

Organisation for Economic Co-operation and Development (2007) *OECD Health Data 2007*. Paris: Organisation for Economic Co-operation and Development.

Pelletier-Fleury, N., Le Vaillant, M., Szidon, P., Marie, P., Raineri, F. and Sicotte, C. (2007) Preventive service delivery: a new insight into French general practice. *Health Policy*, 83: 268–76.

Pollitt, C.G.B. (2000) *Public Management Reform: A Comparative Analysis*. Oxford: Oxford University Press.

Polluste, K., Mannik, G. and Axelsson, R. (2005) Public health reforms in Estonia: impact on the health of the population. *British Medical Journal*, 331: 210–13.

Rechel, B., Wright, S., Barlow, J. and McKee, M. (2010) Hospital capacity planning: from measuring stocks to modelling flows? *Bulletin of the World Health Organization*, 88: 632–6.

Ritsatakis, A. and Järvisalo, J. (2006) Opportunities and challenges for including health components in the policy-making process, in T. Ståhl, M. Wismar, E. Ollia, E. Lahtinen and K. Leppo (eds.) *Health in All Policies: Prospects and Potentials*. Helsinki: Ministry of Social Affairs and Health: 145–68.

Rosen, B. (2003) *Health Care Systems in Transition: Israel*. Copenhagen: European Observatory on Health Care Systems.

Saltman, R.B. (2003) The melting public–private boundary in European health care systems. *European Journal of Public Health*, 13(1): 24–9.

Saltman, R.B. (2008) Decentralization, re-centralization and future European health policy. *European Journal of Public Health*, 18(2): 104–6.

Saltman, R.B. and Bankauskaite, V. (2006) Conceptualizing decentralization in European health systems: a functional perspective. *Health Economics, Policy and Law*, 1(2): 127–47.

Saltman, R.B. and Busse, R. (2002) Balancing regulation and entrepreneurialism in Europe's health sector: theory and practice, in R.B. Saltman, R. Busse and E. Mossialos (eds.) *Regulating Entrepreneurial Behaviour in European Health Care Systems*. Buckingham: Open University Press: 3–52.

Saltman, R.B. and Ferroussier-Davis, O. (2000) The concept of stewardship in health policy. *Bulletin of the World Health Organization*, 78: 732–9.

Saltman, R.B. and Figueras, J. (1997) *European Health Care Reform: Analysis of Current Strategies*. Copenhagen: WHO Regional Office for Europe.

Saltman, R.B. and Figueras, J. (1998) Analyzing the evidence on European health reforms. *Health Affairs*, 17(2): 85–108.

Saltman, R.B., Bankauskaite, V. and Vrangbæk, K. (eds.) (2007) *Decentralization in Health Care: Strategies and Outcomes*. Maidenhead: Open University Press.

Saltman, R.B., Busse, R. and Mossialos, E. (eds.) (2002) *Regulation Entrepreneurial Behaviour in European Health Care Systems*. Buckingham: Open University Press.

Saltman, R.B., Durán, A. and Dubois, H.F.W. (eds.) (In Press) Governing Public Hospitals: Reform Strategies and the Movement towards Institutional Autonomy. Copenhagen: WHO Regional Office for Europe on behalf of the European Observatory on Health Systems and Policies.

Saltman, R.B., Rico, A. and Boerma, W. (eds.) (2006a) *Primary Care in the Driver's Seat?* Maidenhead: Open University Press.

Saltman, R.B., Dubois, H. and Chawla, M. (2006b) The impact of aging on long-term care in Europe and some potential policy responses. *International Journal of Health Services*, 36(4): 719–46.

Schut, F., Gresz, S. and Wasem, J. (2003) Consumer price sensitivity and social health insurer choice in Germany and the Netherlands. *International Journal of Health Care Finance and Economics*, 3(2): 117–39.

Sheiman, I., Langenbrunner, J., Kehler, J., Cashin, C. and Kutzin, J. (2010) Sources of funds and revenue collection: reforms and challenges, in J. Kutzin, C. Cashin and M. Jakab (eds.) *Implementing Health Financing Reform: Lessons from Countries in Transition*. Copenhagen: WHO Regional Office for Europe on behalf of the European Observatory on Health Systems and Policies: 87–118.

Shishkin, S., Kacevicius, G. and Ciocanu, M. (2008) *Evaluation of Moldova's 2004 Health Financing Reform*. Copenhagen: WHO Regional Office for Europe (Health Financing Policy Paper 2008/3).

Simoens, S. and Hurst, J. (2006) *The Supply of Physician Services in OECD Countries*. Paris: Organisation for Economic Co-operation and Development.

Smith, P.C. (2008) England: intended and unintended effects, in M. Wismar, M. McKee, K. Ernst, D. Srivastava and R. Busse (eds.) *Health Targets in Europe: Learning from Experience*. Copenhagen: WHO Regional Office for Europe on behalf of the European Observatory on Health Systems and Policies: 63–82.

Smits, M. and Janssen, R. (2008) Impact of electronic auction on health care markets. *Electronic Markets*, 18(1): 19–29.

Sogoric, S., Rukavina, T.V., Brborovic, O., Vlahugic, A., Zganec, N. and Oreskovic, S. (2005) Counties selecting public health priorities: a 'bottom-up' approach (Croatian experience). *Collegium Antropologicum*, 29: 111–19.

Sorenson, C., Drummond, M. and Kanavos, P. (2008) *Ensuring Value for Money in Health Care: The Role of Health Technology Assessment in the European Union*. Copenhagen: WHO Regional Office for Europe on behalf of the European Observatory on Health Systems and Policies.

Ståhl, T., Wismar, M., Ollia, E., Lahtinen, E. and Leppo, K. (eds.) (2006) *Health in All Policies*. Helsinki: Ministry of Social Affairs and Health.

Starfield, B. (1998) *Primary Care: Balancing Health Needs, Services, and Technology*. New York: Oxford University Press.

Strička, M., Zurlyte, I. and Grabauskas, V. (2006) A local-level HIA in the transport sector: following legal requirements in Lithuania, in M. Wismar, J., Blau, K. Ernst and J. Figueras (eds.) *The Effectiveness of Health Impact Assessment: Scope and Limitations of Supporting Decision-making in Europe*. Copenhagen: WHO Regional Office for Europe on behalf of the European Observatory on Health Systems and Policies: 105–14.

Thomson, S., Foubister, T. and Mossialos, E. (2008) *Health Care Financing in the Context of Social Security*. [Report prepared for the European Parliament: Directorate-General for Internal Policies, Directorate A – Economic and Scientific Policy.] Brussels: European Parliament.

Tragakes, E., Brigis, G., Karaskevica, J. et al. (2008) Latvia: health system review. *Health Systems in Transition*, 10(2): 1–253.

Tresserras, R. and Brugulat, P. (2008) Catalonia: improved intelligence and accountability? in M. Wismar, M. McKee, K. Ernst, D. Srivastava and R. Busse (eds.) *Health Targets in Europe: Learning from Experience*. Copenhagen: WHO Regional Office for Europe on behalf of the European Observatory on Health Systems and Policies: 53–62.

Vagac, L. and Haulikova, L. (2003) *Study on the Social Protection Systems in the 13 Applicant Countries: Latvia Country Report*. Brussels: Commission of the European Communities.

van de Ven, W.P.M.M., Beck, K., van de Voorde, C., Wasem, J. and Zmora, I. (2007) Risk adjustment and risk selection in Europe: six years later. *Health Policy*, 83(2–3): 162–79.

van de Water, H.P.A. and van Herten, L.M. (1998) *Health Policies on Target? Review of Health Target and Priority Setting in 18 European Countries*. Leiden: Nederlandse Organisatie voor Toegepast Natuurwetenschappelijk Onderzoek (TNO).

van Ginnekin, E., Busse, R. and Gericke, C.A. (2008) Universal private health insurance in the Netherlands: the first year. *Journal of Management and Marketing in Health Care*, 1(2): 1–15.

Velasco-Garrido, M. and Busse, R. (2005) *Health Technology Assessment: An Introduction to Objectives, Role of Evidence and Structure in Europe*. Copenhagen: WHO Regional Office for Europe on behalf of the European Observatory on Health Systems and Policies.

Vokó, Z. and Ádány, R. (2008) Hungary: targets driving improved health intelligence, in M. Wismar, M. McKee, K. Ernst, D. Srivastava and R. Busse (eds.) *Health Targets in Europe: Learning from Experience*. Copenhagen: WHO Regional Office for Europe on behalf of the European Observatory on Health Systems and Policies: 137–46.

Vuorenkoski, L. (2007) The government programme for the years 2007–2010. *Health Policy Monitor* 27, http://www.hpm.org/en/Surveys/THL_Finland/10/The_government_programme_for_the_years_2007-2010.html?content_id=251&sortBy=sortCountry&

sortOrder=sortAsc&showDetails=all&lastSortBy=sortCountry&lastSortOrder=sort Asc&language=en&pageOffset=27 (accessed 3 October 2010).

Walley, T. and Mossialos, E. (2004) Financial incentives and prescribing, in E. Mossialos, M. Mrazek and T. Walley (eds.) *Regulating Pharmaceuticals in Europe: Striving for Efficiency, Equity and Quality*. Maidenhead: Open University Press: 177–99.

Wanek, V. (2008) Präventionsgesetz: Leistungsausbau oder Verschiebebahnhof. *Die Krankenversicherung*, 60: 48–52.

Wanless, D. (2002) *Securing Our Future Health: Taking a Long-term View: Final Report*. London: The Stationery Office.

Welteke, R., Menke, R. and Brand, H. (2000) Das NRW-Gesundheitszielkonzept im europäischen und internationalen Vergleich, in R. Geene and E. Luber (eds.) *Gesundheitsziele: Planung in der Gesundheitspolitik*. Frankfurt: Mabuse: 91–106.

White, C. (2006) GP contract settlement under threat. *British Medical Journal*, 332: 10.

WHO Regional Office for Europe (2005). *The Health for All Policy Framework for the WHO European Region – 2005 Update*. Copenhagen: WHO Regional Office for Europe.

WHO Regional Office for Europe (2007) *Health For All Database*. Copenhagen: WHO Regional Office for Europe (European Health for All Series No. 7).

WHO Regional Office for Europe (2010) *Health For All Database*. Copenhagen: WHO Regional Office for Europe.

WHO Regional Office for Europe (2011) Health for All Database. Copenhagen WHO Regional Office for Europe.

Wismar, M. and Busse, R. (2002) Outcome-related health targets – political strategies for better health outcomes: A conceptual and comparative study (part 2) *Health Policy*, 59: 223–41.

Wismar, M., Lahtinen, E., Ståhl, T., Ollia, E. and Leppo, K. (2006a) Introduction, in T. Ståhl, M. Wismar, E. Ollia, E. Lahtinen and K. Leppo (eds.) *Health in All Policies: Prospects and Potentials*. Helsinki: Ministry of Social Affairs and Health: xvii.

Wismar, M., Ernst, K., Srivastava, D. and Busse, R. (2006b) Health targets and (good) governance. *Euro Observer*, 8: 1–8.

Wismar, M., Blau, J., Ernst, K. and Figueras, J. (eds.) (2007) *The Effectiveness of Health Impact Assessment: Scope and Limitations of Supporting Decision-making in Europe*. Copenhagen: WHO Regional Office for Europe on behalf of the European Observatory on Health Systems and Policies.

Wismar, M., Philippi, B. and Klus, H. (2008a) Germany: Targets in a federal system, in M. Wismar, M. McKee, K. Ernst, D. Srivastava and R. Busse (eds.) *Health Targets in Europe: Learning from Experience*. Copenhagen: WHO Regional Office for Europe on behalf of the European Observatory on Health Systems and Policies: 123–36.

Wismar, M., McKee, M., Ernst, K., Srivastava, D. and Busse, R. (eds.) (2008b) *Health Targets in Europe: Learning from Experience*. Copenhagen: WHO Regional Office for Europe on behalf of the European Observatory on Health Systems and Policies.

World Health Organization (2000) *The World Health Report 2000. Health Systems: Improving Performance*. Geneva: World Health Organization. http://www.who.int/whr/2000/en/ (accessed 1 September 2010).

World Health Organization (2011) Global Health Observatory.

Zentner, A., Valasco-Garrido, M. and Busse, R. (2005) *Methods for the Comparative Evaluation of Pharmaceuticals*, 1(Doc09). German Agency for Health Technology Assessment at the German Institute for Medical Documentation and Information.

Zok, K. (1999) *Anforderungen an die Gesetzliche Krankenversicherung: Einschatzungen und Erwartungen aus Sicht der Versicherten*. Bonn: Wissenschaftliches Institut der AOK.

chapter ten

Performance measurement for health system improvement: experiences, challenges and prospects

Peter C. Smith, Elias Mossialos
and Irene Papanicolas

Introduction

Information plays a central role in the ability of a health system to secure improved health effectively and efficiently for its population. It can be used in many diverse ways, such as tracking public health, monitoring health care safety, determining appropriate treatment paths for patients, promoting professional improvement, ensuring managerial control and promoting the accountability of the health system to the public. Underlying all of these efforts is the role performance measurement plays in guiding the decisions that various stakeholders, such as patients, clinicians, managers, governments and the public, make in steering the health system towards better outcomes.

Records of performance-measurement efforts in health systems can be traced back at least 250 years (McIntyre, Rogers and Heier 2001; Loeb 2004). More formal arguments for the collection and publication of information on performance were developed more than 100 years ago, when such pioneers in the field as Florence Nightingale and Ernest Codman campaigned for its widespread use in health care. Until recently, professional, practical and political barriers have prevented these principles from becoming a reality (Spiegelhalter 1999). For example, Nightingale's and Codman's efforts were frustrated by professional resistance and, until recently, information systems have failed to deliver their promised benefits in the form of timely, accurate and comprehensive information.

However, since the early 1980s, health system performance measurement and reporting have grown substantially, thus helping to secure health system improvement. Many factors have contributed to this growth. On the demand side, health systems have come under intense pressure to contain costs. Also, patients now expect to make more informed decisions about their treatment, and strong demands have been made for increased audit and accountability of the health professions and health service institutions (Power 1999; Smith 2005). On the supply side, the great advances in information technology have made it much cheaper and easier to collect, process and disseminate data.

Policy issues

In many respects, the policy agenda is moving away from discussions of whether performance measurement should be undertaken and what data to collect and is moving towards determining the best ways in which to summarize and present such data and how to integrate them successfully into effective structures for governance. Yet, despite the proliferation of performance-measurement initiatives, there remain a large number of unresolved questions about the collection and deployment of such information. Health systems are still experimenting with the concept of performance measurement, and much still needs to be done to realize its full potential.

This chapter reviews some of the main issues emerging in the debate about performance measurement, drawing on and updating the work of Smith et al. (2009), which was prepared for the WHO Ministerial Conference on Health Systems in Tallinn, Estonia in 2008. The chapter first examines the purpose of performance measurement and the different areas for which data are collected. It then examines the different ways in which performance measurement has been presented and used for health system improvement internationally. Finally, the major challenges found in presenting and using performance measures are discussed before the conclusion, which presents the key lessons and future priorities for policy-makers.

Performance measurement

Purpose

Health systems are complex entities with many different stakeholders, including patients, clinicians, health care providers, purchaser organizations, regulators, the government and the broader public. These stakeholders are linked by a series of accountability relationships (Fig. 10.1). Accountability has two broad elements: the rendering of an account (providing information) and the consequent holding to account (sanctions or rewards for the accountable party). Whatever the precise design of the health system, the fundamental role of performance measurement is to help to hold its various agents to account by enabling stakeholders to make informed decisions. It is, therefore, noteworthy that, if the accountability relationships are to function properly, no system of performance information should be viewed in isolation from the broader system design within which the measurement is embedded.

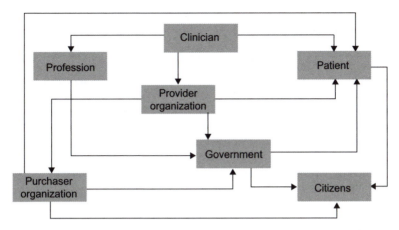

Figure 10.1 Map of some important accountability relationships in the health system

Each of the relationships described in Fig. 10.1 has different needs in terms of the nature of the information, its detail and its timeliness, and the level of aggregation required. For example, in choosing which provider to use, a patient may need detailed comparative data on health outcomes. In contrast, in holding a government to account and in deciding for whom to vote, a citizen may need highly aggregated summaries and trends. Many intermediate needs also arise. In deciding whether providers are performing adequately, a purchaser (such as a social insurer) may need both broad more-aggregated information and detailed assurance of safety aspects. A fundamental challenge for performance measurement is to design information systems that serve these diverse needs. Table 10.1 examines this issue in more detail.

Table 10.1 Information requirements for stakeholders in health care systems

Stakeholder	Examples of needs	Data requirements
Government	Monitoring the health of the nation	Information on performance at national and international levels
	Setting health policy	Information on access and equity of care
	Ensuring that regulatory procedures are working properly	Information on utilization of service and waiting times
	Ensuring that government finances are used as intended	Population health data
	Ensuring that appropriate information and research functions are undertaken	
	Monitoring regulatory effectiveness and efficiency	

(continued)

Table 10.1 Information requirements for stakeholders in health care systems *(cont'd)*

Stakeholder	Examples of needs	Data requirements
Regulators	Protecting patients' safety and welfare Ensuring broader consumer protection Ensuring the market is functioning efficiently	Timely, reliable and continuous information on patient safety and welfare Information on probity and efficiency of financial flows
Payers (taxpayers and members of insurance funds)	Ensuring money is being spent effectively, efficiently and in line with expectations	Aggregate, comparative performance measures Information on productivity and cost-effectiveness Information on access to (and equity of) care
Purchaser organizations	Ensuring that contracts offered to their patients are in line with the objectives the patients expect	Information on patient experiences and patient satisfaction Information on provider performance Information on the cost-effectiveness of treatments
Provider organizations	Monitoring and improving existing services Assessing local needs	Aggregated clinical performance data Information on patient experiences and patient satisfaction Information on access and equity of care Information on utilization of service and waiting times
Physicians	Staying up-to-date with current practice Being able to improve performance	Information on current practice and best practice Performance information benchmarks
Patients	Being able to make a choice of provider when in need Information on alternative treatments	Information on location and quality of nearby emergency health services Information on quality of options for elective care
The public	Being reassured that appropriate services will be available if needed in the future Holding government and other elected officials to account	Broad trends in, and comparisons of, system performance at national and local level Efficiency information Safety information

In practice, the development of performance measurement has rarely been pursued with a clear picture of who the information users are or what their information needs might be. Instead performance-measurement systems have usually sought to inform a variety of users, typically presenting a wide range of data in the hope that some of the information collected will be useful to different parties. Yet, given the diverse information needs of the different stakeholders in health systems, it is unlikely that a single method of reporting performance will be useful for everybody. Instead, data sources should be designed and exploited to satisfy the demands of different users. This may often involve using data from the same sources in different forms. A major challenge for health systems is, therefore, to develop more nuances in the collection and presentation of performance measures for the different stakeholders without imposing a huge burden of new data collection and analysis.

Defining and measuring performance

In general, performance measurement seeks to monitor, evaluate and communicate the extent to which various aspects of the health system meet their key objectives. Usually, those objectives can be summarized under a limited number of headings: for example, health conferred on people by the health system, its responsiveness to public preferences, the financial protection it offers and its productivity. *Health* relates both to the health outcomes secured after treatment and to the broader health status of the population. *Responsiveness* captures aspects of health system behaviour not directly related to health outcomes, such as dignity, communication, autonomy, prompt service, access to social support during care, quality of basic services and choice of provider. *Productivity* refers to the extent to which the resources used by the health system are used efficiently in the pursuit of effectiveness. Besides a concern for the overall attainment in each of these areas, *The World Health Report 2000* (WHR2000; World Health Organization 2000) highlighted the importance of distributional (or equity) issues, expressed in terms of inequity in health outcomes, responsiveness and payment. Table 10.2 summarizes these largely universal aspects of health performance measures.

The degree of progress made in the development of performance measures and data collection techniques varies for the different aspects of health performance. In some areas, such as population health, there are well-established indicators, for example for infant mortality and life expectancy (sometimes adjusted for disability). Even here, however, important further work is needed. A particular difficulty with population health measures is estimating the specific contribution of the health system to health. To address this, researchers are developing new instruments, such as the concept of *avoidable mortality* (Holland 1988; Nolte and McKee 2004; see also Chapter 5).

The contribution of the health system to health care can be more reliably captured in terms of clinical outcomes for patients. Traditionally, this contribution has been examined using post-treatment mortality, which is a blunt instrument. However, interest is increasingly focused on more general measures of improvements in patient health status, often in the form of patient-reported

Table 10.2 Aspects of health performance measures

Measurement area	Description of measure	Examples of indicators
Population health	Measures of aggregated data on the health of the population	Life expectancy Years of life lost Avoidable mortality Disability-adjusted life-years
Individual health outcomes	Measures of individual's health status, which can be relative to the whole population or among groups Indicators that also apply utility rankings to different health states	Generic measures: Short form 36 (SF-36)[a] EQ-5D[b] Disease-specific measures: arthritis impact measurement scales, Parkinson disease questionnaire (PDQ-39)
Clinical quality and appropriateness of care	Measures of the services and care patients receive to achieve desired outcomes Measures used to determine if best practice takes place and whether these actions are carried out in a technologically sound manner	Outcome measures: health status, specific postoperative readmission and mortality rates Process measures: frequency of blood pressure measurement
Responsiveness of health system	Measures of the way individuals are treated and the environment in which they are treated during health system interactions Measures concerned with issues of patient dignity, autonomy, confidentiality, communication, prompt attention, social support and quality of basic amenities	Patient experience measures Patient satisfaction measures
Equity	Measures of the extent to which there is equity in health, access to health care, responsiveness and financing	Utilization measures Rates of access Use-needs ratios Spending thresholds Disaggregated health outcome measures
Productivity	Measures of the productivity of the health care system, health care organizations and individual practitioners	Labour productivity Cost-effectiveness measures (for interventions) Technical efficiency (measures of output/input) Allocative efficiency (measured by willingness to pay)

Notes: [a] SF-36 is a multipurpose, short-form health survey with only 36 questions; [b] EQ-5D is a standardized instrument for measuring the outcome of a wide range of health conditions and treatments. It provides a simple descriptive profile and a single index value for health status that can be used in the clinical and economic evaluation of health care and in population health surveys.

outcome measures. These measures are derived from simple surveys of subjective health status administered directly to patients, often before and after treatment. Numerous instruments have been developed, often in the context of clinical trials. These take the form of detailed condition-specific questionnaires or broad-brush generic measures (Fitzpatrick 2009).

To measure performance when monitoring outcomes from health care interventions over time and between providers, the policy challenge is to identify the most appropriate choice of instrument. In England, for example, the government has recently mandated the use of the generic patient-reported outcome measure instrument EQ-5D for use for all National Health Service patients undergoing four common procedures. This experiment will assess the costs of such routine use and will test whether the resistance of some health professionals to patient-reported outcome measures is sustained. Also, while the relevance of patient-reported outcome measures to acute care is clear, their application to such areas as chronic disease and mental illness remain less well developed.

Although clinical outcome measures are the gold standard for measuring effectiveness in health care, their use can be problematic: for example if the outcomes cannot realistically be assessed in a timely or feasible fashion. This is particularly important for chronic diseases. Measures of the process then become important signals of future success (Donabedian 1966). Process measures are based on actions or structures known to be associated with health system outcomes, in either health or responsiveness. An example of an action might be appropriate prescribing, which is known from research evidence to contribute to good outcomes (Naylor, Iron and Hands 2002). Also, the concept of *effective coverage* is an important population health process measure. Table 10.3 summarizes the basic advantages and disadvantages of using outcome and process indicators and the areas of performance measurement where they are most useful.

Work in the area of responsiveness is inherently challenging, as in principle it requires general surveys of both users and non-users of health services. Also, aggregating diverse areas into usable summary indicators of responsiveness is problematic. The World Health Survey of households in over 70 countries contained a *responsiveness* module that offers some potential for proposing operational solutions to the routine measurement of health system responsiveness (Valentine et al. 2009).

Financial protection from the catastrophic expenditure associated with ill health is a fundamental health system concern. Many high-income countries have introduced universal insurance coverage to address this issue, but even then there are quite large variations in measures of financial protection between countries and over time. The issue, however, is even more acute in many lower-income countries, where there are massive variations in the extent to which households (particularly the poor) are protected from catastrophic expenditure. There is, therefore, increasing interest within WHO and the World Bank to develop reliable and comparable indicators of financial protection (Wagstaff 2009). A major challenge is to move beyond the immediate expenditure on health care to trace the longer-term implications for household wealth and savings.

Table 10.3 Usefulness of structural, outcome and process indicators

Types of indicators	Advantages	Disadvantages	Most useful areas
Outcome	Often more meaningful to stakeholders Attention directed to (and health goals focused on) the patient Encourage long-term health-promotion strategies Not easily manipulated	May be ambiguous and difficult to interpret, as they are the result of many factors that are difficult to disentangle Take time to collect Require a large sample size to detect statistically significant effects Can be difficult to measure, for example wound infection	To measure quality of homogeneous procedures To measure quality of homogeneous diagnoses with strong links between interventions and outcomes interventions done to heterogeneous populations that suffer from a common condition
Process	Easily measured without major bias or error More sensitive to quality of care Easier to interpret Require a smaller sample size to detect statistically significant effects Can often be observed unobtrusively Provide clear pathways for action Capture aspects of care valued by patients (aside from outcomes)	Often too specific, focusing on a particular intervention or condition May quickly become dated as models of care and technology develop May have little value to patients unless they understand how they relate to outcomes May be easily manipulated	To measure quality of care, especially for treatments where technical skill is relatively unimportant To measure quality of care of the homogeneous conditions in different settings

Source: Adapted from Mant 2001; Davies 2005.

Finally, productivity (and efficiency) is perhaps the most challenging measurement area of all, as it seeks to offer a comprehensive framework that links the resources used to the measures of effectiveness described above. The need to develop reliable measures of productivity is obvious, given the policy problems of trying to decide where limited health system financial resources are best spent and of trying to identify inefficient providers. The experience of the WHR2000 (World Health Organization 2000), however, illustrates how difficult this task is at the macro-level. In addition, the accounting challenges of identifying resources consumed become progressively more acute when

Box 10.1   Hospital benchmarking in Finland

Background

In Finland, in 1997, the National Research and Development Centre for Welfare and Health launched a research and development project (Hospital Benchmarking) to produce benchmarking information on hospital performance and productivity (Linna 2006). The main aims of the project were:

- to develop a new measure to describe the output of hospitals that was better than traditional measures, such as admissions or outpatient visits;
- to provide the management of hospitals with benchmarking data for improving and directing activities at hospitals.

Data collection

The project was expanded to cover nearly all publicly delivered specialized health care in Finland and, in 2006, data from the project were integrated into the production of national statistics. Data for the Hospital Benchmarking project are collected annually from hospitals, and they include both inpatient and outpatient care, along with information on diagnoses and procedures. The project produces a wide range of hospital and regional (hospital-, district- and municipality-based) indicators on hospital productivity and costs, by speciality, inpatient wards and diagnosis-related groups. By using uniform personal identity codes, the different episodes of care for the same patient can be linked.

Uses of data

The data allow regional measurement of productivity and costs, which can indicate, for example, how much the costs of a hospital district or a municipality deviate from the national average and how much of this deviation depends on the inefficient delivery of services and the per person use of services.

---

moving to finer levels of detail, such as the meso-level (provider organizations, for example), the clinical department, the practitioner or – most challenging of all – the individual patient or person (Street and Hakkinen 2009). Box 10.1 gives details of the Finnish experience with producing benchmarking data to use for productivity improvement.

The Hospital Benchmarking data in Finland have been used increasingly for appraising and directing hospital activities. Results from the project indicate that productivity of hospitals decreased somewhat during 2001–2005 and that there are significant differences in productivity between hospitals (Finnish National Research and Development Centre for Welfare and Health 2007).

Methodological issues

The diverse uses of health system performance measures necessitate a wide variety of measurement methods, indicators, analytical techniques and approaches to presentation. Also, different methods of data collection – such as national surveys, patient surveys, administrative databases and routinely collected clinical information – are needed to assemble these diverse types of information. The area of performance under scrutiny will determine the most appropriate data collection technique. For example, when measuring responsiveness, household or individual surveys are likely to be the best sources of patient experiences and perspectives; when looking at specific clinical outcomes, clinical registries may be a more informative and cost-effective source of information. In practice, although performance-measurement efforts have progressed over recent years, many health systems still rely on readily available data as a basis for performance measurement.

The first requirement in any performance-measurement system is to develop a robust conceptual framework within which performance measures can be developed. This should ensure that all major areas of health system performance are covered by the measurement system; that priorities for new developments can be identified; and that collection and analysis efforts are not misdirected or duplicated. In short, the eventual requirement is to develop an optimal portfolio of performance-measurement instruments. An example of such a framework is the OECD Health Care Quality Indicators Project, which seeks to assemble a suite of performance indicators that are common to a large number of national performance-measurement schemes (Box 10.2).

Detailed issues about methodology arise when considering the design of individual indicators. An important consideration is the level at which

Box 10.2 The OECD Health Care Quality Indicators Project

Background

Since its beginning, in 2001, the OECD Health Care Quality Indicators Project has aimed to track the quality of health care in a number of countries in order to assess the quality of international health care. This is done by developing a set of indicators based on comparable data that can be used to investigate quality differences in health care among countries.

Indicators

The five areas in which indicators are being collected are:

- patient safety
- quality of mental health care
- quality of health promotion, illness prevention and primary care
- quality of diabetes care
- quality of cardiac care.

The collection of indicators follows a twofold process. Initially, data are gathered from a limited set of new indicators prepared by teams of internationally renowned experts in each of the five areas. Then country experts in all five areas will conduct work that will provide the basis for improving quality data systems across countries.

Source: Organisation for Economic Co-operation and Development Health Care Quality Indicators Project.

to present performance data. Possibilities include the macro-level (such as national life expectancy), the meso-level (such as postoperative mortality rates in hospitals) and the micro-level (such as health outcomes achieved by individual practitioners). Table 10.4 summarizes some of the characteristics of good indicators. The intention is to develop performance measures that exhibit the characteristics of acceptability, feasibility, reliability, sensitivity to change, and validity.

The following sections look more closely at the methodological considerations that need to be taken into account when selecting which indicators to use and how to use and interpret them.

Table 10.4 Characteristics of good performance indicators

Stages	*Characteristics of indicators*
Development of indicators	Face/content validity: the extent to which the indicator accurately measures what it purports to measure
	Reproducibility: the extent to which the indicator would be the same if the method by which it was produced was repeated
Application of indicators	Acceptability: the extent to which the indicator is acceptable to those being assessed and those undertaking the assessment
	Feasibility: the extent to which valid, reliable and consistent data are available for collection
	Reliability: the extent to which there is minimal measurement error or the extent to which findings are reproducible should they be collected again by another organization
	Sensitivity to change: the extent to which the indicator has the ability to detect changes in the unit of measurement
	Predictive validity: the extent to which the indicator has the ability to predict accurately

Source: Adapted from Campbell et al. 2002.

Attribution and causality

Fundamental questions that arise when seeking to interpret many performance data include what has caused the observed performance and to which practitioners, organizations or agencies should variations in performance be attributed. Hauck, Rice and Smith (2003) have shown that there are immense differences in the extent to which the health system influences performance measures, ranging from a very large effect on responsiveness measures (such as waiting time) to a small effect on population mortality, which is heavily influenced by factors outside the health system. Such variations should be considered when holding providers and other stakeholders to account. To guide policy, improve service delivery and ensure accountability, it is critical that the causality of observed measures is attributed to the correct source(s). When using statistical methods to evaluate causal relationships and guide policy, researchers and policy-makers should be careful to control properly for measurement and attribution bias (Terris and Aron 2009). Box 10.3 gives key considerations that users of performance measures need to take into account when addressing causality and attribution bias.

Risk adjustment is an approach widely used to address the problem of attribution. It adjusts outcome data according to differences in resources, case mix and environmental factors, thereby seeking to enhance comparability (Box 10.4). In health care, in particular, variations in patient outcomes will have much to do with variations in patient attributes, such as age or socioeconomic class, and any comorbidities. Similar considerations apply when comparing measures of population health. In such cases, it is essential to employ methods of risk adjustment when using indicators and comparing agents. A key question then is exactly for what is the agent under scrutiny accountable. In the short term, for example, a health system has to deal with the epidemiological patterns and risky behaviour it inherits. This implies a major need for risk adjustment when comparing it with other health systems. In the longer term, one might expect the health system to be accountable for improving epidemiological patterns and health-related behaviour. The need for risk adjustment then becomes less critical, as the health system is responsible for many of the underlying causes of the measured outcomes.

Since early efforts with diagnosis-related groups in the United States, the methods of risk adjustment have been steadily refined over a period of 40 years, particularly in adjusting for outcomes for specific diseases or health care treatments. A key issue remains the quality (particularly the completeness) of the data on which risk adjustment is undertaken, particularly the presence of comorbidities or other complications. Recording these data depends (ultimately) on the practitioners whose performance is being assessed, so there is an ever-present threat to the integrity of the data if the incentives associated with performance comparison are too stark. Also, most risk-adjustment efforts are still works in progress, and there is often a need for careful qualitative clinical commentary on any risk-adjusted data, as there are often technical limitations to any scheme. Risk adjustment, however, is almost always essential if performance measurement is to secure credibility with practitioners, so it is important that efforts to improve on current methodologies are sustained.

Box 10.3 Key considerations when addressing causality and attribution bias

---

Users of performance measures should consider the following recommendations when addressing causality and attribution bias.

Research reports that investigates a possible causal and attributable link between the agents being assessed and the quality outcome proposed should be evaluated with particular attention to:

- the study methodology
- its controls for confounding variables
- the generalizability of the study sample.

Prospective analyses to identify critical pathways involved in the achievement of desired and undesired processes and outcomes of care should be undertaken. These analyses should try to:

- identify possible confounders;
- identify the extent to which agents under assessment are or can be clustered into homogeneous groupings.

In new *performance-measurement initiatives*, sources of random and systematic error in measurement and sampling should be carefully considered when developing the design. Procedures of data collection that maximize the reliability and accuracy of data (both primary and secondary) used for quality assessment should be institutionalized.

Risk-adjustment techniques should be employed when evaluating the relationship between agents under assessment and the quality indicators. Hierarchical models should be used to account for the clustering of data within different levels of the health system under analysis. The use of statistical methods, such as propensity scores or instrumental variables, should be considered.

Causality and attribution bias cannot be completely eliminated, even when utilizing the best available statistical methods. Unintended effects from biases in assessment of performance should be monitored carefully, particularly when reimbursement or other incentives are linked to the measures.

Source: Adapted from Terris and Aron 2009.

A specific issue in the interpretation of many performance data is random variation, which by definition emerges with no systematic pattern and is always present in quantitative data. Statistical methods become central to determining whether an observed variation in performance has arisen by chance rather than from variations in the performance of agents within the health system. As a matter of routine, confidence intervals should be presented alongside performance indicators. In the health care area, a challenge for such methods is to identify genuine outliers in a consistent and timely fashion, without signalling an excessive number of false positives. This is crucial when

Box 10.4 Statistical considerations when performing risk adjustment

Risk adjustment often involves using statistical modelling applied to large databases with information from many providers. The techniques produce weighting schemes for assessing patient risk. The statistical models can then be used to estimate the *expected* outcome for a provider, given its mix of patients or populations. Its actual outcome is then compared with this benchmark. The following should be considered when performing risk adjustment.

- Optimal risk-adjustment models result from a multidisciplinary effort that involves the interaction of clinicians with statisticians, as well as with experts in information systems and data production.
- Different practice patterns, patient characteristics and data specifications may limit the transferability of models across different countries. Before applying a model developed in another setting, clinicians and methodologists should examine its clinical validity and statistical performance.
- Decision-makers should be wary when drawing conclusions about the performance of risk-adjustment models from statistical summary measures (such as coefficient of determination), as these measures may not capture the model's predictive ability for different patient subgroups.
- In cases where it is believed that patient characteristics may also influence differences in the treatment patients receive, it may be more appropriate to apply risk stratification instead of (or alongside) risk adjustment.

Source: Adapted from Iezzoni 2009.

undertaking surveillance of individual practitioners or teams. In dealing with this situation, it must be asked when does a deviation from expected outcomes become a cause for concern and when should a regulator intervene. Statistical methods of squeezing maximum information from time series of data are now reaching an advanced stage of refinement and offer great scope for more focused intervention (Grigg and Spiegelhalter 2009).

Composite measures

Health systems are complex entities with multiple aspects, making performance very difficult to summarize, particularly through a single measure. Yet, when separate performance measures are provided for the many different aspects of the health system under observation – such as efficiency, equity, responsiveness, quality, outcomes and access – the amount of information provided can be overwhelming. Such information overload makes it difficult for the users of performance information to make any sense of the data. In response to these problems, the use of composite indicators has become increasingly popular. Composite indicators combine separate performance indicators into a single index or measure and are often used to rank or compare the performance of different practitioners, organizations or systems by providing a bigger picture and offering a more rounded view of performance (Goddard and Jacobs 2009).

However, if composite indicators are not carefully designed, they may be misleading and could lead to serious failings if used for health system policy-making or planning (Smith 2002). One of the main challenges in creating composite indicators is deciding which measures to include in the indicator and with what weights. As composite indicators aim to offer a comprehensive performance assessment, they should include all important aspects of performance, even if they are difficult to measure. In practice, however, there is often little choice of data, and questionable sources may be used for some components of the indicator. Considerable ingenuity may, therefore, be needed to develop adequate proxy indicators (Smith 2002; Goddard and Jacobs 2009).

Fundamental to composite indicators is the choice of weights (or importance) to be attached to the component measures. All the evidence suggests that there is great variation in the importance different people attach to different aspects of performance, so the specification of a single set of weights is fundamentally a political action. This indicates that the choice of weights requires political legitimacy on the part of the decision-maker. Analysis can, therefore, inform, but should not determine, the choice of weights. There exists a body of economic methodology for inferring weights, which includes methods for calculating willingness to pay, for eliciting patient's preferences from rankings of alternative scenarios and for directing making choices in experiments. These economic methods, however, have not been widely applied to the construction of composite indicators of health system performance (Smith 2002).

Besides capturing effectiveness, a primary benefit of composite indicators is that they allow the construction of measures of the overall productivity (or cost-effectiveness) of a health system. In particular, a composite measure of health system attainment can be assessed alongside expenditure without the need to assign an expenditure to a specific health system activity. This was a principle underlying the WHR2000 (World Health Organization 2000). However, the response to that report emphasized that many aspects of constructing composite attainment and productivity indicators are disputable. Table 10.5 takes a closer look at the advantages and disadvantages of using composite indicators for health performance assessment.

Using performance measurement: key policy levers

Rapid advances in technology and analytical methodology, coupled with changing public and professional attitudes, have made the use of large-scale information systems for performance assessment and improvement increasingly feasible (Power 1999). Experiences with realizing the potential of new data resources to improve system performance, however, have so far shown

Table 10.5 Advantages and disadvantages of composite indicators

Advantages	Disadvantages
Offer a broad assessment of system performance	May disguise failings in specific parts of the health care system
Place system performance at the centre of the policy arena	Make it difficult to determine where poor performance is occurring and, consequently, may make policy and planning more difficult and less effective
Enable judgment and cross-national comparison of health system efficiency	
Offer policy-makers at all levels the freedom to concentrate on areas where improvements are most readily secured, in contrast to piecemeal performance indicators	Often can lead to double counting, because of high positive correlation
	May use feeble data when seeking to cover many areas, which may make the methodological soundness of the entire indicator questionable
Clearly indicate which systems represent the best overall performance and improvement efforts	May make individual measures used contentious and hidden, owing to aggregation of the data
Can stimulate better data collection and analytic efforts across health systems and nations	May ignore aspects of performance that are difficult to measure, leading to adverse behavioural effects
	May only reflect certain preferences when inadequately developed methods for applying weights to composite indicators are used

Source: Adapted from Smith 2002.

inconsistent results, and no consensus exists yet on the best way to proceed. This section looks at some of the experiences in using data for performance improvement and at the lessons learned to date.

Information systems

Many of the earliest efforts to use performance data concentrated on collecting and organizing existing administrative information and disseminating it for management applications. These early efforts focused mainly on cost-containment and resource allocation. Examples include the development of diagnosis-related groups to compare hospital costs in the United States and the release of a suite of performance indicators in England to help managers to understand how their local health systems compared with the rest of the country. Although (from a managerial perspective) such methods are valuable in allowing better exploitation of existing data sources, little attention was given to the use of this information for evaluating external accountability or clinical treatment (Smith 1990).

Later developments, such as the establishment of the Canadian Institute for Health Information in 1994 and the Nordic collaboration in 2000 (Box 10.5),

Box 10.5 The Nordic collaboration

Background

A Nordic Council of Ministers working group, consisting of three to four representatives from each of the Nordic countries (Denmark, Finland, Greenland, Iceland, Norway and Sweden), was established in 2000. Its overall aim was to facilitate collaboration between the Nordic countries through the development of quality indicators and the creation of a foundation for evaluations that should benefit the public, health care professionals and health managers.

Indicators

Six subgroups work on selecting generic and disease-specific indicators and indicators within the areas of patient safety, psychiatry, primary health care, acute somatic care, public health and preventive health care, and patient-experienced health care. So far, the joint quality indicators selected for the Nordic countries fall under the following categories:

1. General and disease-specific indicators (mortality and survival rates for common illnesses)
2. Health promotion and ill health prevention
3. Mental health
4. Primary care
5. Patient safety
6. The patient experience.

Source: Swedish National Board of Health and Welfare 2006.

used large databases of performance measurement in more creative ways to assist with evidence-based decision-making in health planning and with accountability. Initially, performance data were used mostly by federal and provincial institutions. Reports and summary statistics, however, have increasingly been made available to the public, for example, in the form of the Statistics Canada annual reports. The Canadian Institute for Health Information also focused on analysing the data collected to produce reliable summary indicators in order to improve understanding of why trends or patterns emerge and, thus, to guide policy (Wolfson and Alvarez 2002).

Recent technology developments have increased the ability to store a greater volume of information with a greater level of detail, to distribute it more widely and flexibly, and to update it more quickly. In the future, the development of the electronic health record – containing all the information on a patient's health history – offers vast potential for capturing performance in many areas. Many challenges, however, need to be addressed if this potential is to be transformed into reality. First, because of the sheer amount of data and the speed at which it can be processed, auditing its accuracy is becoming increasingly important and challenging; the possibility of error carries with it severe implications if increasing reliance is to be placed on performance data. Second, the constant development of technology calls for continual investment in (and maintenance of) the information infrastructure and entails the need to ensure that the increasing number of information systems are mutually compatible so that their full potential can be exploited. Third, coordination is crucial to ensuring that the information collected is comparable across institutions and settings. Finally, the storage and use of so much information raises ethical concerns about patient privacy (Sequist and Bates 2009).

Public reporting

The placement of information in the public domain, to inform the public and other stakeholders about purchaser and provider performance, is growing. This information often takes the form of *report cards* or *provider profiles* that summarize measures, such as waiting times, patient satisfaction ratings and mortality rates, across providers. Two broad objectives lie behind the public disclosure of information: first, to stimulate quality improvement and, second, to enhance the more general accountability of health system organizations and practitioners to the public who fund and use them. Public reporting can improve quality through two pathways, as illustrated in Fig. 10.2: (1) a selection pathway, whereby consumers become better informed and select providers of higher quality; and (2) a change pathway, whereby information helps providers to identify the areas of underperformance, thus acting as a stimulus for improvement (Berwick, James and Coye 2003).

Both the United Kingdom and the United States have experimented extensively with the use of public disclosure of performance information. The United States has issued report cards for more than 20 years, with its first significant effort led by the federal government agency that administers the Medicare insurance programme. This initiative sought to inform consumer choice and stimulate provider improvement. Following complaints about

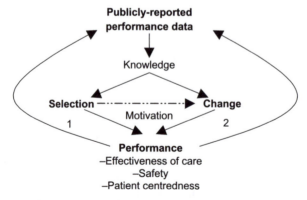

Figure 10.2 Two pathways for improving performance through the release of publicly-reported performance data

Source: Berwick, James and Coye 2003.

the validity of the rankings, it was rapidly withdrawn. However, it has since prompted the development of many other performance reports produced by state and federal governments, employers, consumer advocate groups, the media, private enterprise and business purchasers.

There is considerable evidence that publication of provider performance measures leads to improved performance (Hibbard, Stockard and Tusler 2005). Although the immediate purpose of publishing provider performance measures has often been to facilitate and inform patient choice, there is little evidence that patients make direct use of report cards. However, through their effect on the reputation of providers, report cards do appear to promote performance improvements in providers. Apart from their effect on performance, there are growing public demands to make important outcome information public and, in this respect, report cards can assist regulation and enhance accountability.

Starting in 1992, in the United States, two states (New York and Pennsylvania) began experimenting with public reporting of postoperative mortality rates for coronary artery bypass graft surgery. These rates are risk adjusted and published at the level of both the hospital and the individual surgeon. The associated confidence intervals are also reported, and a number of empirical analyses have examined the effects of these celebrated report-card initiatives. There is no doubt that the schemes have been associated with a marked improvement in risk-adjusted mortality in the two states (Shekelle 2009). However, there is a debate about whether these results necessarily imply that the schemes have been beneficial, and a number of adverse outcomes have also been reported, as follows (Schneider and Epstein 1996; Dranove et al. 2003).

- The coronary artery bypass graft surgery report cards led to increased selection by providers in New York and Pennsylvania, who were more inclined to avoid sicker patients (who might benefit from treatment) and to treat increased numbers of healthier patients (for whom the benefits of treatment are more contested).
- The initiative has led to increased Medicare expenditures with only a small improvement in population health.
- Practitioners were concerned about the absence of quality indicators other than mortality, about inadequate risk adjustment and about the unreliability of data.

In England, all National Health Service health care organizations are issued an annual performance rating – a report-card rating them from zero to three stars, based on about 40 performance indicators. These ratings were strongly promoted by the government and received much media and public attention. Poor performance has put executives' jobs at risk, and the initiative has had a strong effect on reported aspects of health care, such as waiting times. However, it has also induced some unintended behavioural consequences, such as a lack of attention to some aspects of clinical quality that were not being reported. In contrast to the English case, Scotland published a range of important clinical outcome data in the 1990s without any associated publicity. Many governors, clinicians and managers were unaware of the initiative and few incentives were attached to the reports. As a result, these indicators had very little impact on the behaviour of practitioners or organizations (Mannion and Goddard 2001).

Box 10.6   National quality indicators in Norway

Background

Norway started to use national quality indicators for specialized health care services in 2003. By 2006, data for 21 indicators were registered (11 for somatic care and 10 for psychiatric care) and, in addition to the indicators, patient-experience surveys were also included. Data reporting is compulsory, and data are published on the Free Hospital Choice Norway website (Norwegian Health Directorate 2011), along with other initiatives and information on the waiting times for different treatments. Data are presented at the hospital level along with data on national averages and developments over time.

Aims

Some important aims of data collection are:

- to create a base level of quality and generate incentives for health care personnel to improve quality;
- to identify a base level of quality for management;
- to support prioritization of health care services by political and administrative entities;
- to provide the public with information and create transparency in health care services;
- to provide users with information to make decisions.

This experience highlights the need to associate an incentive (which might be financial, reputation or market based) with a public-reporting scheme.

Norway offers another example of public disclosure of performance information. Box 10.6 describes the use of national quality indicators in Norway.

Publicly reported information has had a limited direct effect so far on patients and professionals, probably because it is necessarily aggregated and because the indicators reported are limited and inconsistent (Marshall et al. 2003). However, there is increasing evidence that health care organizations do take notice of these data, which have an important effect on their reputations, and that publication of performance information has led to concrete performance improvements (Marshall et al. 2000a; Shekelle 2009). Notwithstanding doubts about its effectiveness in promoting system improvement, the publication of performance information also serves an important accountability role. There is, therefore, no doubt that increased public reporting of outcomes of care is an irreversible trend in most health systems. However, it can lead to adverse outcomes, if not implemented and monitored with care.

Experience to date suggests that the following should be taken into account when implementing public disclosure of data.

- Careful consideration should be given to the purpose of the disclosure and to the type of information the different health system stakeholders want and are able to use.

- Careful consideration should be given to the effect that public disclosure of information may have on quality of care. Where appropriate, public disclosure of information should be integrated with other quality improvement strategies (Marshall et al. 2000b).
- To enhance their credibility and usefulness, public performance reports should be created in collaboration with physicians and other legitimate interest groups (Schneider and Epstein 1996; Marshall et al. 2000b).
- When reporting data, careful risk adjustment should be implemented to offer accurate comparisons between providers and to ensure that the legitimacy of the comparisons is accepted by professionals (Marshall et al. 2000b; Iezzoni 2009). Detailed information on the risk-adjustment strategies used should be made available alongside the reported information for public scrutiny.

Incentives

There is no doubt that clinicians and other actors in the health system generally respond as expected to financial incentives (Dudley 2005). The incorporation of performance measurement into financial-incentive regimes, therefore, potentially offers a promising avenue for future policy, and a number of experiments that attach financial rewards to reported performance are now under way.

Historically, the use of indirect financial incentives in health care has been proffered through systems of accreditation that offer rewards in the form of access to markets or extra payments once specified structures of care are put in place. Germany has an accreditation system of this type at the regional level, where specific quality indicators are used for accreditation (Der Gemeinsame Bundesausschuss 2011). Accreditation is, however, a very blunt incentive instrument. Policy is now shifting towards much more direct and focused incentives. In particular, the United States has been experimenting with financial incentives in different contexts, such as the *rewarding results* experiment, which uses incentives to improve quality (US National Health Care Purchasing Institute 2002). However, these have so far been small-scale experiments, and the results have been difficult to assess with any confidence.

Many issues need to be considered when designing performance-incentive schemes, including which aspects of performance to target, how to measure attainment, how to set targets, whether to offer incentives at the individual or group level, how strong to make the link between achievement and reward and how much money to attach to an incentive. Also, evaluating such schemes is essential, but challenging. In most instances, a controlled experiment is not practicable, as it is often not feasible to establish a convincing *do-nothing* baseline with which to compare the policy under scrutiny. Moreover, constant monitoring is needed to ensure that unintended responses to incentives (such as cream skimming or other unwanted behavioural responses) are not occurring, that the incentive scheme does not jeopardize the reliability of the performance data on which it relies, and that it does not compromise unrewarded aspects of performance.

The United Kingdom is experimenting with an ambitious financial-reward system for general practitioners, introduced in April 2004, under which about 20% of earnings are directly related to their performance across about 150 quality indicators (Smith and York 2004) (Box 10.7). So far, it has not been possible to attribute any major improvements in practitioner performance,

---

Box 10.7 The contract for general practitioners, United Kingdom

Framework

In April 2004, a new general-practitioner contract took effect in the United Kingdom National Health Service. This new contract more closely linked general practitioners with quality targets for both clinical and organizational activities through the Quality and Outcomes Framework programme. The programme rewards general practitioners for meeting targets in targeted areas, measured by about 150 indicators. Each indicator has a number of points allocated to it, varying according to the amount and difficulty of work required to successfully meet these criteria. A maximum of 1050 points can be earned, and up to 20% of general practitioner income is at risk under the scheme.

Targeted areas

Indicators upon which points are allocated are measured for the following main categories (some smaller categories are omitted):

- clinical areas: 76 indicators (focused on medical records, diagnosis, and initial and ongoing clinical management) and 550 points related to disorders such as coronary heart disease, stroke and transient ischaemic attack, hypertension, hyperthyroidism, diabetes, mental health, chronic obstructive pulmonary disease, asthma, epilepsy and cancer;
- organizational areas: 56 indicators and 184 points for areas such as records and information about patients, communication with patients, education and training, practice management and medicine management;
- patient experience: 4 indicators and 50 points covering items such as appointment length and consulting with patients about other issues;
- additional services: 10 indicators and 36 points for activities such as cervical screening, child health surveillance, maternity services and contraceptive services.

No risk adjustment is undertaken. Instead, practices may exclude certain patients from performance measurement if the required intervention is clinically inappropriate or if the patient refuses to comply.

Findings to date

- In preparation for the 2004 programme, general practitioners in the United Kingdom employed more nurses and administrative staff, established clinics for chronic diseases and increased the use of electronic medical records (Doran et al. 2006). Also, general practitioners are increasingly delegating tasks to other members of clinical staff. For example, a nurse may be asked to specialize in diabetes care (Roland et al. 2006).

- Although the Quality and Outcomes Framework programme was voluntary, in its first year of implementation almost all United Kingdom practices chose the programme, with the median practice scoring 95.5% of the possible points available. In the clinical areas, the median score was 96.7% (Doran et al. 2006). The achievements of years two and three of the contract have been similarly high (Burr 2008).
- Interviews with general practitioners suggested that they were concerned about the programme's focus on biomedical targets, which may lead to a reduced focus on other important aspects of care and may interfere with their ability to treat the patient as a *whole person* (Roland et al. 2006).
- There is little evidence of manipulation of the *prevalence* data on which performance is based. However, some practices do appear to be making excessive use of exception reporting (Gravelle, Sutton and Ma 2007).
- Although there is some evidence that the Quality and Outcomes Framework programme has improved patient care, quality was already improving rapidly in primary care and the specific effect of the programme seems to have been small (Campbell et al. 2007; Hippisley-Cox, Vinogradov and Coupland et al. 2007).

Source: Adapted from Lester and Roland 2009.

or other system improvements, to this bold (and very expensive) experiment. More generally, while performance-based incentive schemes do appear to offer immense potential for system improvement, there is a clear need for more careful research to identify the best mechanisms for harnessing their potential.

Targets

Health system targets are a specific type of performance-measurement and incentive scheme and are a quantitative expression of an objective to be met in the future. Targets have been brought to health policy from the field of business, the main idea being that when goals are explicitly defined as targets, more organized and efficient efforts will be made to meet them. Targets are expected to be SMART: specific, measurable, accurate, realistic and time bound (van Herten and Gunning-Schepers 2000). If well designed, targets can help organizations and practitioners to focus on a manageable number of achievable goals, which thereby lead to system improvements. The governments of many countries have experimented with targets in health care, including European Region Member States (most notably, the United Kingdom), Australia, New Zealand and the United States.

However, evidence is limited on the success of using health system targets (Wismar et al. 2008). They have traditionally been used extensively in public health, but reports of measurable success are rare. The English experience with the 1992 *Health of the Nation* strategy is typical (Department of Health 1992). The strategy was based on the WHO *Health for All* initiative and set a series of ambitious public health targets. However, a careful independent evaluation in 1998 concluded that its 'impact on policy documents peaked as early as 1993; and, by 1997, its impact on local policy-making was negligible' (Department of Health 1998: 1). Hunter (2002) summarized its failings under six broad headings.

1. There appeared to be a lack of leadership in the national government.
2. The policy failed to address the underlying social and structural determinants of health.
3. The targets were not always credible and were not formulated at a local level.
4. The strategy was poorly communicated beyond the health system.
5. The strategy was not sustained.
6. Partnerships between agencies were not encouraged.

Since the late 1990s, targets have been an particularly strong feature of English health care policy. Starting in 1998, the Treasury issued strategic targets, called Public Service Agreements, to all government departments, including the health ministry (Smith 2007). Public Service Agreements were focused primarily on outcomes, such as the improvement of mortality rates, reductions in smoking and obesity and reductions in waiting times. The health ministry used the star rating report cards, described above, as a key instrument to achieve these objectives. In contrast to most national target systems, this proved notably effective in securing some of the targeted objectives in health care (Bevan and Hood 2006). This success can be attributed to the following.

- The targets were precise, short-term objectives, rather than long term and general.
- Targets were based at the local level, rather than the national level.
- Professionals were engaged in the design and implementation of some of the targets. While this ran the risk of leading to so-called capture by professional interests, it also served to increase the awareness of objectives.
- Organizations were given increased financing, information and managerial capacity to respond to challenging targets.
- Concrete incentives were attached to the targets.

However, this success in health care was not replicated in the area of public health, almost certainly because managers felt health care targets were much more amenable to health system intervention.

While targets provide a straightforward way of highlighting key objectives and can be very successful if designed and implemented correctly, there are notable risks associated with their use (Smith 2008). Box 10.8 identifies some of the risks associated with increased reliance on targets. The conclusions from this experience are that, while performance targets offer some latitude for focusing system attention on specific areas of endeavour, they are unlikely

Box 10.8 Risks associated with increased reliance on targets

- Untargeted aspects of the health system may be neglected.
- Managers and practitioners may concentrate on short-term targets directly in their control at the expense of targets that address long-term or less-controllable objectives.
- The complexity of the target system requires a large implementation capacity and may be influenced by professional interests.
- Excessively aggressive targets may undermine the reliability of the data on which they are based.
- Excessively aggressive targets may induce undesirable behavioural responses.
- Targets may encourage a narrow, mercenary attitude, rather than encouraging altruistic professionalism.

Source: Smith 2008.

to secure performance improvements unless implemented carefully alongside other improvement initiatives, such as more general inspection and regulation.

Professional improvement

Most of the uses of performance measurement described above have been concerned with providing some means of external assessment and scrutiny of the health system, as a mechanism for prompting improved performance. However, another important use of performance measurement can be to provide feedback for clinicians on their performance relative to their peers. Databases that serve this purpose exist in many countries. For example, in Sweden they take the form of *quality registers*, where individual-based data on patient characteristics, diagnoses, treatments, experiences and outcomes are all collected voluntarily on the part of the health care providers and shared with other members of the register. The explicit aim of the quality registers is to facilitate the improvement of quality in clinical work through continuous learning and development (Rehnqvist 2002) (Box 10.9). Indeed there is a strong argument that performance measurement should become an inherent part of a clinician's lifelong learning. This suggests the need for a prominent role for performance-measurement principles in early clinical training.

Whether information for professional improvement should be kept anonymous or be made available to the public is widely debated. Evidence suggests that, to be effective, such performance-measurement schemes need to be designed and owned by the professionals who use them (Rowan and Black 2000). It is argued that the most constructive systems are those that encourage positive and cooperative behaviour among clinicians and avoid public threats to their professional or commercial standing, which may encourage defensive behaviour that could lead to cream skimming or other unwanted behavioural responses. Indicators used for professional improvement should therefore:

Box 10.9 Sweden's quality registers

The development of national quality registers has been a major effort in promoting performance improvement. Sweden has about 50 active quality registers, with the first one dating back to 1979. The aim of a national quality register is to encourage good medical practice through the comparison and evaluation of outcome and quality information over time and between providers. A variety of organizational patterns are used, but each is clinically led and typically maintained by a group (usually located in one of the Swedish university hospitals) that collects, assembles, analyses and distributes the data to its members. Several meetings might be organized each year to discuss this material. The participation of clinicians in a registry group is voluntary and in most cases registers develop gradually. When a register is developed, the quality indicators and reporting tools are established on the basis of consensus within the medical specialty and are often refined from year to year. Information on departments is anonymous. However, most well-established registers do present department data publicly. The quality registers provide clinicians with essential information with which to compare performance and facilitate discussion on improvement. Increasingly, data from quality registers have also been used to support decision-making.

Source: Rehnqvist 2002.

- reflect meaningful aspects of clinical practice with a strong scientific underpinning
- ensure risk adjustment of indicators
- allow exclusion of certain patients, such as those who refuse to comply with treatment
- facilitate interpretability
- represent services under a provider's control
- ensure high accuracy
- minimize cost and burden.

Also, as well as measuring the outcomes of care, it is important to seek to measure the extent of inappropriate care (overuse or underuse of treatments).

The requirements of a successful professional-improvement performance-measurement system may, therefore, come into conflict with the requirements of information systems designed to promote accountability and patient choice. This is not to say that the tension between these different needs and demands cannot be resolved. Experiences from Sweden and elsewhere, such as Denmark and the Netherlands, suggest that public and professional needs can be reconciled; for example, some quality registers do publish outcomes on individual practitioners (Danish Institute for Quality and Accreditation in Healthcare 2007). In any case, patients will in all likelihood increasingly demand that more performance data be made available. The challenge for the professions is to ensure that this trend is harnessed to good results, rather than leading to defensive professional behaviour. One solution lies in the careful development of acceptable, statistical, risk-adjustment schemes and in careful presentation of statistical data, so that the public and media are better equipped to understand and interpret the information that is made available to them.

Conclusions

The ultimate goal of any performance-measurement instrument is to promote the achievement of health system objectives. Consequently, its effectiveness should be evaluated not in relation to statistical properties, such as accuracy and validity, but more broadly in relation to the extent to which it promotes or compromises these objectives. Effective performance measurement alone is not enough to ensure effective performance management. The functions of analysis and interpretation of performance data are also crucial. Also, performance measurement is only one (albeit very important) instrument for securing system improvement. To maximize its effect, performance measurement needs to be aligned with other aspects of system design, such as financing, market structure, accountability arrangements and regulation. Finally, a great deal of attention needs to be paid to the political context within which any performance-measurement scheme is implemented. Without careful attention to these broader health system considerations, the best performance-measurement system will be ineffective.

Governments have a major stewardship role to play in harnessing the full potential of performance measurement for improving the health system. The WHR2000 (World Health Organization 2000) defined stewardship as 'defining the vision and direction of health policy, exerting influence through regulation and advocacy, and collecting and using information'. This chapter has sought to outline how performance measurement can help governments to fulfil each of these roles. The discussion has argued that performance measurement offers health systems major opportunities to secure performance improvement and that no health system can be adequately steered without good performance information and intelligence. The overarching role of performance measurement is to enhance the decisions made by actors throughout the health system.

Performance information can help governments directly in formulating and evaluating policy and in undertaking regulation. The broader stewardship role of governments is, however, to ensure that the necessary flow of information is available, functioning properly and aligned with the design of the health system. Performance measurement is a public good that will not occur naturally. Governments, therefore, have a fundamental role to ensure that the maximum benefit is secured from performance measurement, whether through law, regulation, coordination or persuasion. Implementation then requires sustained political and professional leadership at the highest level and also assurance that the necessary analytical capacity is available throughout the health system.

Some of the stewardship responsibilities of government in the area of performance measurement are summarized in Box 10.10.

Given the increasing demand for performance measurement and given the large set of actors and responsibilities, it is important that policy-makers

Box 10.10 Stewardship responsibilities associated with performance measurement

Stewardship responsibilities associated with performance measurement can be summarized under the headings that follow. None of these roles need be undertaken by government itself, but it must be ensured that they all function effectively.

1. Development of a clear conceptual framework and a clear vision of the purpose of the performance-measurement system:
   - alignment with accountability relationships
   - alignment with other health system mechanisms, such as finance, market structure and information technology.
2. Design of data collection mechanisms:
   - detailed specification of individual indicators
   - alignment with international best practice.
3. Information governance:
   - data audit and quality control
   - ensuring public trust in information
   - ensuring well-informed public debate.
4. Development of analytical devices and capacity to help to understand the data:
   - ensuring analysis is undertaken efficiently and effectively
   - ensuring local decision-makers understand the analysis
   - commissioning appropriate research on, for example, risk adjustment, uncertainty and data feedback mechanisms.
5. Development of appropriate data aggregation and presentational methods:
   - ensuring information has appropriate effect on all parties
   - mandating public release of summary comparative information
   - ensuring comparability and consistency.
6. Design of incentives to act on performance measures:
   - monitoring the effect of performance information on behaviour
   - acting to enhance beneficial outcomes and negate any adverse consequences.
7. Proper evaluation of performance-measurement instruments:
   - ensuring money is spent cost-effectively on information resources.
8. Managing the political process:
   - developing and monitoring policy options
   - encouraging healthy political debate
   - ensuring that specific interest groups do not capture the performance-information system.

consider what makes performance indicators effective in improving system performance and accountability. Although there is no conclusive answer to this question, experience has suggested that any policy development should embrace the following elements.

A clear conceptual framework and a clear vision of the purpose of the performance-measurement system should be developed and should be aligned with the accountability relationships inherent in the health system. Performance indicators should attempt to measure performance that is directly attributable to an organization or actor, and not to environmental factors (such as patient attributes or socioeconomic factors). Definitions of performance indicators should be clear and consistent and should fit into the conceptual framework chosen.

Indicators should aim to measure concepts that are relevant to the needs of specific actors and should not focus merely on measuring what is available or easy to measure. They should aim to be statistically sound and should be presented in a way that is straightforward to interpret, thus reducing the likelihood of manipulation or misinterpretation. They should be presented with full acknowledgement of any data limitations, including uncertainty estimates and lack of timeliness. Further exploration of improved processes for handling measurement errors is needed as such errors may confound true performance differences.

More attention should be paid to the presentation of performance data and how this influences their interpretation by patients, providers and provider organizations. In particular, attention should be paid to enhancing the capacity to understand and use information among managers and clinicians. Use of performance data should become an intrinsic part of clinical education and lifelong professional development.

Incentives that act on performance measures should be carefully designed. The impact of performance information on behaviour should be carefully monitored. Actions should be taken to enhance beneficial outcomes and to negate any adverse consequences.

Policy-makers should pay particular attention to the broader health system to ensure that performance measurement is aligned with the design of mechanisms such as finance and market structures, and to recognize the organizational context within which performance data are collected and disseminated.

Performance-measurement systems should be monitored frequently and evaluated to identify opportunities for improvement and any unintended side-effects. The political aspects of performance measurement should be managed effectively. Among other things, this involves ensuring that specific interest groups do not capture the performance information system and also involves encouraging healthy political debate.

In conclusion, health systems are still in an early stage of performance measurement and major steps can still be taken to improve the effectiveness of their measurement systems. Performance measurement, however, offers opportunities for major health system improvements. Advances in technology are likely to increase this potential still further, and the increasing public demands for accountability and information will reinforce current trends. There is, therefore, a policy-making imperative to consider carefully the role of performance measurement in the health system, to implement initiatives of proven effectiveness, to undertake careful trials of less-established mechanisms and to monitor and update performance-measurement systems as new knowledge and capacity emerge.

References

Berwick, D.M., James, B. and Coye, M.J. (2003) Connections between quality measurement and improvement. *Medical Care*, 41(Suppl. 1): 130–8.

Bevan, G. and Hood, C. (2006) Have targets improved performance in the English NHS? *British Medical Journal*, 332: 419–22.

Burr, T. (2008) *NHS Pay Modernisation: New Contracts for General Practice Services in England*. London: National Audit Office, http://web.nao.org.uk/search/search.aspx?Schema= &terms=NHS+Pay+Modernisation (accessed 9 September 2010).

Campbell, S.M., Braspenning, J., Hutchinson, A. and Marshall, M. (2002) Research methods used in developing and applying quality indicators in primary care. *Quality and Safety in Health Care*, 11: 358–64.

Campbell, S.M., Reeves, D., Kontopantelis, E., Middleton, E., Sibbald, B. and Roland, M. (2007) Quality of primary care in England with the introduction of pay for performance. *New England Journal of Medicine*, 357(2): 181–90.

Danish Institute for Quality and Accreditation in Healthcare (2007) *Den Danske Kvalitetsmodels Organisation*. [*The Danish Quality Model Organization*.] Århus: Danish Institute for Quality and Accreditation in Healthcare, http://www.kvalitetsinstitut. dk/sw179.asp (accessed 13 September 2010).

Davies, H. (2005) *Measuring and Reporting the Quality of Health Care: Issues and Evidence from the International Research Literature*. Edinburgh, NHS Quality Improvement Scotland, (http://www.nhshealthquality.org/nhsqis/files/Davies%20Paper.pdf, accessed 8 September 2010).

Department of Health (1992) *The Health of the Nation: A Strategy for Health in England*. London: HMSO.

Department of Health (1998) *The Health of the Nation: A Policy Assessed*. London: HMSO.

Der Gemeinsame Bundesausschuss (2011) [website]. Siegburg: Gemeinsamer Bundesausschuss, http://www.g-ba.de/ (accessed 4 October 2011).

Donabedian, A. (1966) Evaluating the quality of medical care. *Milbank Quarterly*, 44(3): 166–206.

Doran, T., Fullwood, C., Gravelle, H. et al. (2006) Pay-for-performance programs in family practices in the United Kingdom. *New England Journal of Medicine*, 355(4): 375–84.

Dranove, D., Kessler, D., McClellan, M. and Satterthwaite, M. (2003) Is more information better? The effects of 'report cards' on health care providers. *Journal of Political Economy*, 111(3): 555–88.

Dudley, R.A. (2005) Pay-for-performance research: how to learn what clinicians and policy makers need to know. *Journal of the American Medical Association*, 294(14): 1821–3.

Finnish National Research and Development Centre for Welfare and Health (2007) *Sairaaloiden Tuottavuuden Kehitys 2001–2005*, tilastotiedote statistikmeddelande no. 5/2007 [*The Development of Hospitals' Profitability 2001–2005*.], http://www.stakes.fi/ tilastot/tilastotiedotteet/2007/Tt05_07.pdf, accessed 9 September 2010).

Fitzpatrick, R. (2009) Patient-reported outcome measures and performance measurement, in P.C. Smith, E. Mossialos, I. Papanicolas and S. Leatherman (eds.) *Performance Measurement for Health System Improvement: Experiences and Prospects*. Cambridge: Cambridge University Press: 63–86.

Goddard, M. and Jacobs, R. (2009) Using composite indicators to measure performance in health care, in P.C. Smith, E. Mossialos, I. Papanicolas and S. Leatherman (eds.) *Performance Measurement for Health System Improvement: Experiences and Prospects*. Cambridge: Cambridge University Press: 339–68.

Gravelle, H., Sutton, M. and Ma, A. (2007) *Doctor Behaviour under a Pay for Performance Contract: Evidence from the Quality and Outcomes Framework*, research paper no. 28.

York: Centre for Health Economics, University of York, http://www.york.ac.uk/inst/che/pdf/rp28.pdf, accessed 13 September 2010).

Grigg, O. and Spiegelhalter, D. (2009) Clinical surveillance and patient safety, in P.C. Smith, E. Mossialos, I. Papanicolas and S. Leatherman (eds.) *Performance Measurement for Health System Improvement: Experiences and Prospects*. Cambridge: Cambridge University Press: 286–310.

Hauck, K., Rice, N. and Smith, P.C. (2003) The influence of health care organisations on health system performance. *Journal of Health Services Research and Policy*, 8(2): 68–74.

Hibbard, J.H., Stockard, J. and Tusler, M. (2005) Hospital performance reports: impact on quality, market share, and reputation. *Health Affairs*, 24(4): 1150–60.

Hippisley-Cox, J., Vinogradov, Y. and Coupland, C. (2007) *Time Series Analysis for Selected Clinical Indicators from the Quality and Outcomes Framework 2001–2006*. Leeds: The Information Centre for Health and Social Care, http://www.qresearch.org/Public_Documents/Time%20Series%20Analysis%20for%20selected%20clinical.pdf (accessed 13 September 2010).

Holland, W. (1988) *European Community Atlas of 'Avoidable Death'*. Oxford: Oxford University Press.

Hunter, D. (2002) England, in Marinker, M. (ed.) *Health Targets in Europe: Polity, Progress and Promise*. London: BMJ Books: 148–64.

Iezzoni, L. (2009) Risk adjustment for performance measurement, in P.C. Smith, E. Mossialos, I. Papanicolas and S. Leatherman (eds.) *Performance Measurement for Health System Improvement: Experiences and Prospects*. Cambridge: Cambridge University Press: 251–85.

Lester, H., Roland, M. (2009) Performance measurement in primary care, in P.C. Smith, E. Mossialos, I. Papanicolas and S. Leatherman (eds.) *Performance Measurement for Health System Improvement: Experiences and Prospects*. Cambridge: Cambridge University Press: 371–405.

Linna, M. (2006) Benchmarking hospital productivity. *Health Policy Monitor*, 26 April http://www.hpm.org/survey/fi/a7/4 (accessed 14 September 2010).

Loeb, J.M. (2004) The current state of performance measurement in health care. *International Journal for Quality in Health Care*, 16(Suppl. 1): i5–9.

Mannion, R. and Goddard, M. (2001) Impact of published clinical outcomes data: case study in NHS hospital trusts. *British Medical Journal*, 323: 260–3.

Mant, J. (2001) Process versus outcome indicators in the assessment of quality of health care. *International Journal for Quality in Health Care*, 13(6): 475–80.

Marshall, M.N., Shekelle, P.G., Davies, H.T.O. and Smith, P.C. (2003) Public reporting on quality in the United States and the United Kingdom. *Health Affairs*, 22(3): 134–48.

Marshall, M.N., Shekelle, P.G., Leatherman, S. and Brook, R.H. (2000a) The public release of performance data: what do we expect to gain? A review of the evidence. *Journal of the American Medical Association*, 283(14): 1866–74.

Marshall, M.N., Shekelle, P.G., Leatherman, S. and Brook, R.H. (2000b) Public disclosure of performance data: learning from the US experience. *Quality in Health Care*, 9: 53–7.

McIntyre, D., Rogers, L. and Heier, E.J. (2001) Overview, history, and objectives of performance measurement. *Health Care Financing Review*, 22: 7–43.

Naylor, D.C., Iron, K. and Hands, K. (2002) Measuring health system performance: problems and opportunities in the era of assessment and accountability, in P.C. Smith (ed.) *Measuring Up: Improving Health System Performance in OECD countries*. Paris, Organisation for Economic Co-operation and Development, 13–34.

Nolte, E. and McKee, M. (2004) *Does Healthcare Save Lives? Avoidable Mortality Revisited*. London: The Nuffield Trust.

Norwegian Health Directorate (2011) [website] *Fritt Sykehusvalg Norge [Free Hospital Choice Norway]*. Oslo: Social- og Helsdirektoratet, http://www.frittsykehusvalg.no (accessed 4 October 2011).

Organisation for Economic Co-operation and Development. *Health Care Quality Indicators Project* [website]. Paris: Organisation for Economic Co-operation and Development, http://www.oecd.org/health/hcqi (accessed 10 September 2010).

Power, M. (1999) *The Audit Society: Rituals of Verification*, 2nd edn. Oxford: Oxford University Press.

Rehnqvist, N. (2002) Improving accountability in a decentralized system: a Swedish perspective, in P.C. Smith (ed.) *Measuring Up: Improving the Performance of Health Systems in OECD Countries*. Paris, Organisation for Economic Co-operation and Development: 87–96.

Roland, M.O., Campbell, S., Bailey, N., Whalley, D. and Sibbald, B. (2006) Financial incentives to improve the quality of primary care in the UK: predicting the consequences of change. *Primary Health Care Research and Development*, 7(1): 18–26.

Rowan, K. and Black, N. (2000) A bottom-up approach to performance indicators through clinician networks. *Health Care UK*, Spring: 42–6.

Schneider, E.C. and Epstein, A.M. (1996) Influence of cardiac-surgery performance reports on referral practices and access to care. *New England Journal of Medicine*, 335(4): 251–6.

Sequist, T. and Bates, D. (2009) Developing information technology capacity for performance measurement, in P.C. Smith, E. Mossialos, I. Papanicolas and S. Leatherman (eds.) *Performance Measurement for Health System Improvement: Experiences and Prospects*. Cambridge: Cambridge University Press: 552–81.

Shekelle, P.G. (2009) Public performance reporting on quality information, in P.C. Smith, E. Mossialos, I. Papanicolas and S. Leatherman (eds.) *Performance Measurement for Health System Improvement: Experiences and Prospects*. Cambridge: Cambridge University Press: 537–51.

Smith, P.C. (1990) The use of performance indicators in the public sector. *Journal of the Royal Statistical Society*, 153(1): 53–72.

Smith, P.C. (2002) Developing composite indicators for assessing health system efficiency, in P.C. Smith (ed.) *Measuring Up: Improving the Performance of Health Systems in OECD Countries*. Paris, Organisation for Economic Co-operation and Development: 295–316.

Smith, P.C. (2005) Performance measurement in health care: history, challenges and prospects. *Public Money and Management*, 25(4): 213–20.

Smith, P.C. (2007) Performance budgeting in England: public service agreements, in Robinson, M. (ed.) *Performance Budgeting: Linking Funding and Results*. Houndmills: Palgrave McMillan: 211–33.

Smith, P.C. (2008) England: intended and unintended effects, in M. Wismar, M. McKee, K. Ernst, D. Srivastava and R. Busse (eds.) *Health Targets in Europe, Learning from Experience*. Copenhagen: WHO Regional Office for Europe on behalf of the European Observatory on Health Systems and Policies: 63–81.

Smith, P.C. and York, N. (2004) Quality incentives: the case of UK general practitioners. *Health Affairs*, 22(3): 112–18.

Smith, P.C., Mossialos, E., Papanicolas, I. and Leatherman, S. (eds.) (2010) *Performance Measurement for Health System Improvement: Experiences, Challenges and Prospects*. Cambridge: Cambridge University Press.

Spiegelhalter, D.J. (1999) Surgical audit: statistical lessons from Nightingale and Codman. *Journal of the Royal Statistical Society*, 162(1): 45–58.

Street, A. and Hakkinen, U. (2009) Health system productivity and efficiency, in P.C. Smith, E. Mossialos, I. Papanicolas and S. Leatherman (eds.) *Performance Measurement for Health System Improvement: Experiences and Prospects*. Cambridge: Cambridge University Press: 222–48.

Swedish National Board of Health and Welfare (2006) *Nationella kvalitetsindikatorer inom hälso- och sjukvården* [*National Quality Indicators in the Health Care System*]. Stockholm: National Board of Health and Welfare, http://www.socialstyrelsen.se/publikationer2006/2006-107-13 (accessed 15 September 2010).

Terris, D.D. and Aron, D.C. (2009) Attribution and causality in health care performance measurement, in P.C. Smith, E. Mossialos, I. Papanicolas and S. Leatherman (eds.) *Performance Measurement for Health System Improvement: Experiences and Prospects.* Cambridge: Cambridge University Press: 311–38.

US National Health Care Purchasing Institute (2002) *Ensuring Quality Providers: A Purchaser's Toolkit for Using Incentives.* Washington, DC: National Health Care Purchasing Institute.

Valentine, N., Prasad, A., Rice, N., Robone, S. and Chatterji, S. (2009) Health systems responsiveness: a measure of the acceptability of health-care processes and systems from the user's perspective, in P.C. Smith, E. Mossialos, I. Papanicolas and S. Leatherman (eds.) *Performance Measurement for Health System Improvement: Experiences and Prospects.* Cambridge: Cambridge University Press: 138–86.

van Herten, L.M. and Gunning-Schepers, L.J. (2000) Targets as a tool in health policy. Part 1: lessons learned. *Health Policy,* 53(1): 1–11.

Wagstaff, A. (2009) Measuring financial protection in health, in P.C. Smith, E. Mossialos, I. Papanicolas and S. Leatherman (eds.) *Performance Measurement for Health System Improvement: Experiences and Prospects.* Cambridge: Cambridge University Press: 114–37.

Wismar, M., McKee, M., Ernst, K., Srivastava, D. and Busse, R. (eds.) (2008) *Health Targets in Europe, Learning from Experience.* Copenhagen: WHO Regional Office for Europe on behalf of the European Observatory on Health Systems and Policies.

Wolfson, M. and Alvarez, R. (2002) Towards integrated and coherent health information systems for performance monitoring: the Canadian experience, in P.C. Smith (ed.) *Measuring Up: Improving the Performance of Health Systems in OECD Countries.* Paris, Organisation for Economic Co-operation and Development: 133–55.

World Health Organization (2000) *The World Health Report 2000. Health Systems: Improving Performance.* Geneva: World Health Organization. http://www.who.int/whr/2000/en/ (accessed 1 September 2010).

chapter eleven

Investing in health systems: drawing the lessons

*Martin McKee, Suszy Lessof
and Josep Figueras*

Health policy-makers face enormous pressure to ensure cost-containment and financial sustainability, particularly in those countries whose governments have chosen to pursue stringent austerity measures in the wake of the 2008 economic crisis. This book is not the place to discuss the wisdom of the cutbacks being proposed in some countries, except to note that leading economists are divided about their consequences for the long-term growth of the economy (Stuckler et al. 2010a) and that the cutbacks are likely to have considerable consequences for public health (Stuckler et al. 2009; Stuckler, Basu and McKee 2010b). Instead, we recognize that they are a political reality that must be confronted by those responsible for health policy.

The evidence reviewed in this volume recasts health systems not as a drain on resources but as an opportunity to invest in the health of the population and, crucially, in economic growth. It does not attempt to offer definitive answers or be prescriptive about 'how much' to invest or 'what' to invest in. Rather, the volume sets out a framework outlining the central issues; synthesizes key evidence; and structures it so that policy-makers can assess investment decisions whatever their values or socioeconomic context. The issues are wide ranging and the evidence on many interventions is still limited. Nonetheless, the document shows that strengthening health systems has the potential to improve the health and well-being of Europe's people significantly, provided of course that investment is underpinned by evidence on cost-effectiveness, not least against alternative interventions inside and beyond the health system, and by rigorous performance assessment.

The chapters in this volume summarize the main evidence on the three sides of the conceptual triangle of health systems, health and wealth and the interaction with the central goal of societal well-being. They focus on the contribution of health to economic growth and well-being and the impact of health systems on health improvement, population health, equity and responsiveness; but also address the dynamic relationships between wealth and health and the size and shape of the health system. In addition, they highlight the importance of performance measurement in making the case for investment and in ensuring better performance and value for money.

Chapters 1 and 2 show how health systems, health and wealth are inextricably linked in a set of mutually reinforcing and dynamic relationships. This new paradigm offers an opportunity for a fundamental reassessment of the role of health systems in society. It poses three key questions which are addressed in the subsequent chapters.

- How can we improve health, wealth and societal well-being by investing in health systems?
- How can we ensure that health systems are sustained in the future?
- How can we monitor, manage and improve performance so that health systems are as effective and efficient as possible?

Chapter 2 addresses the definitions, boundaries, functions and goals of health systems. After a review of various approaches it concludes that the health systems framework set out in the *World Health Report 2000* (World Health Organization 2000) offers a solid conceptual basis to understand health systems and facilitate policy and managerial action, performance measurement and accountability. The authors, however, acknowledge a number of implementation challenges such as the practical operationalization of health system goals, accounting and measuring health system activities, the variability of ministerial responsibilities and the quality of available data. Nonetheless, all things considered, the advantages of adopting this framework far outnumber the problems.

Therefore, the health system definition set out in this chapter (and adopted in the volume as a whole) builds on that of the WHR 2000 but expands the role of stewardship beyond health actions whose primary activity is to improve health. It includes:

- delivery of health services (both personal and population based);
- activities to enable the delivery of health services (specifically finance, resource generation and stewardship);
- stewardship activities that aim to influence what other sectors do when it is relevant to health, even where the primary purpose of those sectors is not health improvement.

This approach emphasizes the scope of health systems beyond health care. It is the role of health ministries as the stewards of the health of their people, to take responsibility for all three of the points and to be accountable for the health sector and for influencing action in other sectors that impact on health.

The chapter showed how the health systems framework builds on a broader public health strategy and demonstrated that the Essential Public Health Functions (EPHF) (Pan American Health Organization/World Health Organization 1998) can be incorporated within the health system functions. Moreover, it argued that health systems and its stewards have an essential role to play influencing other non health sectors to act on health determinants – Health in All

Policies. However, the ultimate responsibility for health governance and health lies with the government, and indeed with society, as a whole.

Chapter 3 examines the upward cost pressures on health expenditure. Health services are too easily portrayed as a burden, absorbing increasingly more resources. The ageing of Europe's population, the emergence of new and more expensive technologies and the growth of citizens' expectations all add to the upward pressure on health care. However, it is increasingly clear that this assessment is too simple; demographic (and other) trends do not necessarily or inevitably translate into higher societal costs.

Ageing need not pose a huge challenge to health systems, particularly if the health system and those outside it that influence health adopt evidence-based policies which promote healthy ageing, and if societies arrange their employment policies (including retirement age) in ways that ensure that older people can remain economically active. While simple cross-sectional analyses suggest that health care costs increase with age, this does not mean that ageing populations will be more expensive. It is now clear that cost is a function of proximity to death and not simply of being older. There is now evidence from several countries that older people are healthier than ever and experience compressed morbidity, in part as a result of healthier lifestyles and in part because of access to safe and effective treatments.

The introduction of new technologies *can* be managed in ways that secure their benefits while limiting aggregate costs. Proactive and adequately resourced health technology assessment systems, coupled with mechanisms such as regulation and payment systems to ensure compliance, can reduce the risk of inappropriate use of technology and promote cost-effective care. Similarly, initiatives to engage with citizens can manage expectations, offsetting some of the pressures to provide potentially inappropriate technologies, and balancing responsiveness with efficiency.

In summary, increased expenditure on health systems is not inevitable. Governments can control it and. with the judicious use of policy levers and management tools, ameliorate the impact of spending pressures.

Chapter 4 serves as a reminder that health has a value in and of itself. It matters to individuals and societies across Europe. This value can be expressed in monetary terms based on the decisions that individuals make in their everyday lives, such as whether to undertake a dangerous job for a higher salary. Methods such as this do have drawbacks; nonetheless, the evidence demonstrates conclusively that people attach huge importance to the notion and enjoyment of health, regardless of cultural or economic differences.

Health also has a significant impact on economic productivity. Development economists have long recognized the importance of the right mix of physical and human capital. However, when thinking about the latter, they have traditionally focused on education and not health. This changed with a publication by the Commission on Macroeconomics and Health in 2001, which found that poor health dragged down economic growth in developing countries. Later work showed how the same was true in high- and middle-income countries. People in poor health are less likely to work and, when in work, are less productive. They are less likely to invest in their own education or to save for retirement, and so to support the wider economy. The economic position of countries today owes much to the extent to which they were able to achieve better health historically. The current economic and labour market context, social security arrangements, retirement age and the interactions between them will need to be taken into account in addressing the economic benefits of better health in the future. The evidence is clear: a healthy population including healthy older people can contribute very substantially to the economy.

Health status also clearly influences health expenditure. If no one was ill there would be no need for health services. Analyses undertaken in several countries suggest that policies which promote healthy lifestyles and early use of preventive care may be able to reduce future demands on the health system. As already noted, ageing populations need not necessarily place greater demands on health systems. This does not, however, offset all the pressures to increase overall spending, nor does it reflect the likely increases in demand for social care.

Policy-makers must demonstrate that health systems have a discernible and positive impact on health, and contribute to equity and overall societal 'responsiveness' if they are to justify investment in health systems in annual budget rounds. They need to show that investments in health system interventions constitute value for money and fare positively against alternative interventions within the broader public health realm acting on health determinants in other sectors. The impact of health systems is assessed in Chapters 5 to 8.

Chapter 5 on the contribution of health care to population health shows, the evidence is unequivocal: much ill health can be tackled by health care services. Around a half of the gains in life expectancy in recent decades stem from improved health care. What is more, there remains significant mortality from causes amenable to health care, suggesting that appropriate investment will have direct and tangible benefits in the future.

Chapter 6 provides compelling evidence of the value of wider public health interventions both within the health sector and across sector boundaries. Moreover, the cost-effectiveness of these often compares favourably with clinical services. There is particular scope for interventions on key risk factors, such as legislation on salt and saturated fats to address diet-related risks, fiscal and regulatory changes to influence tobacco use, or traffic control measures to prevent accidents. These demonstrate how important it is that public health action takes place across sectors. Furthermore, there is a need to have a comprehensive perspective and combine 'upstream' and 'downstream' measures so that macro-level initiatives shape determinants, while downstream measures help individuals to modify behaviours.

There is still debate around which public health measures are the best value for money or how exactly to bundle them most effectively to reflect the national context of disease burden and risk. What is no longer debatable is the major impact on health status of these measures within the health system or beyond in other sectors. They do make a difference and there is a powerful case for investing in them.

Chapter 7 explores the wide inequalities in health that persist in Europe. Life expectancy at birth is over 15 years longer in the best-performing country in Europe than in the worst. There is also a gap of 10 years in life expectancy within countries, including in the wealthier ones. In many countries, inequalities are widening as those who are better off benefit from lifestyle changes and improved health care, while the poor are left behind. Health inequalities have high economic costs. They undermine economic performance, increase social costs and diminish societal well-being. If the existing gaps could be narrowed, there would be substantial gains in national income, coupled with reductions in the costs of health care as demands for ambulatory and inpatient care reduced. Similarly, there would be substantial savings in unemployment and disability benefits. Societal well-being and social cohesion would also increase as health was distributed more equitably.

This calls for effective action on the social determinants of health and in particular upstream interventions, such as changes in taxation and benefits. It is, however, essential to link these policies with downstream ones, directly tackling risk factors such as smoking and poor diet. This will often involve taking on powerful vested interests. Finally, there is a need to ensure that health systems promote equity by removing the barriers to access and to effective and responsive care that are faced by those who are already disadvantaged. In these ways, health systems can reduce the health gap within countries, uphold the values of European societies and make inroads into the economic costs of the unequal distribution of health.

Chapter 8 considers the concept of responsiveness to legitimate expectations by the public, a fundamental goal of health systems. It is not, however, easy to capture because patient expectations vary according to culture, age and class, and because it is difficult to disentangle their experience from other factors that affect their perceptions of the health system.

Policy-makers have a range of tools they can use, from training staff to respect patients' dignity and autonomy to improving facilities. They may use the levers of pay, regulation or contracting to specify what is expected and afford patients defined rights through service guarantees or ombudsman schemes. They need, however, to be clear about the trade-offs involved. The issue of choice highlights the potential tensions between responsiveness and other health system goals. While 'choice' may be politically attractive, it favours the knowledgeable and articulate and may increase inequalities. Similarly, while it may promote patient autonomy, choice can also allow for ineffective therapies or fragmentation of care, both of which will impact adversely on health. Those responsible for health policy have to balance these tensions. While challenging, helping populations to access and interpret transparent, valid and meaningful data related to performance can support an informed debate, provided that there are effective safeguards against manipulation of data or patients' and health professionals' behaviour.

Chapter 9 reviews the experience of the waves of health system reform that have taken place in Europe in recent decades. No countries have been exempt. Reforms have reflected wider societal debates, the search for efficiencies and, in many cases, wholesale political and social change. They have also consistently sought to enhance the performance of one or more health system function.

Reforms of health services delivery have often been prompted by concerns about costs or efficiency, but they may also reflect concerns about responsiveness and equity. Reforms have sought to integrate care, to substitute across levels of care and to strengthen primary care, including giving this sector more responsibility for public health programmes. Some reforms have focused on quality, introducing a wide range of initiatives at all levels. Others have been linked to new public management strategies that blur the boundaries between public and private. The more effective reforms have been aligned with corresponding adjustments in resource generation and financing.

Reforms of resource generation try to secure the right mix of human resources, fixed capital and technology. Human resource policies have been developed against a background of staff shortages and typically seek to match skills to new types of service delivery; to give increased emphasis to primary care, public health and teamwork; and to ensure quality through continuing education and certification. Generation of physical resources has undergone less extensive reform; examples include the use of private financing to construct hospitals. Investment in new technologies, particularly pharmaceuticals, has been shaped by health technology assessment, regulatory measures and the promotion of generic products.

Financing reforms have perhaps been the most dominant and apparent because of concerns about costs and the levers that funding offers for improving other functions. Challenges to sustainability and solidarity have been met with reforms of revenue collection and pooling, while efficiency has stimulated reforms of purchasing. In broad terms, collection and pooling reforms have involved the introduction of health insurance, particularly in eastern Europe, have tried to strengthen links between revenue collection and expenditure by decentralizing responsibilities, or have sought to shift the burden of financing to individuals through co-payments or complementary insurance. The issues of fragmentation of funds, risk selection and funding for population health have been addressed, in part, by regulation, improved public pooling mechanisms and the creation of dedicated health promotion funds. Funding long-term care remains a challenge.

Purchasing reforms address the issue of how to allocate pooled resources in order to lever the changes that policy-makers want. They often involve more explicit market elements that allow fund holders to specify volume, timeliness and quality of care. These include strategic purchasing, the introduction of a purchaser–provider split, contracting, case-based or performance-related payments, and sometimes more explicit market elements such as provider competition or selective contracting. These mechanisms give purchasers leverage over priorities but have associated risks, not least that providers will focus only on specific targets to the detriment of other areas. The success of purchasing reforms and management of potential adverse affects depends heavily on information to assess what is being purchased and on performance measurement.

Stewardship reforms have sought to ensure better governed, more-accountable and more-responsive health systems. Nonetheless, the stewardship function still faces significant challenges, if only because of the complex overlap between health system functions and goals. The environments within which health systems exist are highly complex, demanding coordination between branches of government (executive, legislature and judiciary), levels of government (central and regional) and increasingly between the public and private sectors.

There is an important distinction to be drawn between the capacity to make an impact and actually making it. If health systems are to secure the investment needed to realize their potential, they must be seen to be efficient and effective, and it is here that performance measurement is crucial. This was addressed in Chapter 10. Whereas policy-makers in the past often reformed without critically evaluating their efforts, they now need to define expectations, track resources and demonstrate outcomes. Performance measurement makes possible a structured assessment of how health systems are doing and flags up what can be done better.

The capacity to measure health system performance has increased in some countries in recent years, although from a very low starting-point. Information technology (if successfully implemented) can facilitate data collection and analysis and can allow better scrutiny of costs, outputs and outcomes. However, the way information is marshalled and presented can usually be improved, particularly in terms of integrating findings with governance mechanisms. If performance measures are to improve performance, information must be readily accessible at the level where decisions are made.

Systems must be designed to take basic data, interrogate them and present them to different audiences so that patients, planners and health professionals can find what they need when they need it and in good time. Achieving this is not straightforward, particularly given the need to track a range of functions and to link inputs and outputs. Selecting indicators that are valid, reliable and responsive to change is crucial (vital if they are to guide management action), but very challenging. There have been attempts to combine disparate indicators into a single composite index to show overall performance, but these have not been successful. Such efforts do succeed, however, in flagging up the importance of transparency. They also touch on the value of intermediate or instrumental objectives in signposting (and measuring) progress towards ultimate goals. Well-chosen and defined indicators, provided that they are specific and amenable to action, can map how far a function is moving along a critical pathway and can help to signpost the steps that are to be taken to improve performance.

The effectiveness of performance measurement depends on how far it helps to achieve health system objectives, and it must, therefore, be linked to policy levers that promote real improvement. Public reporting of performance is a tool that can be effective, if undertaken with great care, whether through informing the public or by prompting providers to react to the implied threat of scrutiny. Explicit financial incentives to reward providers achieving predefined standards can also act as levers for change, as can health system targets that lend themselves to work across sectors. As there is a risk in all these approaches that providers will focus on narrow goals without enhancing patient care, vigilance is required. Vigilance is also needed in the design and application of performance measures to avoid a short-term focus or a stifling of innovation. Policy-makers need to take an active role in ensuring that the whole approach to performance measurement is embedded in governance systems. This means aligning it with the political context and providing for the proper integration of financing mechanisms, market structures and regulation. It is also part of the stewardship role of ministries of health to foster the collection of relevant and appropriate data, ensure transparent analysis, promote the systematic application of evidence in planning and evaluation, and encourage an informed public policy debate. The combination of all these factors can best support the achievement of health system goals and the managing of any trade-offs between them. Health system stewards are responsible not just for assessing performance but ultimately for ensuring that performance measures lead to better performance.

There is no correct level of health system investment; it is for societies, through the democratic process, to chose how and how much to invest. However, the weight and range of evidence makes it clear that societies should be investing in health systems as part of societal efforts to enhance health and wealth and to achieve societal well-being. Particularly at a time of economic difficulty, health policy-makers can be assertive in arguing for resources, provided of course that they have the performance measurement systems in place to demonstrate that they are using investment efficiently and to good effect.

References

Commission on Macroeconomics and Health (2001) *Macroeconomics and Health: Investing in Health for Economic Development.* Geneva: World Health Organization Commission on Macroeconomics and Health.

Pan American Health Organization/World Health Organization (1998) *Essential Public Health Functions (EPHP).* World Health Statistics Quarterly, 51(1): 44–54. http://www.paho.org/english/dpm/shd/hp/EPHF.htm (accessed 2 September 2010).

Stuckler, D., Basu, S., Suhrcke, M., Coutts, A. and McKee, M. (2009) The public health effect of economic crises and alternative policy responses in Europe: an empirical analysis. *Lancet,* 374: 315–23.

Stuckler, D., Basu, S., McKee, M. and Suhrcke, M. (2010a) Responding to the economic crisis: a primer for public health professionals. *Journal of Public Health,* 32: 298–306.

Stuckler, D., Basu, S. and McKee, M. (2010b) Budget crises, health, and social welfare programmes. *British Medical Journal,* 340: c3311.

World Health Organization (2000) *The World Health Report 2000. Health Systems: Improving Performance.* Geneva: World Health Organization. http://www.who.int/whr/2000/en/ (accessed 1 September 2010).

Index

Page references to Boxes, Figures or Tables are in *italic* print, while references to Notes are denoted by the letter 'n' and note number appearing after the page number.

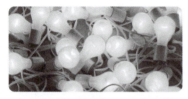
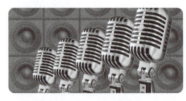
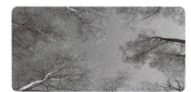
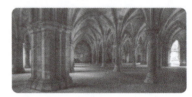
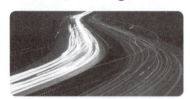
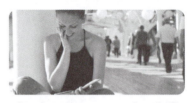
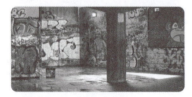